PULMONARY HYPERTENSION

A PATIENT'S SURVIVAL GUIDE

THIRD EDITION, Revised in March 2008

GAIL BOYER HAYES

MEDICAL EDITOR: RONALD J. OUDIZ, M.D.

Director, Liu Center for Pulmonary Hypertension, Harbor-UCLA Medical Center

CHAPTER ON NUTRITION: MAUREEN KEANE, M.S.

A Publication of the Pulmonary Hypertension Association
801 Roeder Road, Suite 400
Silver Spring, Maryland 20910
United States
800-748-7274 (support line)
301-565-3004 (PHA administration)
pha@PHAssociation.org
www.PHAssociation.org

YOU NEED A PH DOC, NOT JUST A BOOK

This manual is not intended to provide personal medical advice. Pulmonary hypertension is a serious condition and treatment must be individualized. Readers should seek medical advice from physicians with expertise in the field. PHA will not be responsible for readers' actions taken as a result of their interpretation of information contained in this book.

Published by the Pulmonary Hypertension Association in the United States of America.

ISBN: 0975898701

Library of Congress Control Number: 2004094560

Illustration on page 16: Copyright © 2002 Mayo Foundation for Medical Education and Research. All rights reserved. Used with permission from the *Mayo Clinic Health Letter* newsletter.

Figures on pages 81 and 144: Rubin, LJ, et al., "Bosentan Therapy for Pulmonary Arterial Hypertension," *The New England Journal of Medicine*, 346(896-903), Mar. 21, 2002. Copyright © 2002 Massachusetts Medical Society. All rights reserved.

Algorithm on page 14 adapted from Gaine SP, Rubin LJ, "Primary Pulmonary Hypertension," *Lancet*, 352:719-725. Copyright ©1998 with permission from Elsevier, and from Data Medica, publisher of *Advances in Pulmonary Hypertension*.

Photographs on pages 6 and 10, and the figures on pages 94 and 145 are from *Advances in Pulmonary Hypertension*, Copyright ©2002, 2003 by Pulmonary Hypertension Association and DataMedica, and are used with permission. All rights reserved.

Chest gave PHA special permission to use material in advance of publication (July 2004) for their guideline: "Diagnosis and Management of Pulmonary Arterial Hypertension: ACCP Evidence-Based Clinical Practice Guideline." This supplement is a must-read for the proactive PH patient.

To maintain its objectivity, *Pulmonary Hypertension: A Patient's Survival Guide*, is produced by volunteers and PHA, without direct financial support from any person or group with a monetary interest in PH-related products or services. The names of some patients have been changed to protect their privacy, but all stories are true. Because of the devastating nature of this disease, some of the patients may have since died, but their voices live on in these pages.

For additional copies of this book, or for permission to reprint any part or to translate, contact the Pulmonary Hypertension Association, 801 Roeder Rd., Suite 400, Silver Spring, MD 20910. Phone: 301-565-3004. Fax: 301-565-3994. pha@PHAssociation.org. The book may also be ordered on the web at www.PHAssociation.org. Or call PHA's support line: 800-748-7274. The price is $15 for PHA members living in the U.S., $25 for nonmembers or those living outside the U.S.

Contents

The Magic of PHA

The formation of the Pulmonary Hypertension Association might be the first time that patients, doctors, and researchers joined together in a synergistic swarm to learn so much so fast about a fatal disease thought to affect so few people. PHA has both generated this energy and directed it into productive channels.

This is how it began. A mere 18 years ago, in 1990, Pat Paton, a PH patient, and her sister Judy Simpson, a nurse, asked the National Organization for Rare Disorders (NORD) to help them locate other PH patients. As a result, Pat, Dorothy Olson, Theresa Knazik, and Shirley Brown—all PH patients—became pen pals. Theresa began *Pathlight* in May of 1990 and dubbed the group the United Patients' Association for Pulmonary Hypertension (UPAPH). Shirley became very ill and succumbed to PH, but the others incorporated UPAPH in November 1990. Husbands (Ed Simpson, Harry Olson, Bob Knazik, and Jerry Paton) also helped out with money, labor, and love.

At that time, PH was thought to be an exceedingly rare disease, and few general practitioners or even specialists were familiar with it. Showing great foresight, UPAPH ferreted out doctors and scientists with expertise in the disease and enlisted their help. The organization quickly metamorphosed into PHA, which now has over 9,000 patient and professional members (that's not counting the members of our more than 160 support groups worldwide). PHA raises about $1.5 million a year (the amount is increasing each year) to combat this dreadful disease and improve the lives of PH patients. Although PHA now has a permanent office and professional staff, patients remain the beating heart of the organization. They help with much of the work: putting out publications, organizing and staffing conferences, running support groups, answering calls to PHA's help line, and serving on PHA's Board of Trustees. They also put their lives on the line to help researchers find a cure. Another of the founders, Theresa, has since passed on, but Pat, Dorothy, Judy, Jerry, Ed, and Harry are still active in PHA.

Awareness of PH has grown right along with PHA. We now know there are 40,000 to 200,000 patients in the U.S. alone, which means PH is more common than some better-known lung diseases, such as cystic fibrosis. PHA uses its medical journal, *Advances in Pulmonary Hypertension*; its newsletter, *Pathlight*; its website (www.PHAssociation.org); biennial international conferences; support groups; and many other means to get out the word on PH. Much of PHA's budget goes to support scientific research.

What was once a hopeless disease is no longer so. Thanks to new medicines and raised awareness, it is estimated that over the last decade at least 5 to 6 years has been added to a typical PH patient's life. In 1990, there was no accepted treatment for PH, only palliative medications. Today we have many options to discuss with our doctors. Some PH patients now live long lives. We've got the ball rolling. Medical breakthroughs come along with increasing frequency, hence the need for a third edition in just a decade! We can beat this thing.

Gail Boyer Hayes

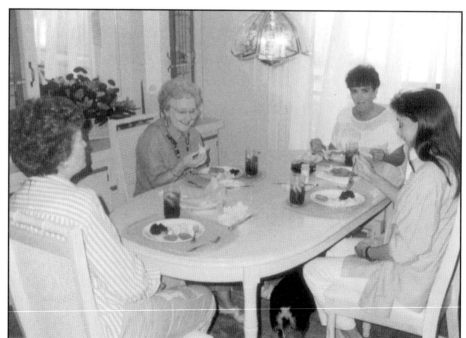

A "kitchen table" gathering in Indiantown, Florida, December 1990, at which organizational plans for PHA were discussed. From left: Judy Simpson, Dorothy Olson, Pat Paton, and Teresa Knazik

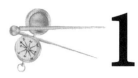

How Do I Know I've Really Got PH?

"I have *what?*" is the new patient's first question. "Are you *sure?*" is the second. After months or years of wondering why you don't feel well, you are relieved that you finally know why: you have high blood pressure inside your lungs, and the disorder has a name, pulmonary hypertension (PH). But when your doctor told you what was wrong with you, his or her face was grave. You might have been told that *without treatment,* pulmonary hypertension is usually a rapidly fatal disease. If your doctor wasn't up to speed, you might even have been told there was nothing to stop PH, and to "get your affairs in order." So, along with the relief, you also feel scared, confused, and angry. We've been there; we know.

With the right treatment, PH patients can now hope to live a long time. The treatments and your options are complicated, however, so you need to know which symptoms to keep an eye on, how the disease makes you sick, what kinds of treatments are available, and how to live well in spite of PH. Most of us like to be active participants in these decisions—it's *our* lives that are at stake. **PHA hopes this book will raise questions to be discussed with your physician, but it is not intended to give medical advice or to set a standard for the care of pulmonary hypertension patients.**

If you are a typical PH patient, your illness was probably misdiagnosed (often more than once) before your persistence and intelligence got you into the hands of a physician familiar with PH. Congratulations on already having leaped a major hurdle on the road to feeling better!

Because PH symptoms are the same as the symptoms of a lot of other diseases, PH has traditionally been diagnosed through a process of exclusion—by looking for and ruling out those other diseases. There are many doctors who still don't have PH on their lists of possibilities, and many more who have never (to their knowledge) encountered someone with the disease. Asthma and "too much stress in your life" are common misdiagnoses. Another reason that PH is hard to diagnose is that no two patients seem to have exactly the same disease or symptoms. As discussed later, improvements in echocardiograms now make it easier for a doctor who suspects PH to look for it directly, earlier in the diagnostic process.

What Does PH *Feel* Like?

The symptoms for all types of PH (see below) are pretty much the same. If a doctor can find no other obvious cause for them, PH should be suspected and a chest x-ray and echocardiogram done. Lots of things other than PH can cause these symptoms, of course (including some conditions that themselves cause PH). There is a direct correlation between the severity of symptoms and the progression of PH. In other words, the worse you feel, the sicker you probably are—and vice versa. Some women find that their symptoms get a lot worse just before, or during, their menses. Very few patients have ALL of these symptoms:

Breathlessness, also called shortness of breath, air hunger, or *dyspnea* (pronounced either DISP-nee-uh , disp-NEE-uh, sometimes with a silent "p") is the key symptom. If you peek at your chart when the doctor is out of the room and see "SOB," it does not reflect your doctor's opinion of your character; it's just an abbreviation for this symptom. Some of us experience shortness of breath with exertion, or even during or after meals.

Chest pain, also called *angina pectoris* (AN-jin-ah PEK-ta-ris), especially if you have it during physical exertion (there may also be a pounding in the chest during exertion). About a third of PH patients have this symptom.

Dizziness upon standing, or climbing stairs, or straightening up from a bent position; some patients feel dizzy just sitting in a chair.

Fainting, or *syncope* (SIN-ko-pee) happens when your brain doesn't get enough oxygen and goes "off the air" because of a lack of blood flow to it (see the discussion below on why we faint). Children are particularly prone to fainting upon exertion. On the other hand, many patients never lose consciousness.

Chronic fatigue—if you don't know what this is, you don't have the symptom. The author hasn't the energy to explain.

Swollen ankles and legs (*edema*, pronounced eh-DEE-muh) are very common. If you press into the flesh of your lower leg, it may briefly leave a dent.

Depression. Fatigue may cause this, as may some medications, or the (very real) stresses of coping with PH.

Dry cough. Many patients have a dry cough. Your sputum may contain drops of blood (*hemoptysis*). It's hard to say what causes the cough: maybe an enlarged heart pressing on a nerve, or some blood pressure medicines, or increased fluid retention.

Raynaud's (RAY-nose) **phenomenon** means you are prone to chilly blue fingers. This disorder is especially common in persons who got PH because of connective tissue disease, but many primary pulmonary hypertension patients also get it.

Symptoms of severe PH. If pressures inside the lungs increase, demanding more work from the heart, then symptoms get worse: fatigue increases, there is a throbbing in the neck, a feeling of fullness in the neck and abdomen, ankles and the lower extremities swell even more, and fluid may collect in the areas around the lungs and around the abdominal organs (this is called *ascites*, pronounced a-SIGH-tees—the "a" sounds like the "a" in "alone"). You might need more than one pillow at night to elevate your head and lungs. A few PH patients also get a buildup of fluid in the thin layer of tissue around the heart (*pericardial effusion*).

Breathlessness when lying down, called *orthopnea* (or-THOP-nee-uh), can be caused by fluid in the lungs and is a classic sign of left-heart failure. PH patients, of course, experience *right*-heart failure, and it is less clear why they may have orthopnea. Some patients say it feels like choking, others call it "air hunger." Your liver may feel tender. Lips and fingernails may take on a bluish tint (*cyanosis*, pronounced sigh-uh-NO-sis). A lack of oxygen to your brain can cause memory lapses. A decrease in appetite is common; some patients lose weight and hair. Menstruation may become irregular or even stop.

A bit more about that potentially serious chest pain. Chest pain has many possible causes, some of them unrelated to the heart and lungs. It might be heartburn, a pulled muscle, bruised rib, or anxiety. But it might really be your heart—or the high pressure in your pulmonary arteries, or a pulmonary embolism—so get on the phone and tell your doc about any new or severe chest discomfort. Be as specific as you can about the nature, location, and duration of the discomfort. Notice if the pain seems to happen when you exercise, are upset, or whatever. Some PH patients say their chest pain is dull and deep, some say it is sharp and stabbing. Some may have uncomfortable heartbeat sensations (*palpitations*); it may feel as if your heart is pounding, fluttering, flip-flopping, skipping a heartbeat, or racing. One woman describes palpitations as "an empty elevator crashing down inside me."

Why do some of us pass out? There is more than one cause of fainting in PH patients. (Many things unrelated to PH can also cause fainting.) Too little blood flowing to the brain because a heart can't pump well, or has rhythm problems, or is beating too fast or too slow may cause fainting. Strong emotion or pain can activate the nervous system and cause fainting. Anxiety and other things can lead to hyperventilation, which can lead to fainting (a decrease in the carbon dioxide level in your blood causes vessels in the brain to constrict). If you stand still for a long time and your leg muscles aren't being used, blood may pool in your veins, your blood pressure falls, and you plop. Some PH patients faint when they sit up or stand up too quickly (*orthostatic hypotension*). This can be caused or made worse by vasodilator drugs, which lower the blood pressure all over your body.

Exertional fainting happens when your body can't keep up with your need for extra oxygen and blood flow when you are exercising. More than one of us has passed out just beyond the *top* of a flight of stairs! This is why: you might faint after you *stop* exercising, because your blood vessels are still dilated to accommodate the extra blood flow, but your heart rate has begun to fall back. Your blood pressure falls, and so do you.

Most of us who are prone to fainting have some warning before we black out. Because of

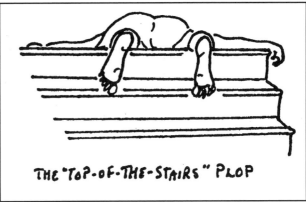

THE "TOP-OF-THE-STAIRS" PLOP

the many possible causes of fainting, whether you have warning does not usually relate to the severity of your PH. If heart rhythm problems cause you to faint, there may be no warning before you pass out. On the other hand, you usually do have warning before passing out from hyperventilation: chest discomfort, dizziness, and a pins-and-needles sensation.

Tell your family not to keep you upright if you faint; it's best to be lying down, to allow the blood to get to your brain and heart. Elevating the legs while lying down can speed recovery.

The mystery of good days and bad days. A typical PH patient has good days and bad days. Why this is so is one of the great mysteries. Some days you might dash up a flight of stairs with little trouble, but other days it's all you can do to operate the TV remote. The good days are a good sign, because they suggest that your blood vessels are still flexible, which means the potential for reversing the damage is better.

A message from Linda on the PHA message board vividly captures the difference between good and bad days: "Have you ever had one of those days where your neck starts to build up pressure, you feel like the top of your head is being screwed on tighter and tighter, and the rest of your head is going to explode? Then your feet start to burn and ache, and your legs start to hurt, and you can't seem to get enough air in, and when you bend over to tie your shoe laces then [try] to walk out to your car, you think you might die on the way....Then you have to walk into the gas station to pay for your gas, and on the way you see gray spots start to roll across your eyeballs and you say to yourself, 'Oh, no, not now.'...Then there are those good days. Thank God for them. The weather is pleasant, you get up in the morning and feel well rested....You get the shopping done quickly, an oil change in the car, the bed sheets changed, and [mail] your packages at the post office."

Functional Classifications of PH

You will hear references to *classes* of PH patients. Functional classifications for PH are based on either a modified version of the New York Heart Association (NYHA) categories for left-heart failure, or on a more recently developed World Health Organization (WHO) system. They are almost identical.

Class I: PH patients in this category have no symptoms during ordinary physical activity. Their hearts function normally.

Class II: Although these patients are comfortable at rest, ordinary physical activity is somewhat limited by undue breathlessness, chest pain, fatigue, or near fainting.

Class III: These PH patients usually have no symptoms at rest, but their physical activity is greatly limited by breathlessness, chest pain, fatigue, or near fainting while doing routine things.

Class IV: These PH patients are often breathless and tired even while resting and can't do any physical activity without symptoms. They show signs of right-heart failure. Under the WHO system, anyone who is prone to fainting goes into this class.

Don't panic if your doctor says you are Class III or IV. Because our medical system often fails to detect PH in its early stages, many, if not most, patients are already in the higher classes when diagnosed. Until then, our symptoms could indicate so many common diseases that they do not prompt doctors to

think of the more unusual disease of PH. (Patients themselves may think it is nothing particularly serious, and that they are just "out of shape.") With treatment, you may well drop down to a lower class.

Types of PH

An early attempt to classify PH patients divided them into those with primary pulmonary hypertension (PPH) and those with secondary pulmonary hypertension (SPH). The term "*primary*" means unexplained (*idiopathic*). It's just a label doctors use when they don't know what caused a disease. The new term, which we use in most places in this book instead of PPH, is IPAH (idiopathic pulmonary arterial hypertension). When PH is known to be caused by another disease (such as scleroderma, chronic bronchitis, emphysema, or interstitial fibrosis), it is called *secondary,* because it happened as a result of the other disease.

The PPH/SPH distinction often doesn't make much sense. For example, the term PPH is used, especially in older publications, when PH is known to have been triggered by diet pills, street drugs, or other known diseases that are not directly associated with the heart and lungs, such as liver disease. Furthermore, once the gene for the type of PH that runs in families was discovered, it didn't really make sense to say the cause of familial PH was unknown.

When the poobahs of the PH world gather for a World Symposium on PH every few years, they tinker with how they classify various types of PH in order to bring the classifications up-to-date with current science. The latest classification was proposed in July 2003 and is published in a July 2004 supplement to *JACC*. It groups types of PH in a way that is more helpful to doctors trying to figure out how to treat particular PH patients. This new way of talking about types of PH is discussed in Chapter 3. *In this book, the term PH is used to include all types of PH, unless otherwise indicated.* Especially in older studies, researchers focused only on what they loosely defined as PPH patients, to simplify research results. So when this book discusses the results of those studies, it also limits them to "PPH" patients, unless it is obvious that newer terms can be substituted. Some of you who have PH that is associated with another known disease (such as scleroderma or interstitial lung disease) might feel as if you're left hanging, wondering if what was learned also applies to you. It often might, but in many instances more research is needed.

What Tests Will My Doctor Do To Tell If It's PH?

The following are typical approaches used by PH specialists, but the diagnostic procedure will vary from doctor to doctor.

Physical exam. A routine checkup seldom discovers PH, so it often goes undiagnosed. Because the symptoms of PH are common to many diseases, personal and family medical histories are important. Your doctor will use a stethoscope to listen for **unusual heart sounds** such as an increase in the pulmonic component of the second heart sound (the sound the pulmonic valve makes when it snaps shut), an ejection click, systolic murmurs (whooshing sounds due to the leakage of blood backwards across the tricuspid valve), and for a gallop (a soft thud during the time the right ventricle is filling, which indicates that ventricle is weak). Okay, this is pretty technical stuff, but a patient who asks, "Hey, doc, hear a systolic murmur?" is more likely to be treated as an intelligent participant in his or her own medical treatment.

Your doctor will also feel for a right ventricular or parasternal lift, for an enlarged (or even throbbing) liver, and for fluid in your abdomen (*ascites*). Your ankles and lower legs will be checked for swelling (*edema*), and the jugular vein in your neck examined for swelling. The doctor will probably look at your fingers, because a long period of low concentrations of oxygen in the blood sometimes causes nail beds to take on a bluish tint (*cyanosis*) or fingers to form a small bulge at the end (*clubbing*).

Electrocardiogram (ECG). This is one of the first tests done on a potential PH patient. Electrodes are stuck to your skin and a recording is made of the electrical impulses of your heart. The results may indicate that the right side of the heart is thickened due to the unusual stress of high pressure, but an ECG cannot, by itself, diagnose PH. You may be asked to take an ECG stress test, where you pedal a stationary bike or walk on a treadmill while you are hooked up to an ECG machine. There is a very small risk of a heart attack or serious rhythm problem during such a test, but trained people stand by ready to handle such emergencies (if your doctor thinks you'll have such problems, he/she won't order the test).

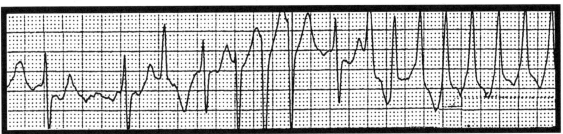

The author's ECG prior to beginning treatment for her PH--not a pretty sight.

There's a whole science to reading ECGs, so we won't attempt to explain the peaks and valleys in these jittery lines.

Blood tests are done to check on how much oxygen there is in your blood (*arterial blood gases*), how your liver and kidneys are functioning (back pressure or limited cardiac output from severe PH can hurt them), and to find whether you have collagen vascular disease (like lupus or scleroderma—more on this later), thyroid problems, signs of infections, or HIV antibodies. If you have too many red blood cells (*polycythemia*), your body may be trying to compensate for getting too little oxygen. If a lot of carbon dioxide (CO_2) is found, a reduced rate and depth of breathing (*hypoventilation*) may be the cause. (Hypoventilation can cause a decreased concentration of oxygen in the blood that can, in turn, cause PH or make it worse.) If your blood doesn't coagulate normally (if it's too "thin," and you bleed too much) and you are not taking a blood thinner, this may suggest liver disease, as does a low albumin level.

Low oxygen saturations may or may not be found in PH patients; they are more commonly found in the sickest patients. Low oxygen saturation in a PH patient may mean the patient's heart is shunting blood from the right side back to the left side, or bypassing the air sacs of the lungs. It is possible, however, for someone with severe PH to have normal oxygen saturation. If low saturation is found, it can be caused by several things, including the presence of interstitial lung disease (chronic inflammation and disruption of the walls of the air sacs), and holes in the heart, which may lower the oxygen saturation even if the patient has only mild PH.

The oxygen saturation of your blood can also be measured by putting a clothespin-like clip (a *pulse oximeter*) over your fingertip. It sends a light through your skin that lets a gizmo determine how red your blood is. More red means more oxygen in the red blood cells, the Certs-shaped blood cells that haul around the oxygen. Sometimes an overnight sleep study with a pulse oximeter will be done. Kids having such a test may say they have "an E.T. finger."

Even if the blood gas or oximeter test shows normal oxygen levels, your doctor may want to take a closer look and see how your oxygen saturation is while you are exercising or sleeping. Many PH patients who have normal oxygen saturations at rest will require supplemental oxygen when up and about, when doing more strenuous activities, or while sleeping.

At the PHA conference in 2002, a patient asked a panel of doctors why, when she was well saturated with oxygen, she was still short of breath. The doctors said that although a lack of oxygen can make you short of breath, shortness of breath is usually related more to right-heart failure and cardiac output than to how much oxygen is bound to the red blood cells. For example, when you start climbing a flight of stairs, even if your blood is "fully loaded" with all the oxygen it needs, the blood stream doesn't deliver the oxygen to where it is needed in time to prevent breathlessness.

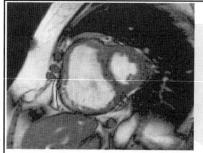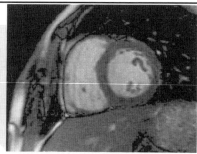

These MRI scans show how the right ventricle of a person with severe PH (the photo on the left, above) has thick, muscular walls and is larger than normal. It has pushed the left ventricle into a D shape. In the healthy person (photo on right) the right ventricle is thin-walled and C-shaped.

Photo from Advances in Pulmonary Hypertension, *Vol.2, No.4.*

Chest x-rays can reveal an enlarged right ventricle and enlarged pulmonary arteries (the main pulmonary artery leading from the right ventricle of the heart to the lungs, and the first left and right branches of that artery).

If the smaller, peripheral blood vessels are not visible in the lungs in an x-ray (or angiogram), "pruning" of the vasculature tree might have occurred, which is a sign of PH. This means that as the vessels go further out from the right heart towards the lungs, they quickly taper (narrow down).

Your doctor can also look at the x-ray for clues that suggest emphysema or interstitial fibrous disease of the lungs. PH caused by chronic blood clots can be suggested by triangular or wedge-shaped patches of scar tissue in the lungs downstream from suspected clots where almost no blood vessels are seen on the x-ray.

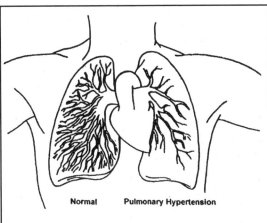

The "pruning" effect of PH on small arteries in the lungs. (A PH patient would usually have pruning in both lungs.)
Illustration by Andrea Rich.

Doppler Echocardiogram. This procedure is painless and is often used both to make a preliminary diagnosis and to later monitor a patient's condition. In their February 2002 *Journal of Respiratory Diseases* article, "A Systematic Approach to Pulmonary Hypertension," Gordon Yung and Lewis Rubin (both at UC San Diego) emphasize that a chest x-ray and echocardiography should be done "whenever this [PH] diagnosis is suspected."

Doppler-echocardiography can also show that a patient has congenital heart disease, which may have caused the patient's PH.

Here's what to expect: a technician will put some sticky-backed electrodes (*patches*) on your skin. You lie on your side in a darkened room while the technician uses bouncing sound waves (sonar, or ultrasound) to make a moving image of your heart (the machine works a lot like a fisherman's depth and fish finder, and is the same machine that obstetricians use to take pictures of a fetus developing in a mother's uterus). A chilly "transducer" (it looks like a microphone attached to a cable) is pressed against your chest, along with some clear jelly to enhance the transducer's ability to pick up sound waves. The microphone first sends the sound waves into your body and then picks up their echoes when they hit internal surfaces like a heart valve.

Because some PH patients may have an elevated PAP only while exercising, many experts do exercise echoes while their patient is exercising, usually on a semi-erect or supine bicycle. When an exercise echo is done immediately after the patient stops exercising, the results are less accurate.

As far as is known, it does not harm the body to have these high-frequency sound waves pass through it. No x-rays or needles are involved in this procedure. This is why the procedure is called "noninvasive."

During the echo, a record is made of things like whether the right chambers of the heart are enlarged, the thickness of the wall of the right ventricle, any structural heart abnormalities (such as narrowed heart valves or congenital heart disease), or any abnormal amounts of fluid around the heart.

As mentioned, in PH patients, the right chambers of the heart are often enlarged and weakened. The muscular walls of the right ventricle are thicker than normal because it is working too hard. If the dividing wall between the two ventricles bows into the space of the left ventricle, this is another indication that the PH is severe (see the MRI scan illustration on p. 6). A *smaller*-than-normal *left* ventricle is also a sign of severe PH.

An echo can reveal whether the right ventricle is contracting well or poorly. Cardiac output can be estimated from an echo, although the measurement is not always accurate.

The echo also measures the amount of blood flowing through the heart valves. For example, when the right ventricle of a person with PH contracts, some blood does not go into the pulmonary artery, as it should, but leaks (*jets*) backwards through the tricuspid valve, into the right atrium (*tricuspid regurgitation*). The Doppler principle (the same principle that explains why the sound from a train's horn coming toward you is different from the sound when it is going away from you) allows an estimation to be made of the severity of the PH. The speed with which blood cells jet backwards through the tricuspid valve depends on the pressure difference between the ventricle and atrium. This pressure difference is a reflection of the pressure in the pulmonary artery.

After the test, mathematical calculations usually allow an expert to estimate your systolic pulmonary artery pressure (PAP). It cannot be measured on everyone. Note that echocardiograms give an estimate of *systolic* PAP, which is often 30 to 50 percent higher than your *mean* PAP. To calculate your mean PAP you need to know your diastolic PAP as well, which is only obtainable from an echo if there is leakage in the pulmonary valve (much less common than tricuspid regurgitation).

Even then, it is not always reliable. The only way to get exact measurements is with a cardiac catheterization (see below).

How does your echo compare to those of other PH patients? A study at the University of Michigan of 51 PPH patients who had echoes found that, at the time of their diagnosis, 96 percent already had a systolic PAP of over 60 mg Hg, 92 percent had an enlarged right atrium, 98 percent an enlarged right ventricle, and 76 percent had reduced right ventricle systolic function (a weakened right heart).

Echocardiograms are pretty accurate for most patients, but not as precise as cardiac catheterizations. The echo numbers may be off slightly or by a great degree. When pressures are really high (above 100 mmHg) they may be more likely to deviate. Because echoes are less risky—and more pleasant for the patient than catheterizations—some doctors may use them to monitor a PH patient. There are situations, however, where repeated catheterizations are essential.

If an echocardiogram is done by a technician without special training and/or experience with PH patients, the results can be way off. Anecdotes abound of patients who were falsely told they did or did not have PH on the basis of poorly done echoes. This means you need to ask about the technician's training and experience (and also that of the doctor who will be interpreting the tests). An echo cannot be properly interpreted without clinical information from your specialist.

Experts can also use these echoes to look for heart disease that may have contributed to your PH. For instance, if your left atrium is too big, it may be that you have high pulmonary venous pressures. You might have heart valve problems, or congenital heart disease. To look for the latter, you'll probably have a "bubble" study done during your echo, which uses agitated salt water, pushed into your veins via an IV, to look for blood flowing through places that it shouldn't (such as holes in the heart). This is called *shunting*.

If shunting looks likely, your doctor may order **transesophageal echocardiography** to get better pictures of what is going on, because the esophagus (the tube from your throat to your stomach) is close to your heart. This isn't a whole lot of fun, because you have to swallow a probe, a long narrow tube with a small echo microphone on the end. It's very low risk, however, and the use of sedation and local anesthesia can make you comfortable during the procedure. If it's your child undergoing this, plan a treat like ice cream afterwards— *after* the throat-numbing medicine wears off!

Computed tomography (CT or CAT scans) uses a computer hooked up to an x-ray machine that rapidly rotates around you taking pictures from many angles. The computer translates these images into detailed, 3-D "slices" of your body, revealing much that can't be seen by an ordinary x-ray. CT scans are getting better and better as a diagnostic tool, and can detect blood clots in the large arteries of your lungs, yield information about your heart, and diagnose lung disease. CT scans can sometimes find other causes for your symptoms, such as pulmonary fibrosis or emphysema (these diseases can lead to PH). A CT scan may reveal blood clot (*chronic thromboembolic*) problems (although a negative scan doesn't completely rule out such clots), blocked pulmonary veins (*veno-occlusive disease*), tumors, inflamed vessels, or mediastinal fibrosis (there's more on these causes of PH in Chapter 3). Some PH specialists are now using ultrafast CT scans (called electron-beam tomography or EBT) in addition to echocardiograms, to monitor changes in the size of a patient's right atrium and right ventricle. These scanners take their pictures faster than conventional CT scanners and thus can better "freeze" the heart in motion.

Magnetic resonance imaging (MRI) scans for PH have also improved. Like CT scans, they are noninvasive (nothing goes inside your body). Magnetic fields and radio waves produce pictures of your heart and arteries; no radiation is involved and the procedure is not thought to involve any risk. It's painless, but expensive. The pictures look sort of like x-rays, but can often show some tissues x-rays miss.

An MRI might be ordered to look for large blood clots (although it can't totally rule them out), problems with the structure of pulmonary arteries, the size and shape of the right ventricle, the thickness of the wall of the right ventricle (which correlates, in an MRI, with mean PAP) and other relevant things. Your mean PAP can be estimated from information obtained with an MRI.

Here's what happens: you lie inside a big white tube to have the test, and listen to queer noises, some of which sound like tennis shoes tumbling in a dryer. Some machines' walls are open on the side, and some are closed. If your facility has one of the latter and you get claustrophobic, it helps to put on a sleep mask or drape a folded towel across your eyes. Remove all metal objects before the test; the magnets used are *powerful.* They will rip earrings from your ears and you will not be able to pull them off the magnet. Also, don't get within 50 feet of the magnet with your credit cards—they will be instantly demagnetized. If you have a pacemaker or war shrapnel buried inside you, you can't have this test. By accompanying her daughter to such a scan, one mom learned for the first time about her daughter's body piercings.

Nuclear scan (a.k.a. ventilation / perfusion scan or V/Q scan). This is done to take a look at the plumbing in your lungs and see if the trouble could lie in the large or the small vessels. **The Q of V/Q:** a radioactive isotope is injected into a peripheral vein, and your chest is then scanned for radioactivity. It is usually

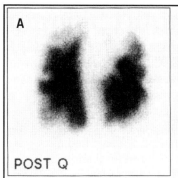
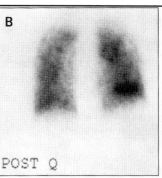

Figure A shows a perfusion scan in a patient with chronic thromboembolic PH. It has many bilateral, segmental perfusion defects. In Figure B, which is a scan of a "PPH" patient, there is a "mottled" look to the lungs without any segmental perfusion defects.

From Advances in Pulmonary Hypertension, *Vol. 2, No.1.*

done on an outpatient basis. The isotope's movement in the pulmonary arteries is tracked from outside your body by special cameras (sort of like Geiger counters). Your doctor looks for areas where blood flow is blocked or reduced by clots. If none are found, it means the problem is probably in the small vessels. If significant blockages (clots) are found in the larger arteries, this can be good news, because chronic thromboembolic disease can often be cured by surgery. Therefore, these clots should be looked for in all PH patients. If your V/Q scan is normal, you can usually (not always) rule out chronic thromboembolic disease.

The V of V/Q: in this procedure you breathe in a little radioactive gas and let it fill the airways of your lungs. Doctors can then compare the blood flow in your lungs' arteries with the airflow through adjacent airways. If it's PH that's causing your problems, the airflow will probably be fairly normal in areas where blood flow is low due to occluded arteries.

Occasionally, what looks like thromboembolic disease on a V/Q scan may turn out to be a tumor or inflammation in a pulmonary artery, something pressing on an artery, or pulmonary veno-occlusive disease (a rare disease where fibers gunk up small pulmonary veins).

Pulmonary function tests. These tests measure how much air your lungs can hold,

how much air moves in and out of them, and their ability to exchange oxygen and carbon dioxide. They may be done to assess the severity of your PH and glean clues as to its cause.

In one test, you breathe in until it hurts, then expel that breath as fast and thoroughly as you can. This reveals your lung volume. The lungs of many persons with PH process a slightly smaller volume of air, probably because the PH makes them stiffer. (If the volume found is less than 70 percent of normal, something other than PH may be causing the reduction in volume.)

In another test, you breathe in and out as deep and fast as you can. It can be quite stressful, especially when the technician is yelling at you to try harder.

Pulmonary function tests can also tell if there is a blockage in the trachea, a nerve problem, or a muscular weakness that contributes to breathing difficulties, and whether you hyperventilate (blow off too much carbon dioxide, making you lightheaded).

Carbon monoxide diffusing capacity test (DLCO). A DLCO estimates how well oxygen is transferred from your lungs' air sacs into your blood. Because it's hard to measure this movement using oxygen itself, carbon monoxide (CO) is substituted. You breathe in

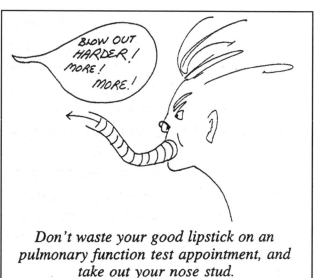

Don't waste your good lipstick on an pulmonary function test appointment, and take out your nose stud.

a little CO, hold your breath for 10 seconds, and then exhale into a CO detector. If no CO is detected, it means it was well absorbed by your lungs (and that oxygen would be well absorbed, too). If CO is still found in the air you breathe out, then it wasn't transferred well from the lungs' air sacs into the blood vessels surrounding them. Patients with IPAH, familial PH, or PH due to chronic thromboembolism often do not exchange quite as much oxygen as they should. However, many lung diseases other than PH can also cause a poor diffusing capacity. A normal test strongly suggests that a patient's PH is not caused by pulmonary fibrosis, emphysema, etc. Your ability to exchange oxygen usually correlates with your pulmonary vascular resistance, NYHA or WHO class, and your ability to do physical work, but not necessarily with the severity of your pulmonary artery pressures. Researchers at Harbor-UCLA Medical Center say that measuring DLCO (and, to a lesser extent, lung volume) can help specialists evaluate patients who complain of breathlessness and fatigue. If a patient is not exchanging oxygen well, it can make a doctor think more seriously about PH, so that PH may be discovered several years earlier than it might otherwise be.

If you have limited systemic sclerosis or scleroderma (see Chapter 3), the higher your PAP, the lower you can expect your DLCO to be. Your doctor will probably want to repeat a DLCO test once or twice a year to see if your pulmonary vessels are becoming more damaged.

Exercise tolerance tests. Your doctor might ask you to walk on a treadmill or give you a **6-minute walk test** to find your exercise tolerance level. A healthy person should be able to walk at least 500 meters in 6 minutes; someone with moderate PH might manage only 300-400 meters. Children might be asked to ride a stationary bicycle.

Because our symptoms vary from day-to-day, are these tests accurate? Doctors say that if you haven't just gotten off an airplane from a flight to Australia, or stood in line for hours the day before, the test results are reproducible to within about a 15 percent variation. If you are being tested as a participant in a drug trial, you will be given a series of exercise tolerance tests to get an accurate baseline. Your weight, physical conditioning (or lack thereof), lack of effort, and PH may all affect how well you do on the tests.

Cardiopulmonary exercise testing (CPET). CPET is used to tell your specialist how sick you are, and also to see what effects treatments have had upon your condition. In a CPET, you breathe into a mouthpiece (maybe while riding a stationary bicycle or walking on a treadmill) while an ECG is being done. Although not painful, it's not a glamorous procedure. Wear exercise clothes and sneakers. Because your nose is pinched shut and your mouth is clenched around a tube, you may drool a lot. The bicycle seat can be politely described as uncomfortable in spots. Ask for a gel pad if the seat is too hard. If you feel panicky about having to breathe through a mouth tube, try pretending you are snorkeling.

If you are feeling tired the day you take exercise tests, you may find them exhausting in more than one sense, and may want to arrange for somebody to drive you home afterwards.

Polysomnogram. This is a combination of tests done if sleep apnea is suspected. (Sleep apnea is when you episodically stop breathing at night.) The tests monitor brain wave activity (with an electroencephalogram or EEG), the amount of oxygen in your blood (with a pulse oximeter), the movement of air in and out a nostril as you breathe, and the up and down movement of your chest wall.

Right-heart catheterization. This is still one of the most accurate and useful tests for PH, and the only test that directly measures the pressure inside the pulmonary arteries. It should be done in all patients at least once, to get a definitive diagnosis (unless there is some special safety reason for not doing so). If your doctor has good reason to suspect PH, but PH didn't show up on a resting or exercise echo, then a right-heart catheterization might be called for. Because of the accuracy of this test, some doctors use it not only to diagnose, but also to monitor their PH patients. When combined with the injection of contrast dye (pulmonary angiography) it can tell whether chronic thromboembolic disease is causing your PH.

A right-heart catheterization, vasodilator study, and maybe an angiogram are usually done while you are awake, because the docs need your cooperation in taking deep breaths and such. Children and some adults might be sedated to make them less anxious. You have to spend a long time lying on a hard table (thus earning the appellation "patient") but most find the procedures more uncomfortable than painful.

I was allowed to watch from behind a clear plastic "lead" screen, to protect from x-rays, while Lisa had her catheter put in. She was covered from head to toe with sterile paper and cloth drapes; only her pink face was visible. Even the machines close to her were covered with sterile plastic. The doctor at the University of Washington worked fast and confidently. He used a small portable x-ray machine called a fluoroscope that let him see exactly where the catheter was going. The catheter, a thin, flexible tube with a small inflatable balloon on the tip (a *Swan-Ganz catheter*) was inserted into Lisa through a vein in her neck (often a groin vein is used) and threaded all the way through the right side of her heart and into her pulmonary artery, where it immediately started measuring her pressures (*hemodynamics*). Lisa said the experience felt more like tugging and pressure than pain.

A cardiac cath gives your doctor your systolic, diastolic, and mean PAP, right atrial pressure, cardiac output, and pulmonary capillary wedge pressure. (The narrowing of the small arteries may make wedge pressures inaccurate, however.) *Pulmonary vascular resistance* (PVR) is then calculated from the other numbers and is an index of how much resistance to blood flow through pulmonary blood vessels is present.

Cardiac caths are also a way of finding congenital defects in the heart, such as a hole between heart chambers or the large arteries that isn't supposed to be there. (Unfortunately, a cardiac cath does not detect every type of congenital heart disease.)

For a **pulmonary angiogram**, sometimes done at the same time as the cardiac cath, x-ray dye is injected through the catheter and then an x-ray is taken of the pulmonary arteries to see whether the vascular tree has been "pruned" or blocked by blood clots. This is the very best way to define the anatomy of such clots. (If a lung scan or CT scan has excluded clots in the lungs as a cause, an angiogram is often not necessary.)

Left-heart catheterization. Similar to a right-heart cath, but with the catheter inserted via an artery rather than a vein, this test allows measurements of pressures on the left side of the heart, and is also done to take pictures of the heart and the coronary arteries (a *coronary antiogram*). In PH patients it is usually done to exclude the possibility that abnormal pressures in the left heart are causing, or contributing to, the elevation of a patient's PAP.

Heart catheterizations are usually safe if done by a physician with experience working on PH patients. But there are risks involved. Although most complications are minor, and most hospitals are well equipped to deal with them, there is still a tiny risk of infection (less than one in a thousand), and of various uncommon problems (including heart attack, stroke, bleeding, or even death). The 1993 and 2000 editions of the *Mayo Clinic Heart Book* discuss cardiac caths in general as well as the somewhat greater risks associated with catheterizing arteries (where the blood pressure is higher than in veins), which include bleeding, bruising, clotting, and the risk of a hole being accidentally poked through the artery or the heart.

Talk over the risks and the benefits with your doctor. Ask how many **PH** patients he or she has catheterized. If a doctor has little experience doing right-heart caths, the risk of complications may be higher than with a more experienced doc.

Vasodilator study (a.k.a. acute vasodilator challenge). If you have **PH**, you'd much rather take a pill (such as a calcium channel blocker, or CCB) than undergo more complicated therapy. Therefore, while the catheter is still in place, doctors can evaluate your response to drugs that relax your pulmonary arteries. Sometimes, some doctors will skip this step on certain types of patients who are unlikely to respond well and/or are unlikely to tolerate CCBs: those who have connective tissue disease, advanced Class IV symptoms, significant right ventricular failure, or who are rapidly deteriorating.

There is a lot of heated discussion over which drug is best to use for the vasodilator test. Epoprostenol, iloprost, nitric oxide, adenosine (a potent vasodilator with biochemical features virtually identical to epoprostenol), sildenafil, and CCBs have all been used. Nitric oxide, iloprost, and even epoprostenol can easily be administered through a facemask or nasal cannula. Because inhaled gases affect only your pulmonary system and quickly leave your body, they are increasingly being used (although inhaled epoprostenol is an "off-label" use). The other

PH drugs enter your body through an IV, although CCBs may also be given as pills. *CCBs are seldom used any more in this test because they hang around in the system too long and are more likely to cause shock or prolonged hypotension in those who don't respond well.* Although most patients who respond well to one vasodilator will also respond well to the others, there are exceptions. Some patients who do not respond to nitric oxide may respond to prostacyclin. Some who do not respond to CCBs may respond to prostacyclin, adenosine, or nitric oxide. If you do respond well to prostacyclin, adenosine, or nitric oxide, you are more likely to respond well to CCB pills.

The test drug is tried in higher and higher doses, pausing at each dose to see how you are reacting. When a significant response occurs, or the side effects get bad, the test is considered complete. By noting changes in lung pressures and cardiac output in response to a vasodilator, your doctor can determine the best drug for you and the best starting dose. Even if you do not respond well to these drugs during the short test, over a longer period you might benefit from epoprostenol or bosentan just as much as someone who does respond.

Doctors can't agree on what constitutes "vasoreactivity" or a good ("acute") response. In the past, it has been somewhere in the neighborhood of a 15-30 percent decline in PVR. But recently, Dr. Olivier Sitbon in (Université Paris-Sud, Clamart, France) showed that for a patient to have a really good response, their mean PAP should fall to 40 mm Hg or even lower while being given the vasodilator.

If you are being tested at a facility that is not a PH center (PHA doesn't recommend this), make sure your doctors know that a decrease in your PVR might not be accompanied by a decrease in your PAP if your cardiac output goes up. Maybe 10 to 15 percent of IPAH patients have a good response to a vasodilator. Even fewer patients with secondary PH have a good response. But among children, 30 to 35 percent are vasoreactive.

Not surprisingly, the lucky few are called "responders." Why do they respond? It is thought that in the early stages of PH, the structural changes to pulmonary arteries are likely to be less, and you are more likely to respond well. If you have really severe PH, the damage to your small pulmonary arteries probably goes well beyond the muscle layer of the vessels, which relaxes in response to vasodilators. The vessel wall becomes stiff and less able to relax.

Responders are usually sent home with CCB pills. The Mayo Clinic sends home 10 to 15 percent of the PH patients they test with such pills. (Sometimes, before they go home and while the cath is still in place, their dose is adjusted.) But responders with right-heart failure and high right-atrial pressures (equal to or greater than 20 mm Hg) are often started on epoprostenol or bosentan in spite of their good hemodynamic response. After being sent home, responders are carefully monitored. Over time (weeks, months) the dose is usually gradually increased if the patient can tolerate it.

Lung biopsies are only done now in special circumstances, because they yield too little information for the risk involved.

New tests for PH in the future? If you've read this far, you're probably thinking that better ways are needed to diagnose PH and determine the disease's likely course in different patients. You are right. We need a test that is easy, that can be done in a standard way at any treatment center with reproducible results, that correlates well with survival, that doesn't hurt much, and that doesn't cost a lot. That's wishing for a lot, and is probably more than any one test could ever do given all the types of PH. But improvements over the present diagnostic system are both needed and possible.

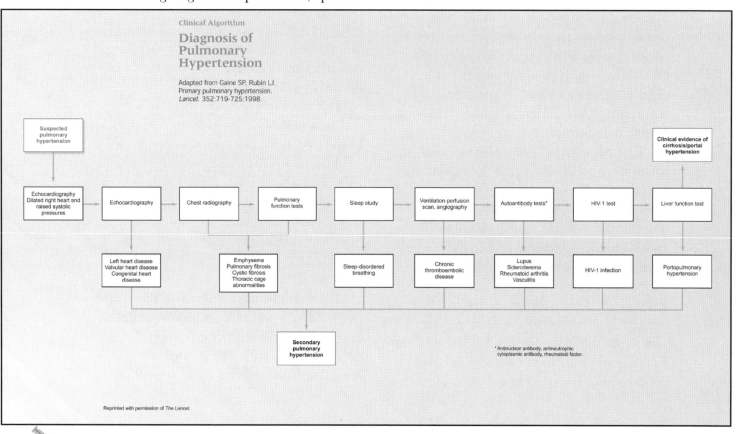

Clinical Algorithm

Diagnosis of Pulmonary Hypertension

Adapted from Gaine SP, Rubin LJ. Primary pulmonary hypertension. Lancet. 352:719-725;1998.

Reprinted with permission of The Lancet.

PH: the *Other* High Blood Pressure

Pulmonary hypertension means high blood pressure *inside the lungs* (*pulmonary* means concerning or involving the lungs). The blood pressure measured by a cuff on your arm is called the "systemic" blood pressure, and reflects the pressure between the left side of your heart and the rest of your body (excluding your lungs). The lay term "high blood pressure" typically refers to systemic hypertension, which is easily measured and relatively easy to treat. Pulmonary hypertension, on the other hand, is more difficult to diagnose and more challenging to treat.

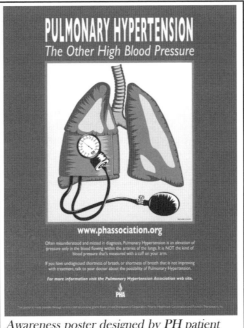

Awareness poster designed by PH patient Michelle Smith.

The circulation of blood in your lungs encounters only a fifth of the resistance that circulating blood encounters elsewhere in your body. The vessels in your lungs are very sensitive to increases in pressure: they don't like it, and they respond in complex ways. This response initiates the PH process. PH affects your heart as well as your lungs, but unless your PH is caused by another disease, it appears to start in your lungs. The walls of the small blood vessels within the lungs get thicker and often constrict. This shrinks (or blocks off) the opening inside them and makes them unable to carry as much blood. It's kind of like what happens when you attach a nozzle to a garden hose: instead of water just sliding out of the hose and falling to the ground, it squirts out with such force that it can knock the leaves off a plant 6 feet away. It can do damage.

As you tighten the nozzle, you might notice the hose itself getting stiffer because of back pressure. This is like what happens when blood can't get through your lungs easily—the pressure backs up all the way to your heart, which pumps harder and harder to try to push the blood through. Eventually, your heart just can't keep up, and there is less blood circulating through your lungs to pick up oxygen. You become tired, dizzy, and short of breath.

How Scientists Are Learning about PH

The mystery of PH is only beginning to be solved. There are several ways scientists learn about PH: (1) by conducting clinical trials; (2) by epidemiological studies (looking at various groups of people to find unusual clusters or absences of disease and then trying to identify factors that are responsible); and (3) by uncovering the step-by-step processes in the body that lead to PH. The third way is the realm of basic research, and is the subject of this section

PH is a disease of the *blood vessels* of the lungs. Long-time PH researcher Dr. Norbert F. Voelkel (University of Colorado, Denver) says that one of the great mysteries of PH is "why conditions as diverse as viral infection, shear stress, portal hypertension, and drug use all basically generate the same pulmonary vascular lesions." (*Shear stress* refers to the effect of fast-moving blood sliding along vessel walls, and *portal* refers to the vein leading to the liver from the gut. *Lesions* are areas of diseased or injured tissue.) Dr. Bruce Brundage has also worked with PH patients for decades. PH is not a single disease, he says, but a final common pathway that many different disease processes lead to. (Dr. Brundage was recently Chair of PHA's Board of Trustees. He no longer sees patients, but is medical director at the Heart Institute of the Cascades at St. Charles Medical Center in Bend, Oregon.)

with one another and with substances made elsewhere in the body in exceedingly complex ways—sometimes in long chains of reactions (*cascades*), which scientists are just beginning to understand (more on this later).

First, you need to know how blood travels throughout your body. Blood entering the right side of your heart through the systemic veins carries very little oxygen—the red blood cells are like empty rubber rafts floating downstream. The right side of your heart pumps the blood into the arteries of your lungs. (Here's a factoid to impress your friends: the only place in the body where arterial blood is blue is in these arteries!) Pulmonary arteries grow smaller and become *arterioles*. Arterioles are about the size of a hair—so small that red blood cells have to go through them one or two at a time as they approach the even tinier *capillaries*, the vessels snuggled around the air sacs in your lungs. When the rafts reach the air sacs, they take aboard a load of oxygen. (As we breathe in oxygen—which is helpfully made for us by plants—we breathe out carbon dioxide waste, which is created by our bodies when the

The Inside Story on Pulmonary Vessels

Blood vessels in our lungs make important chemical compounds. One important thing these compounds do is to make blood vessels expand or contract. A second thing they do—that now appears to be even more important—is to make, repair, and destroy cells in the vessel walls. What's harming us, in part, may be too much, or too little, of some of these substances. They interact

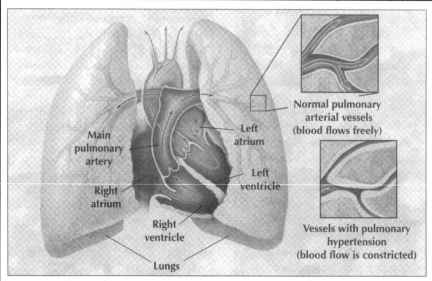

When the tiny arteries in your lungs become constricted or obstructed over time, there's increased resistance to blood flow through the lungs. This causes increased pressure within these arteries — pulmonary hypertension.
Illustration used with permission of the Mayo Foundation (see copyright page).

oxygen is used.) The oxygen is hauled out of the lungs through the pulmonary veins and flows back to the left side of the heart. It is then pumped out to the rest of the body, where the rafts slowly empty as their oxygen is used to fuel body cells. The blood and carbon dioxide waste then return to the right side of the heart, and the circulatory cycle repeats itself.

Usually it's problems in the pulmonary arterioles that cause PH (but sometimes the blockage occurs in the pulmonary veins). The walls of the arterioles have three layers: an inner layer of endothelial tissue, a middle layer of smooth muscle and elastic connective tissue, and an outer layer of fibrous connective tissue. Arterioles can expand or constrict as they do their job of carrying blood to the air sacs in the lung. We don't yet know for certain how blame for PH should be allocated among the three layers in the walls of arterioles.

When too little *oxygen* is getting to the lungs (as happens when PH is secondary to chronic obstructive lung disease or some forms of interstitial fibrosis), then the trouble seems to start in the smooth muscle layer, which bulks up because low oxygen levels cause it to constrict. (The

A Microscope's View of Some Changes That Can Occur in "PPH"

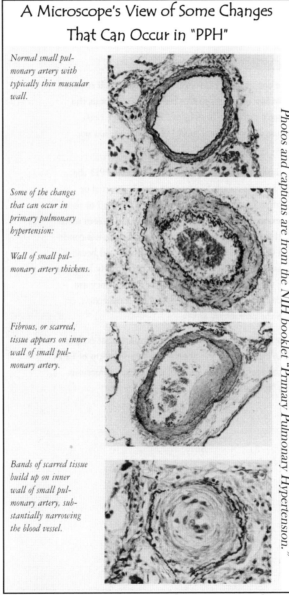

Normal small pulmonary artery with typically thin muscular wall.

Some of the changes that can occur in primary pulmonary hypertension:

Wall of small pulmonary artery thickens.

Fibrous, or scarred, tissue appears on inner wall of small pulmonary artery.

Bands of scarred tissue build up on inner wall of small pulmonary artery, substantially narrowing the blood vessel.

Photos and captions are from the NIH booklet "Primary Pulmonary Hypertension."

diseases mentioned in this chapter are explained in more detail in Chapter 3.)

The new focus on the endothelium. In most forms of PH (including PH associated with collagen vascular disease, portal hypertension, and HIV), the trouble appears to begin not with vasoconstriction, but in the single layer of cells (the *endothelium)* that lines the arterioles. The endothelium releases natural substances that can relax *(vasodilate)* or tighten up *(vasoconstrict)* an arteriole's walls. In healthy arterioles, the substances also provide a "Teflon" surface that red blood cells and other cells can't stick to and jam up things inside the vessel. Some years ago, researchers shifted their attention from looking mainly at vasodilation to a harder look at vascular occlusive disease — at how arterioles get clogged and stiffened by the proliferation of cells. A great deal of research now focuses on the endothelium.

The drama of endothelial research! Because little pulmonary vessels are unique, researchers can't just snatch an umbilical cord from a newborn and dash with it to a laboratory while the cells are still alive. Cells from an umbilical cord might behave differently from cells coming from a lung's blood vessels.

Pulmonary arterioles are very thin and delicate, and endothelial cells from them are extremely hard to grow in a Petri dish. Lungs taken out of PH patients during a transplant are an obvious source, but the right cells have to be preserved by freezing, and not by the usual practices of quickly tossing them into formalin or encasing them in paraffin. Most lung transplants seem to happen in the middle of the night and are tense clock-ticking situations focused on the well-being of a particular patient, not on the needs of a scientist lurking around hoping for a fresh scrap of vessel. Fortunately for us, the scientists are sometimes lucky and get the scraps they need.

The war of the clones. The endothelium of a PH patient looks and behaves differently from the endothelium of a healthy person. Researchers are beginning to learn what turns a healthy endothelium into a sick one. The fault in the endothelium can often involve a genetic mutation. One or more genetic factors make the endothelial cells in "PPH" patients more vulnerable to mutation. [A reminder: although the new term for unexplained PH is idiopathic pulmonary hypertension (IPAH), the older, looser term "PPH" is sometimes used in this book, in quotes, because that is the term that researchers doing particular studies used in the past. Such studies might have included patients with familial PH or PH caused by certain drugs or the HIV virus. Because "PPH" is now such a familiar term, it will probably be some years before it really washes out of the medical literature.]

In people with severe "PPH," a cell in the endothelium apparently mutates in a way that gives it a reproductive advantage over other endothelial cells. The mutated cell then makes too many copies of itself. One theory says that because all the copies come from the same original cell, and are identical, they are *monoclonal*. (IPAH, diet pill-associated PAH,

and familial PAH may be associated with monoclonal cells.) The cell can mutate in response to an injury from some unknown mechanical factor (possibly a burst of hypertension), or in response to various chemicals the body produces when under cardiovascular stress. It might also mutate because of exposure to ingredients in certain diet pills, or possibly because of exposure to the HHV-8 virus. This proliferation of monoclonal cells in "PPH" may be similar to what happens in the growth of tumors.

In people with PH associated with other diseases, the proliferation of endothelial cells seems to happen in response to some known outside injury, such as the high shear stress that results from blood flowing too fast through a vessel, a virus, or inflammation. More than one cell mutates and goes on a reproductive frenzy. These colonies of cells are *polyclonal*—they are not identical, and do not all grow from a single cell. High shear stress can both speed up cell division and cause the production of more growth factors.

Both monoclonal and polyclonal colonies of cells produce chemicals that help them to expand their turf.

What do the "sick" parts look like? The colony of mutated cells forms a "wounded" area inside the vessel (a *plexiform lesion)*. Under a microscope, the lesions look like a mess of out-of-control blood vessels mixed up with lots of weird spindle-shaped endothelial cells, smooth muscle cells, and other cellular matter.

Between 20 and 80 percent of people with "PPH" have such lesions. They resemble the skin lesions of Kaposi's sarcoma, which you may have heard about in connection with stories about AIDS patients. The cells in the plexiform lesions make the wrong amounts of various chemical substances that react with blood vessels, and this makes the situation even worse.

The plexiform lesions clog the insides of the little arteries and solidify over time, causing scarring (*fibrosis*) of the inner and maybe the middle layers of artery walls. Scar tissue is stiff, and makes the blood vessels less able to contract or expand. This process is sometimes called *vascular remodeling*. (When PH is treated with some drugs the reversal of this process—the undoing of some damage—sometimes seems to occur. This is also referred to as vascular remodeling.)

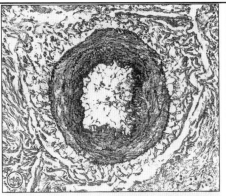

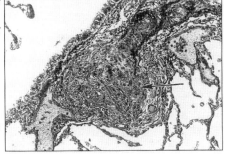

Figure A shows a cross section of a muscular pulmonary artery (enlarged to 100 times its real size) with medial hypertrophy (overgrowth of the middle layer of the vessel's wall). The media occupies 30% of the cross-sectional area.

Figure B shows a side view of plexiform lesions (arrow) arising from a constricted muscular pulmonary artery and feeding into dilated thin-walled arteries. The lesions are shown 100 times their actual size.

Both figures are reprinted with permission from the book edited by Dr. Lewis J. Rubin and Dr. Stuart Rich, Primary Pulmonary Hypertension. Marcel Dekker,1977.)

The lesions that form in PH are not the same thing as atherosclerosis, fatty deposits that form in and on the artery walls of many people. Angioplasty—a treatment used for atherosclerosis—is seldom a treatment for PH, because the arterioles involved in PH are too small and numerous to work on. However this procedure has been tried in thromboembolic PH.

A disease that feeds on itself. In PH, injured endothelial cells also signal the smooth muscle cells they are attached to, and tell them to contract more than normal. As in any exercised muscle, the smooth muscle cells bulk up. It appears that the middle and outside layers of the vessel walls get thicker in all types of PH, whether or not the disease is severe.

Unfortunately, once the process begins, it becomes a vicious cycle that feeds on itself. Blood circulation is restricted and clots are more likely to form. This injures even more endothelial cells. Think again about water going through the nozzle on a hose: because there is less space in the nozzle than in the hose, pressure builds and the water flows faster through the narrowed area, so that the shear stress causes even more irritation of the blood vessel wall. Eventually, the blood flow to some small arteries is entirely cut off.

Chemical Substances That Are Out of Whack in PH

In calling these substances good guys or bad guys, this applies only in terms of what they do to those of us with PH. They are made inside our bodies and are essential to life, in appropriate quantities. It is likely, of course, that somewhat different things go wrong in different PH patients. Growth factors and chemicals that relax and constrict pulmonary blood vessels interact in all sorts of complicated ways, and a single chemical might play the roles of both hero and villain in the PH drama.

To follow the discussion below, it helps to know that an *enzyme* is the chemical equivalent of a matchmaker. It brings other chemicals together so they can join up, forming something new, then ducks out and looks around for other chemicals to bring together. If you are reading abstracts on PubMed and come across a chemical with a name that ends in "ase," it's probably an enzyme.

If you find all this complicated and confusing, you are not alone. Most medical students find organic chemistry their most difficult subject.

Vasodilators (good guys): prostacyclin and **nitric oxide** are two important ones, because they relax the walls of the little arteries. Some research suggests PH patients have too little **prostacyclin** in relation to the amounts they have of a vasoconstrictor called **thromboxane A2**. (Thromboxanes are involved when platelets clump together to form blood clots). Dr. Voelkel's group at the University of Colorado Health Sciences Center has found that an enzyme called **PGI2-synthase** (PGI2 is prostacyclin) helps pulmonary blood vessels respond to a lack of oxygen, and that PH patients don't make enough PGI2-synthase in their endothelial cells. In addition to being a vasodilator, prostacyclin may inhibit the proliferation of smooth muscle cells. Different sizes of pulmonary arteries express prostacyclin differently; the loss of the ability to make prostacyclin is something that happens in severe PH.

PH patients also have low levels of **nitric oxide (NO)** in their lung tissues. Some of the NO in our bodies is made right inside our lungs. An enzyme makes it out of another substance, **arginine**. Researchers at the Cleveland Clinic Foundation compared "PPH" patients with healthy folks and found that the higher the pulmonary artery pressures, and the longer the time since diagnosis, the less NO the "PPH" patients had in their lung tissues.

Bradykinin is another vasodilator, but it's a complicated fellow that does lots of other things, too, such as playing a role in inflammation. Not much is yet known about its role in PH.

"Black hat" chemicals (bad guys): in addition to causing vessels to tighten up, these chemicals may also sometimes stimulate cell growth and proliferation, and inflammation. Released by cells in the endothelium, **endothelins** are the most potent mammalian vasoconstrictors known. Several groups of researchers have found too much endothelin in the blood and urine of PH patients. (Endothelin was discovered by Dr. Masahi Yanagisawa of Japan only in the late 1980's.) **Endothelin-I (ET-1)**, in particular, is a prime suspect in PH. It constricts, inflames, promotes fibrosis, and might cause cells to divide. The production of ET-1 is stimulated by many different chemicals that our bodies make in response to cardiovascular stress, including **angiotensin II, norepinephrine, vasopressin, bradykinin, thrombin,** and **cytokines** (e.g. tumor necrosis factor alpha and transforming growth factor beta). Angiotensin II-converting enzyme and norepinephrine are themselves vasoconstrictors, as is **serotonin** (a neurotransmitter involved in sleep, memory, and depression).

The mineral **potassium** is also involved in the development of PH. Potassium channels are like small doors in cell walls that let potassium in and out of cells. Sometimes the doors don't work properly in PH patients' lung vessel cells, and bad things happen, such as vasoconstriction. Including potassium in your diet does *not* worsen your PH, however, and is often essential if you use diuretics.

A group of German researchers has found that the low levels of NO (a good vasodilator) in the blood of "PPH" patients may be related to an excess of **ADMA** (asymmetric dimethylarginine, if you must know), a substance that slows down the enzyme that makes NO out of arginine.

Chemicals related to blood clotting. Many PH patients have problems with blood clots forming in the arteries of their lungs, so chemicals related to this process interest researchers. Blood clots are known to release the growth factor **thrombin,** which acts on fibrinogen to form fibrin. Fibrin forms networks of fibers inside vessels that trap red blood cells and platelets, forming clots. Another growth factor comes from **platelets.** Platelets are tiny disks of protoplasm found in our blood that help it to clot. They may cause tiny clots to form in the lungs of many **PH** patients. Making platelets less sticky may be one of the good things prostacyclin does.

There is continued research into the role of **angiotensin II. Angiotensin-converting enzyme (ACE)** hangs around in the endothelium bringing together chemicals that turn angiotensin I into angiotensin II. Angiotensin II causes vasoconstriction and remodeling in vessels and the heart muscle. If this conversion can be blocked (by using a converting enzyme inhibitor), it may be possible to prevent proliferation. Such drugs already exist and are used to treat systemic hypertension and left-heart failure. But there is no proof yet that they help in **PH.** Researchers at the University of Colorado have found that persons with severe "PPH" have a significantly higher incidence of a particular oddity in a part of the ACE gene than do people in normal control groups. (This genetic oddity also seems, however, to help the right ventricles of "PPH" patients' hearts pump well!)

Serine elastase inhibitor. Dr. Marlene Rabinovitch and her group at the Hospital for Sick Children (Toronto, Canada) injected rats with the alkaloid toxin monocrotaline, which injured their pulmonary endothelial cells and gave the rats PH. She then gave the rats an oral drug that blocks an enzyme called serine elastase. (Increased serine elastase activity is associated with **PH.**) The blocking drug stopped smooth muscle cells in the rats' pulmonary arteries from growing into parts of the vessels where they didn't belong. Even more wonderful, the already out-of-place smooth muscle cells were killed off (*myocyte*

apoptosis). The success of this experiment gives more reason to hope that damaged pulmonary arteries can be repaired. These blockers are also being studied as a treatment for cancer. Unfortunately, there is no such elastase-blocking substance now available for safe use in humans. Dr. Rabinovitch is now at Stanford University, studying how these findings relate to the genetic aspects of PH and other vascular diseases.

Your Overworked Heart

The heart is divided into four pumping chambers. It is the right side of a PH patient's heart that usually has problems. The bottom chamber, called the *right ventricle*, pumps deoxygenated blood through the pulmonary valve and into the pulmonary artery, which divides and carries blood to both lungs. If you have PH, your right ventricle has to work so hard to force blood through blocked lung vessels that it bulks up. The right ventricle is not designed to do such hard work; normally the pressure inside it is only 20 to 25 percent of that in the left ventricle.

When pressures remain too high for too long, the right ventricle becomes so stretched out that it cannot contract effectively. This is called *congestive right-heart failure* or *cor pulmonale.* ("Failure" does not mean that the heart has stopped, only that it can't pump out all the blood in it into the lungs.) When your right ventricle fails, there is a backup of pressure into veins throughout your body, and you swell with fluid, especially in your legs, liver, abdomen, and the spaces in your chest surrounding your lungs. In PAH, your right atrium also tends to get bigger, because of back pressure from the right ventricle.

There is good news: when the pressures in your lungs lessen (because of successful treatment with medications, treatment of the condition that caused the PH, or the transplantation of a new lung or lungs), your heart tends to return to its normal size. Your body has little tricks that also automatically kick in to help your heart work well. So, after treatment, you may no longer have congestive heart failure. But if your heart has been stressed so long that scar tissue has formed in its structure, it is still damaged. If, in spite of treatments, you continue to collect fluids in your spongy tissues, etc., it is said that you have *decompensated heart failure*.

What Is "Mean Pulmonary Artery Pressure"?

PH patients often compare their mean pulmonary artery pressures (mean PAPs). Your PAP is measured in mm Hg (millimeters of mercury). The mean PAP of a resting healthy person is around 14 mm Hg. If you have PH, your mean pressure is above 25 mm Hg at rest. There are cases, however, where pressures are normal at rest and the PH shows up only during exercise; this is why, if your doc suspects PH, but it doesn't show up when you're resting, you might also need to be tested while exercising.

Don't confuse your *mean* PAP with your *systolic* PAP, which is higher. If you're comparing pressures with your PH buddy, be sure you're talking about the same thing. The systolic pressure is measured when the heart is squeezing blood out; the diastolic pressure is measured when the heart is relaxed. To find your mean PAP, multiply your diastolic artery pressure by two, add the product to your systolic artery pressure, and divide the total by three. (Or just ask your PH specialist.)

Most "PPH" patients start to notice symptoms of the disease when their mean PAP is around 30 to 35 mm Hg at rest, but some do not have any symptoms even when their pressure is much higher. There is no magic cut-off PAP number above which someone will die. A few patients with systolic pressures over 120 can still function quite well, while others have little energy with pressures around 50. There is not a uniformly accepted way to grade PH as mild, moderate, or severe, but this is how at least some doctors define the disease in terms of *mean* PAP pressure:

> Mild: 26-35 mm Hg mean PAP
> Moderate: 36-45 mm Hg mean PAP
> Severe: above 45 mm Hg mean PAP

Or, in terms of *systolic* PAP pressure:

> Mild: 40-55 mm Hg
> Moderate: 55-75 mm Hg
> Severe: above 75 mm Hg

Please don't take these classifications as gospel. Cardiac output, right atrial pressure, exercise capacity, functional status, and other factors also indicate how well a patient is doing, so two patients with the same mean PAP might have very different qualities of life and chances of survival.

What is "Cardiac Output"?

Your *cardiac output* is the amount of blood your heart pumps out each minute. It's determined by multiplying the stroke volume by the number of times your heart beats each minute (*heart rate*). *Stroke volume* is the portion of the blood held in your ventricle that is squeezed out with each beat. It is measured during your heart catheterization with a Swan-Ganz catheter. Some physicians estimate it with the echocardiogram, but others feel this method is not sufficiently accurate.

A normal cardiac output is around 5 quarts a minute. When a person has severe PH, their heart pumps only about half the normal amount of blood. Sometimes calcium channel blockers given to treat PH have the unwanted side effect of lowering stroke volume. When your cardiac output is low, you may have lower systemic blood pressure (the kind measured by a cuff on your arm), and feel dizzy.

It is usually a patient's cardiac output, and not their mean PAP, that correlates the best with their symptoms. Think of it this way: the pressure inside your lungs is like your municipal water pressure—how forceful is it? And the resistance inside your lungs is like the diameter of the pipes in your house. Small, clogged pipes carry less water. If you divide the pressure by the resistance, you get the flow (cardiac output). Therefore, the only way to keep cardiac output up when resistance is increased is to increase the pressure—which is just what happens in our bodies. As discussed earlier, in the self-feeding loop that is one of the great dangers of PH, the tension against the artery walls increases as pressure rises, leading to vascular changes that worsen PH.

If you are blessed with a strong heart, for a while it can keep up the flow by enlarging and pumping harder and more often (against the higher pressure). As the disease progresses, and the resistance grows, the heart can't keep up. Fluid begins to seep out of your vessels and into spongy tissues. Legs and ankles swell, fluid may collect in your abdomen, your liver might get enlarged.

When the stroke volume is maxed out because the heart can't pump any more strongly, then it begins to beat more often. A rising pulse rate can be bad news. Some doctors say that a resting pulse rate that has climbed to over 100 beats per minute is a sign of worsening PH.

Fortunately, there are drugs available today that can do much to improve the flow of blood through your lungs. See Chapter 5 for details.

Who Gets PH?

We all want to know why me? Was it something I ate? Something I was exposed to? Something my mother was exposed to while she was pregnant? Something I might pass on to my children? There aren't many answers yet, only educated guesses. It does seem that those of us with PH have pulmonary blood vessels that are ultra-sensitive to one or more things. Although PH can often be triggered by another, known disease, the way that the triggering disease is linked to the PH is still usually unknown. Why, for example, does emphysema lead to PH in some persons but not in others?

Incidence of PH in the U.S.

The true incidence of either idiopathic PAH (IPAH) or PH secondary to other diseases hasn't been determined. In 1998, the National Hospital Discharge Survey by the Centers for Disease Control and Prevention (CDC) found that 67,497 men and 107,357 women were hospitalized with PH in the U.S. For every 10,000 Americans there were almost 7 hospitalizations for the disease. Still citing the CDC, in 1998 there were about 3.1 PH-related deaths per 100,000 Americans that year.

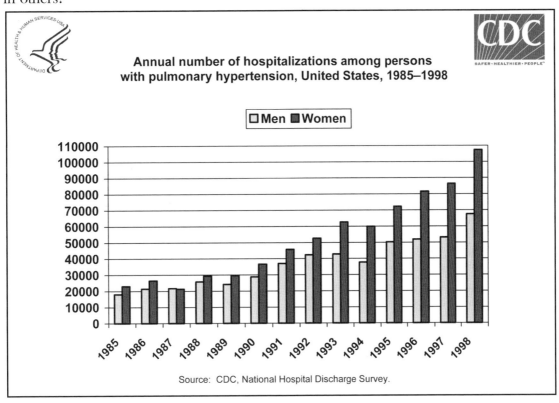

Annual number of hospitalizations among persons with pulmonary hypertension, United States, 1985–1998

Source: CDC, National Hospital Discharge Survey.

In the early 1990's, only one or two persons out of a million were thought to have IPAH or FPAH, and it was believed that PH in general was a rare disease. Then the fen-phen scandal broke in the U.S., drawing more attention to PH. Today, the CDC views PH as an underdiagnosed chronic disease. Far more people have PH triggered by another disease than have IPAH or FPAH. One estimate is that when you consider everyone who has troublesome PH of any sort, it adds up to 30 to 50 people out of a million.

PH can pop up at any age, even at birth or after retirement. It affects persons of all races and ethnic backgrounds. Many were surprised when an examination of CDC mortality data found that what the CDC called PPH (which included FPAH and PAH caused by anorectic diet pills as well as IPAH) appeared to be more frequent in blacks than in whites and in older adults than in younger ones. An accurate estimate of the presence of various forms of PH in the population is hard to get, and more study is needed.

Risk Factors & Mysteries

PH is definitely linked to **gender**. The forms of PH called idiopathic (IPAH) and familial (FPAH) under the new classification (see below) are roughly two-and–a-half times more common in women than in men (at PH centers across the U.S. it ranges from being twice as common in women to nine times as common). For unknown reasons, females of childbearing years are more likely to get **IPAH** or **FPAH**. Other types of PH also occur more often in women, although the difference between men and women may not be as great.

If others in your family have PH, your chances of developing PH are greater. **Pregnancy** and **systemic hypertension** are other possible risk factors suggested by registries, expert opinion, and case series (research papers comparing several patients

with PH with people who do not have PH but are otherwise like the PH patients in age, gender, etc.). **Obesity** alone is *not* believed to be a risk factor. But if it is combined with **obstructive sleep apnea** (so that oxygen levels fall while you're sleeping) it might cause mild PH. A clue, in obese patients with PAH, is the swelling of both legs. If present, it might make a doc wonder about whether the patient has obstructive sleep apnea. Also, if you're overweight, your heart has to pump harder to send blood to all parts of a bigger body, which increases your cardiac output; there are studies showing that a **chronically high cardiac output** might trigger PAH. The theory that PH might be caused by **chronic levels of high stress**, and the resulting high levels of catecholamines and epinephrine produced in the body, is not in fashion. But it is believed that stress can significantly aggravate existing PH.

Links between PH and diseases in addition to those discussed below will

---

Clinical Incidence of "PPH" among Various Groups*

In the general population . . . . .1 in 500,000 . . . .(0.0002%)
Familial IPAH . . . . .191 in 1,920 . . . .(9.9 %)
  (as % of all IPAH patients)
Connective tissue diseases . . . . .1 in 10-1,000 . . .(0.1-10%)
HIV infected . . . . .5 in 1,000 . . . . . .(0.5%)
Cirrhosis/portal hypertension . .5-8 in 1,000 . . . .(0.5-0.8 %)
  (as % of all liver disease patients)
Took appetite suppressants
  for over 3 months . . . . .1 in 17,000 . . . . .(0.006 %)
Took appetite suppressants
  for over 6 months . . . . .1 in 10,000 . . . .(0.01%)
People with atrial septal defects . . . .(4-6%)
  not operated on
People with ventricular septal defects . . . .(10%)
  not operated on**

* This data was taken from Nazzareno Galiè et al., "Primary Pulmonary Hypertension: Insights into Pathogenesis from Epidemiology," Chest, 114(3 Suppl.): 184S-194S (Sept. 11, 1998). Echocardiograms show a higher incidence of PH in those with connective tissue disease (15-35%) and in those with cirrhosis/portal hypertension (2%).
** There are no reliable estimates of the risk of developing PH for a child born with a ventricular septal defect (VSD) because such children are at an increased risk of death during early childhood. Only 10 % of adults with untreated VSDs have severe PH.

undoubtedly be discovered. Even when a link is known to exist, *why* it exists often remains a mystery. For example, it isn't really known why PH appears more often in folks with thyroid problems (see below). When PH is secondary to another disease, there does not seem to be any correlation between the severity of that other disease and the development of PH—the sickest are no more likely to get PH than the less sick.

Those of us who have PAH appear more likely than most to also have a problem with our immune systems (we often have autoimmune diseases, in which cells produced by own body attack our body's own tissues), and it is possible that abnormalities in such systems play a role in the development of PAH (see the discussion under 1.3, APAH, on autoimmune disease).

It's time for a pop-up refresher course on immunities. An *antigen* is a substance capable of triggering an immune response in our bodies, which results in the creation of a specific *antibody*, a protein that helps protect our bodies from infection and disease. An *autoantibody* is an antibody that reacts against your own tissue. An *antinuclear antibody (ANA)* is an autoantibody directed against normal parts of a cell's nucleus.

In many IPAH patients, autoantibodies against the thyroid gland and nonspecific antinuclear antibodies are found, but their role in making us sick is unknown. In patients who develop secondary PAH from specific autoimmunities—such as systemic lupus erythematous, scleroderma, and juvenile rheumatoid arthritis—the PAH develops more frequently than in a control population, but this does not appear to be linked to the levels of circulating antibodies. Although persons who have their spleens removed might be more likely to develop PAH (see below), another puzzle is why some IPAH patients have such **low platelet counts**. At the PHA

conference in the year 2000, a PH patient with the exceedingly rare **Castleman's** disease (noncancerous growths develop in lymph node tissue) spoke at one of the sessions, surprising a couple of docs who thought they had the only PH patient with this disease. Also, some people with **Gaucher's disease** (an inability to metabolize fat well) develop PH for unknown reasons. One doctor had a case where it appeared that PH was triggered by the **POEMS syndrome** (polyneuropathy [many inflamed nerves], organomegaly [enlarged organs], endocrinoopathy [a disorder of the endocrine glands], monoclonal gammopathy [too hard to explain here], and skin changes).

Updated (Again) Diagnostic Classifications

A new way of classifying types of PH was proposed at the World Health Organization's World Symposium on PPH in Evian, France, in the fall of 1998 (the classification included in the Second Edition of the *Survival Guide*). These categories were further refined at the WHO World Symposium on PAH in Venice, Italy, in 2003. It's a pain learning new terms every couple of years. But each time, the categories make more sense, and make it possible to speak more clearly about the disease. Because of the "final common pathway" that the disease often takes, many treatments for PH work for all groups in a category. By generalizing therapies, larger pools of patients are available for drug trials, which can speed the search for a cure. The chart on the next page contains the official, jargon-laden categories. Explanations in plain English are on the following pages.

Category 1: Pulmonary Arterial Hypertension (PAH)

This means high blood pressure occurs in the *arteries* of the lungs, that it is not the result of pulmonary venous hypertension, hypoxemia, or thromboembolic disease. It is also called "pre-capillary PH," because it is the disease of the pulmonary arteries themselves that causes the problem, and is not related to anything going on downstream from the arteries (i.e. the lung air sacs, the pulmonary veins, or the left heart).

1.1. Idiopathic (IPAH)

Idiopathic means unexplained, or, as some jokers put it, that "doctors are idiots" because they don't know what causes a disease. This is the most baffling form of PH, but the category shrinks year by year as more causes are found. As explained earlier, it used to be included in the category called primary pulmonary hypertension (PPH), and some articles still use the old term. Much of the research on "PPH" actually included patients who had familial PAH (FPAH), or PH triggered by the HIV virus, anorectic diet pills, etc. IPAH looks just the same under the microscope as FPAH (see below), and patients have the same symptoms, the same gender ratio, and mortality rates. Even some of the same genetic mutations appear to be involved in both.

A small percentage of IPAH is thought to be due to DNA errors that were not inherited, but acquired some time after birth. The rest are called *sporadic* IPAH. This is the most poorly understood type of PH. *Sporadic* means that the disease just popped up out of

---

Revised Clinical Classification of Pulmonary Hypertension (WHO World Symposium on PAH Venice 2003)

(This material appeared in a larger context in an article by Dr. Lewis Rubin in the Journal of the American College of Cardiology in July 2004. Used with special permission.)

1. Pulmonary Arterial Hypertension (PAH)
  1.1. Idiopathic (IPAH)
  1.2. Familial (FPAH)
  1.3. Associated with (APAH):
    1.3.1. Collagen Vascular Disease
    1.3.2. Congenital systemic to pulmonary shunts**
    1.3.3. Portal hypertension
    1.3.4. HIV infection
    1.3.5. Drugs and toxins
    1.3.6. Other (Thyroid disorders, Glycogen Storage Disease, Gaucher's Disease, Hereditary Hemorrhagic Telangiectasia, Hemoglobinopathies, Myeloproliferative Disorders, Splenectomy)
  1.4. Associated with significant venous or capillary involvement
    1.4.1. Pulmonary veno-occlusive disease (PVO)
    1.4.2. Pulmonary capillary hemangiomatosis (PCH)
  1.5. Persistent pulmonary hypertension of the Newborn

2. Pulmonary Venous Hypertension
  2.1. Left-sided atrial or ventricular heart disease
  2.2. Left-sided valvular heart disease

3. Pulmonary Hypertension associated with hypoxemia
  3.1. Chronic obstructive pulmonary disease
  3.2. Interstitial lung disease
  3.3. Sleep-disordered breathing
  3.4. Alveolar hypoventilation disorders
  3.5. Chronic exposure to high altitude
  3.6. Developmental abnormalities

4. Pulmonary Hypertension due to chronic thrombotic and/or embolic disease
  4.1. Thromboembolic obstruction of proximal pulmonary arteries
  4.2. Thromboembolic obstruction of distal pulmonary arteries
  4.3. Non-thrombotic pulmonary embolism (tumor, parasites, foreign material)

5. Miscellaneous
  Sarcoidosis, Histiocytosis X, Lymphangiomatosis, Compression of pulmonary vessels (adenopathy, tumor, fibrosing mediastinitis)

---

the blue in somebody with no family history of the disease.

About 10 to 20 percent of what *appears* to be sporadic IPAH is really FPAH. Because so many people who carry the FPAH gene never develop PH, it's easy to overlook the presence of the gene in a family. When researchers at the University of Leicester, UK, looked at the PH genes of 50 IPAH patients with no family history of the disease, they found 11 different mutations in the BMPR2 gene of 13 of the patients. The researchers then looked at the parents of those 13 patients, and found three parents who carried a mutation. In other words, over a quarter of the patients sampled had inherited a PH gene, even though no one else in their family was known to have PH.

The Vanderbilt PH research team explored the ancestry of five PH families with 394 known members spanning seven generations and traced them all back to a single founding couple in the mid-1800s! Only 20 family members have been diagnosed with PH; 12 of those 20 (sixty percent) were originally thought to have sporadic PH.

Dr. Greg Elliott at the LDS Hospital, University of Utah, in Salt Lake City has collected DNA samples from persons with sporadic IPAH. He uses the genealogy records kept by the LDS church to (successfully) search for unknown family connections between PH patients. (You don't have to be Mormon to participate in his study—most participants are not.) Dr. Elliott attends PHA conferences with his needles and swabs in hand. He calls the synergism at the conferences among patients and doctors phenomenal and unique, and is grateful for the help we have given him.

Will you pass on your "sporadic" PH to your kids? If your PH is really a result of a mutation in a germinal cell (egg or sperm), then you might. Otherwise, you won't.

1.2. Familial (FPAH)

If more than one person in your family has PAH, you are said to have "familial" FPAH. PAH is inherited in at least 6 to 10 percent of cases of PAH. More accurately, the *predisposition* to PAH is inherited; only about 20 percent of persons who inherit the genetic predisposition actually develop the disease.

The human genome is often compared to a book containing a set of instructions that your body has to read to carry out a process. Other instructions outside the book tell the body how to go about reading it. Both sets of instructions can be altered in ways that cause problems.

Matt Ridley, the author of *Genome*, takes the analogy further: the book has 23 chapters (*chromosomes*). Each chapter has a couple thousand stories (*genes*); each story is given a title (the name of the gene). The stories are made up of paragraphs (*exons*), which are interrupted by advertisements (*introns*). Each paragraph is made up of words (*codons*), and the words are written in letters *(bases)*.

Every cell in your body contains a complete book *except* for your sex cells (a.k.a. *germ cells*—ova or sperm). They carry only a half set of chromosomes, which are eager to become whole by merging with a half set from your mate.

All you really need to know for the pop quiz is that each gene carries instructions for making a particular protein (proteins are complex chemical compounds like enzymes, hormones, immunoglobulins, etc.). If even a single "letter" in the entire gene is changed or out of place (*mutated*), the product the gene makes is different and the wrong instructions are sometimes sent. The copying process in our bodies makes faithful copies of the mutated gene, so the change is permanent. (Sometimes, of course, mutations are beneficial and make it more likely that an organism will survive. This is the basis of the evolution of living things.)

Many things can cause mutations including radiation, ultraviolet light (in skin), certain medicines and other chemicals, and copying mistakes in DNA when cells divide. If a mutation happens to a cell in most parts of your body, it affects only you and is not passed on to your children. But if it occurs in a sex cell, it might be passed along to your children. This is called a *germ-line* mutation. FPAH can be caused by both germ-cell mutations and by as yet unidentified genetic predispositions. Scientists looking at whole lung tissue or DNA from blood samples can tell if it comes from patients with familial or non-familial PAH.

It is believed that a single gene out of the roughly 30,000 on the human genome is responsible for most cases of inherited FPAH. The FPAH gene was discovered in July 2000 by two independent research teams. One team was based at Columbia University (New York, NY). The other group included PH researchers from both the U.S. (Vanderbilt University) and Europe: the International PPH Consortium.

The FPAH gene is on chromosome 2. It codes for a protein called "**bone morphogenetic protein receptor 2**" (**BMPR2**). It is part of the transforming growth factor beta (TGF-beta) family. Don't let the name fool you: these "bone morphogenetic" proteins were first identified as helping to regulate the growth of bone and cartilage, but more recent studies have shown they also help regulate the growth, differentiation, and destruction of other types of cells. BMPR2 affects the growth and differentiation of cells that line the blood vessels of the lungs. It does not appear to control vasodilatation or vasoconstriction.

The Columbia researchers found at least five different mutations on the gene that may make it more likely someone will get FPAH. (Since then, mutations have been found in all but one of the 13 exons that make up the

gene.) Because only 9 of the 19 families in this study had mutations that are likely to disrupt the functioning of the receptor, it is possible that the entire gene might not have been screened, or that other genes are also directly involved in the disease.

There is still much to learn about precisely why the mutations cause FPAH. As Dr. Nazzareno Galiè says, "We have the disease on one side and the mutation on the other—what lies between is still unknown, yet critical to the understanding of the disease." (Dr. Galiè is at the University of Bologna, Italy, and

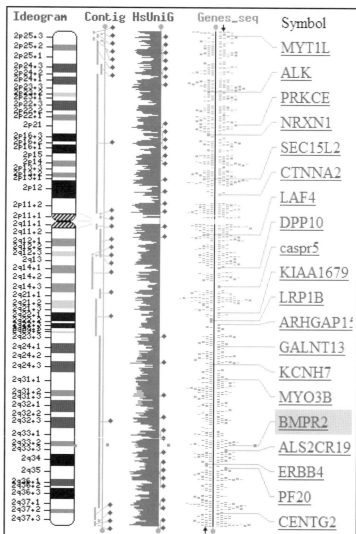

Location of BMPR2 on chromosone 2.
From National Center for Biotechnology Information
U.S. National Library of Medicine gene map viewer at
www.ncbi.nlm.nih.gov.

has authored or coauthored over 280 papers related to PH.)

More recently, researchers at the University of California in San Diego have discovered that a gene (**angiopoietin-1**) that grows smooth muscle cells is active in FPAH patients. Normally, this gene is only turned on in embryos. It appears to interact in complicated ways with the BMPR2 gene. Defects in the signaling pathway involving angiopoietin-1, TIE2 (the endothelial-specific receptor for angiopoietin-1), BMPR1A and BMPR2 appear to apply to all forms of PH.

Why was it important to find a gene that causes FPAH? Learning how a gene responsible for FPAH differs from normal genes in what it does is our best shot at truly understanding what is going on inside our blood vessels and finding a cure for all types of PH, not just the inherited variety. Because a gene responsible for FPAH has been identified, it is possible to search more directly for the basic mechanism of the disease.

What is already known about the gene? The gene is autosomal dominant with incomplete penetrance. Autosomal means it's not on the sex-determining X or Y chromosome. *Dominant* means it takes only one parent—either mom or dad—to pass it on. (So those of us with familial FPAH have one good gene paired with one near-twin faulty one on chromosome 2.) *Incomplete penetrance* means that even though you carry the gene you may not develop FPAH. Such persons are called *obligate* carriers, because when you study a family tree showing who has FPAH, and who hasn't, the laws of genetics say that some healthy family members *must* carry the gene. The disease, but not the gene, sometimes skips a generation.

If I have the gene will I get FPAH? Even if you are a carrier, your chance of developing FPAH is only about 10 to 20 percent. (It's possible that the rate is higher or lower for various types of mutations, but this is not yet determined.) There are carriers who have lived into their nineties without developing PH (but who have children or grandchildren with the disease). So it's clear that something more—some broader genetic factor or environmental factor—is also needed to trigger the disease.

In actuality, the FPAH gene does not have just "incomplete" penetrance, but "markedly reduced" penetrance. Researchers speculate that a second, autosomal, mutation along the BMPR2 signaling pathway may be required for IPAH to develop. Or the lack of penetrance may be due to a mutation in the signaling pathway (either germinal or autosomal) *combined with* an environmental insult (like an HIV infection or exposure to certain diet pills). Thirdly, the reduced penetrance might be caused by the presence of "good" modifier genes (either autosomal or sex-linked) that act to reduce the harmfulness of the "bad" gene.

Some researchers have observed that FPAH seems to be more severe and to occur at earlier and earlier ages in successive generations (*genetic anticipation*). It may be, however, that the disease is just being diagnosed earlier, or that there are now more environmental triggers around. The mean age of onset is 36 years.

Females with the gene appear more likely to develop the disease than do males. The reason isn't known. Men and women both have chromosome 2. It's possible that alterations on the x (female) chromosome influence the development of the disease, or that sex hormones play a role. If you carry the gene, you are somewhat more likely than normal to give birth to a female child. This might be because male fetuses die more often before they are born; it is possible that the FPAH gene plays a role in embryologic development.

To learn more about genetics and the

human genome, check out Uncle Sam's awesome Human Genome Project website: www.ornl.gov/hgmis.

National Registry for Familial FPAH. Dr. Jim Loyd and Dr. John

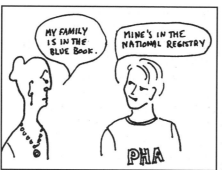

Newman (Vanderbilt University) realized early on that there might be a "PH gene." Back in 1980 the science of molecular genetics hadn't advanced far enough to look for such a gene. Believing that such a day would come, the scientists—who had no funding to support this activity— started collecting and saving cells from members of families with PH. Vanderbilt University still keeps a list of families with hereditary PAH, and is researching the genetic aspects of the disease. The Registry can be contacted by calling Lisa Wheeler at 1-800-288-0378. Nearly 100 U.S. families have been identified with two to eight FPAH patients per family, and one to seven generations involved. (Columbia University has also collected about 100 PH families. Overlap is likely, so there are maybe 150 or so PH families in the U.S.) Over two-thirds of the patients are female. Even though an FPAH gene has been found, the registry expects to enroll families at least through 2008. They will happily accept a DNA sample from families living anywhere in the world who have more than one member with FPAH. So far all enrollees are of European or Japanese descent, but there are cases in the literature of FPAH running in African-American families. Any DNA information is coded and the identity of the individual is never shared or published. This protection is ensured by agreements with the Institutional Board for the Protection of Human Subjects at each medical center.

Genetic samples are needed from as many family members as possible—not only those sick with PAH—to see which parts of the gene are shared between those who got the disease and those who have not. Maybe healthy carriers have another mutation that protects them, or maybe they were not exposed to an environmental factor that triggered the IPAH in their relative.

Registries abroad. At the University of Leicester in Leicester, UK, Dr. Richard Trembath is collecting DNA samples (he had found 25 families at the time this was written). Dr. Marc Humbert is collecting in France. You can reach him through Service de Pneumologie et Réanimation Respiratoire, UPRES 2705 (Maladies Vasculaire Pulmomaires), Hôpital Antoine Béclerè, Université Paris-Sud, Clamart, France. In Italy Dr. Nazzareno Galiè at the Instituto di Bologna is doing the same (he is interested in hearing from anybody with IPAH, not just familial cases). In Germany, Prof. Werner Seeger maintains a registry: Ambulanz für Pulmonale Hypertonie, Abt. Pneumologie der Med. Klinik II, Klinikstrasse 36, D- 35392 Giessen, Deutschland. Tel.: 0641-99 42534 oder 42500.

REVEAL registry. The REVEAL (Registry to Evaluate Early and Long Term PAH Disease Management) registry, sponsored by Actelion was launched in March 2006. This is a US based, multi-center registry. It hopes to collect data from WHO Group I PH patients who will be followed for 5 years. The registry's goals are to : (1) characterize demographics and clinical course of PAH patients, (2) evaluate and compare patient outcomes, (3) identify factors that predict short-term and long-term clinical outcomes, (4) assess the relationship between medications and outcomes, and (5) collect data in the hopes of addressing the evolving research needs of the PAH community.

Private genetic testing. Even if you gave a DNA sample for genetic studies, you will not automatically be told if you have an FPAH gene. To underline the distinction between research efforts and clinical testing, most research groups will take fresh DNA samples from those who want to know.

Genetic testing in a clinical setting is now possible. But the gene is so large, and has so many possibly relevant mutation sites that routine testing of all PH patients isn't feasible. When genetic testing is done clinically, it may be put on your medical chart, so insurance companies and others can often get access to it. Talk to your doctor or the researcher about this concern. You may decide not to submit an insurance claim for the test, so your doctor does not have to reveal the fact you took the test or the results. Or you might ask a lab about being tested anonymously, using a pseudonym or a number, as is sometimes done for HIV.

Testing is complicated because so many different mutations on the FPAH gene are involved. Furthermore, mutations have only been found, so far, in about 75 percent of the families in which FPAH is known to run. (It's even possible that other genes might be involved in some families as well as other mutations on the known FPAH gene.)

It is theoretically possible to test a fetus for PH, although the author couldn't find any cases where this had been done. Because not everyone with the gene gets PH, because PH doesn't affect intelligence, and because many of us with PH are able to live good lives, terminating a pregnancy because of a PH gene would be a wrenching decision.

The consensus is that you should get counseling prior to getting a genetic test. During this counseling ask about anything you don't understand or that troubles you about the test, and also grill the testers on how they will protect your family's privacy; it's the entire family's privacy that's at stake, not just that of the person being tested.

Why would you want to know? If one of your parents has FPAH, you might or might not have the gene that predisposes you to PH. Learning you don't have it would let you stop worrying every time you feel a little tired or short of breath. In the future we may know things to do (or avoid exposure to) that can keep carriers from developing the disease. You may be more alert for symptoms of PH in yourself or your child and get treatment earlier, which can be lifesaving. Knowing that you do or do not have the gene may allow you to do more informed financial, family, and estate planning.

Why would you not want to know? Maybe you think you would worry yourself to death if you knew for sure you had the gene, or had passed it on to a child. Or you might be concerned that if an employer or insurance company learns you have the PH gene they will discriminate against you. Although federal law prevents genetic discrimination by federal employers, there is no similar protection against discrimination by private employers. About half the states have some sort of privacy or genetic discrimination law, but they vary a lot. Also, because only about 20 percent of persons who carry the FPAH mutation ever get the disease, many choose to get regular echoes as a screen for PH rather than go through genetic testing.

All major diseases—not just PH—have a genetic component. Because the human genome has now been decoded, many disease-causing mutations will be found. So it seems possible that Congress will eventually pass laws preventing discrimination by private employers solely on the basis of one's genetic inheritance.

Warning: if you decide against genetic testing and you have a first-degree relative with familial IPAH, then you should get an echocardiogram every 3 to 5 years to screen for IPAH. If symptoms appear, get an echo right away.

How you can help. PHA members played a BIG role in finding out about the FPAH gene. Many of us enrolled in the National Registry, and most of us who went to PHA's international conferences donated blood and shared our medical and family histories. If you have not already done so, please help out the researchers when they next approach you. If you are scared of needles, a swab can be taken of cells from inside your cheek.

PH can run in your family even if you don't know it. By diving into genealogy, researchers have found unexpected family links between PH patients who didn't even know each other. If you think that great-uncle Hogwash might have died of PH even though his death certificate lists another cause, if an autopsy report or a biopsy sample of *any part* of him is still around it could reveal whether he truly had FPAH. (A crime lab sample could do the same, if he was that sort of fellow, and might still be stashed in an evidence room.) Nobody is going to ask you to dig up Hogwash himself, although it is technically possible to even get DNA from mummies.

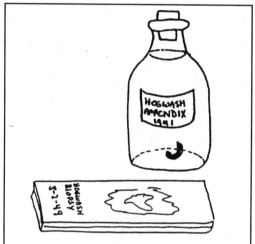

Unanswered questions. At the 2002 PHA conference, Dr. Greg Elliott suggested some areas for more research: Why does the PH gene only lead to disease in *pulmonary* arteries? Why is there incomplete penetrance? What other mutations might exist that relate to PH? How does a patient's genetic makeup relate to how his/her PH manifests itself, and how he/she reacts to various treatments?

One day scientists might be able to peek at someone's genes and say, "You should take a prostanoid, not an endothelin antagonist, and better avoid those Brussels sprouts unless you take a baby aspirin with them. And by the way, marry Sally, not Betty, if you want healthier kids."

1.3. PAH Associated with Other Diseases or Things (APAH)

PAH (including IPAH and FPAH) is strongly associated with various autoimmune diseases. An autoimmune disease happens when something causes your immune system to make antibodies that attack your body's own normal tissues. In other words, you are under friendly fire. The battle causes a lot of inflammation, which can cause further damage. There are more than 80 known autoimmune disorders, but they all have many features in common. About 8.5 million people in the U.S. have an autoimmune disease, and 80 percent of them are women. The different hormones in men and women might cause this lopsidedness. A new theory is that a pregnant woman exchanges cells with her fetus, and these cells can persist in either the mother or the newborn's circulation for decades, and may, on rare occasions, trigger an autoimmune disease.

Autoimmune disorders that seem to appear in families of PH patients, or in the patients themselves, include the connective tissue diseases discussed below. None of these diseases are contagious.

Unfortunately, some doctors who treat autoimmune disease patients aren't as familiar as they should be with PH. Jessica found this out when she went to a lupus convention where a doctor spoke about lupus and how it affects the heart. She noticed he'd been looking at her off and on during his speech (Jessica was wearing oxygen), and when he had finished she raised her hand and asked him to explain about lupus and PH, a problem he hadn't mentioned. (Go girl!) He was caught totally off guard and stumbled through an explanation that didn't earn him a passing grade. You can bet he'll be better prepared in the future, and Jessica might have prolonged lives in that room.

1.3.1. Connective Tissue Disease (a.k.a. Collagen Vascular Disease)

Collagen is the strong fibrous stuff found in connective tissue. *Connective tissue*, as its name implies, connects and supports parts of the body. It is usually dense with blood vessels. This group of immunologic, rheumatic diseases includes scleroderma, CREST syndrome, rheumatoid arthritis, systemic lupus erythematous (SLE), vasculitis, and mixed connective-tissue disease. A quick description of each follows. Several other connective tissue diseases, such as **dermatomyositis/polymyositis** (a skin rash associated with inflamed muscles), and **Sjögren's syndrome** (slowly progressive dryness of the eyes and mouth and recurrent salivary gland enlargement) are, for unknown reasons, associated with PH. Knowing a bit about these diseases can help you understand what some members of your support group have to cope with in addition to their PH.

There is no simple test to tell you if you have one of these diseases, but nearly all patients who have connective tissue disease have autoantibodies in their blood.

Scleroderma. Scleroderma means "hard skin," but this same hardening can happen to an organ or tissue because of the growth of too much collagen. The disease affects mainly the small blood vessels and the collagen-producing cells throughout the body. It sometimes causes only very mild symptoms, but it can kill as well. When it does, it is most often due to pulmonary disease. Because collagen is affected, patients can develop taut, shiny skin and mask-like expressions. When the small vessels in the fingers narrow, shutting off the supply of blood, patients are very apt to get chilly, bluish fingers when they are exposed to cold (*Raynaud's phenomenon*—see below). The cause of scleroderma is unknown, and there is not presently a cure. About 150,000 to 300,000 persons in the U.S. have the disease, and it strikes around four times as many women as men.

Scleroderma can lead to PH because it can cause scar tissue to build up in the lungs or heart, but it overlaps with PAH because this fibrosis can be missing or mild in the lungs, but severe in the pulmonary vessels (as in PH, cells proliferate in the inside layer of vessels making the muscle layer thicker).

Dr. Jane Morse (Columbia University, New York, NY) and others did genetic tests on scleroderma/PAH patients and concluded that their diseases were *not* associated with mutations of the BMPR2 gene. As with IPAH, there is probably a "susceptibility gene" for scleroderma that makes you more vulnerable.

Among the connective tissue diseases, PH is most frequently associated with chronic sclerosis, which affects the entire body (*systemic sclerosis*), sometimes including the heart and lungs. There is also what's called *localized* scleroderma, which affects just some skin areas and usually not internal organs or blood vessels, and is not associated with PH. By looking at the antibodies in your blood, a doctor can tell a lot about the type of scleroderma you have.

Roughly a third of systemic scleroderma patients develop at least mild PH. It isn't known how often the mild PH detected in many scleroderma patients grows into serious PH. A yearly echocardiogram is recommended to screen for PH. Doctors still miss a lot of PH in scleroderma cases, and it often goes undetected until it is more difficult to treat. The good news is that scleroderma / PAH can remain mild for many years, not progressing. Increasing shortness of breath is a clue that it's getting worse.

Many specialists think that yearly diffusing capacity tests should be done on scleroderma patients. If a patient has a diffusing capacity that is less than 55 percent of predicted, they probably have PAH. It is also thought appropriate to get a baseline echocardiogram on all scleroderma patients, and repeat this test periodically. If mild PH is found, it can be wise to undergo a catheterization to rule out false positives that generate a lot of needless worry. It's unlikely that a cath will find that a scleroderma patient is responsive to vasodilators, but it might reveal blood shunting to where it shouldn't, or left ventricle problems, or valve problems that are contributing to the PH.

Systemic scleroderma is further divided into *limited* and *diffuse scleroderma*. The distinction depends on the degree of skin involvement and specific antibodies. Limited scleroderma is discussed below. Diffuse scleroderma affects 50 to 60 percent of scleroderma patients and tends to spread beyond the entire skin. Symptoms include a sudden, severe onset, thickening skin, bad joint pains, and more frequent and severe interstitial lung disease (inflammation and disruption of the walls of air sacs in the lungs, making it harder for them to transfer oxygen).

Limited scleroderma (formerly known as CREST syndrome) is a special form of scleroderma affecting mostly the skin (*cutaneous sclerosis with calcinosis*). This is what the letters in CREST stand for:

C=calcinosis (abnormal deposits of calcium in the skin and other soft tissues)
R=Raynaud's phenomenon (see paragraph below)
E=esophageal reflux (felt as heartburn)
S=sclerodactyl (tight thick skin on the fingers, or "sausage fingers")
T=telangiectasia (spider veins—red spot in the skin)

Any one of these symptoms can be found in other diseases, or even in healthy blokes. If you have all five symptoms, it's probably accurate to say you have limited sclerosis. If you only have two or three signs, you may have a different disease.

Limited sclerosis is *not* the same thing as localized scleroderma, as explained above. The terms used are maddeningly confusing. About 40 to 50 percent of scleroderma patients have the limited form of the disease. Autoantibodies against centromeres (parts of the chromosomes in the nucleus of cells) are commonly (but not always) found in limited scleroderma. They are not found in the "diffuse" form of scleroderma. The absence or presence of these antibodies does not relate to the probability of a patient getting PH. Although limited scleroderma is less likely to damage internal organs, about 60 percent of affected persons get PH (which is a much higher incidence than with diffuse scleroderma). It is possible for interstitial lung disease to occur in limited scleroderma patients, but this is independent of the severity of PH. It often shows up when someone has had limited scleroderma for about a decade. When limited scleroderma patients die, it is often due to right-heart failure caused by their secondary PAH.

The onset of limited scleroderma is less dramatic than the onset of diffuse scleroderma. It can start with Raynaud's symptoms for 5 to 15 years, then puffy fingers, a sore that won't heal on a finger, and shortness of breath. Stomach and bowel problems are more frequent, as well as skin ulcers on the thighs.

A retrospective study at Ospedale Maggiore and the University of Milan (Italy) concluded that being postmenopausal is the biggest risk factor that a female limited scleroderma patient has for developing PH. (Being haplotype HLA-B35 adds to the risk.) The researchers speculate that hormone replacement therapy might be useful in preventing PH in this situation.

One study found that all patients with limited scleroderma/PH had Raynaud's phenomenon, while only 68 percent without PH had cold fingers.

Rheumatoid arthritis is one of the most common forms of arthritis (5 percent of U.S. adults over 65 have it), but the cause is still unknown. One study found that 21 percent of people with rheumatoid arthritis (and no other pulmonary or cardiac disease) have mild PH. Still to be determined is how this mild PH affects patients' longevity or quality of life. It is suspected that virus-like agents can trigger the disease in people with a genetic susceptibility. Joints become chronically inflamed, especially those of the hands, feet, or ankles. The linings of internal organs can also be inflamed, and in a few cases blood vessels are inflamed. The disease has active and passive periods. Sometimes it just goes away; sometimes the pain and swelling leads to destruction of joints. Women are two or three times more likely to have it than men.

Systemic lupus erythematous (SLE, lupus). This is another autoimmune disease. About 1.4 million people in the U.S. have lupus. It affects more women than men (surprise!); in this case, nine times more, and the women are usually of childbearing age. Like PH, lupus requires both a trigger and a genetic vulnerability. A prime suspect is the Epstein-Barr virus (one of the herpesviruses), which is linked to several other diseases. Most people have been infected with the virus, but only a few develop lupus.

SLE patients have off-and-on inflammation of their joints, tendons, other connective tissues, and organs. A butterfly-shaped rash often develops over the nose and cheeks. Lupus can be mild or fatal. It is possible for lupus to affect only the blood vessels in the lungs, so it looks just like IPAH/FPAH. Patients with this version respond nicely to epoprostenol (Flolan).

A survey done at Shanghai Second Medical University of 84 Chinese patients with SLE found that 11 percent of them also had PH, and that more severe PH was associated with higher levels of endothelin in the blood and more active lupus. Estimates of the percentage of SLE patients with PH are all over the map, however. It's probably in the ballpark to say that about 4 to 14 percent of lupus patients develop PH.

As mentioned, SLE can involve the tiny blood vessels. It can also cause pneumonitis, or an inflammation of the lung tissue itself. This type of lupus can come and go, along with symptoms of PH. In addition, SLE can cause an inflammation of the lining that covers the outside of the lungs and heart and the inside of the chest cavity. Rarely, a diffuse interstitial lung disease develops as a chronic form of lupus pneumonitis. It scars the lung tissue, making it hard for oxygen to get into the blood. The respiratory muscles and diaphragm can be affected, making breathing difficult. Lupus is also associated with more blood clots than some other collagen vascular diseases, and it inflames the heart muscle and heart valves.

Recent research by a team at the Oklahoma Medical Research Foundation has found that certain antibodies for lupus are present in the blood of someone years before they develop symptoms. This discovery might lead to early identification or patients who might benefit from therapies to prevent the disease from developing.

Vasculitis. This means an inflammation of blood or lymph vessels. The process can be either systemic or localized in one part of the body. Vasculitis is not really a disease, but something that happens along with some autoimmune connective tissue diseases. It can also happen in the absence of such disease. Any blood vessel can be involved, but when the inflammation happens in the small vessels of the lungs it can lead to fibrosis and excessive growth of the innermost layer of the blood vessels, which may, in turn, lead to PH. The most common form of vasculitis in lung vessels is the vasculitis due to a syndrome called Wegener's granulomatosis. These patients very rarely develop PH.

Mixed connective tissue disease (MCTD). People with this have symptoms of more than one type of connective disease (often they have mostly SLE or scleroderma complicated by myositis [inflammation of muscles]). The same name (MCTD) is sometimes used for "Sharp's syndrome," which is a specific type of MCTD with quite specific antibodies. Raynaud's phenomenon (see below) is very common, as are achy joints, swollen hands, weak muscles, a butterfly-shaped rash on the face, trouble swallowing, and shortness of breath. The true incidence of PH in people with MCTD isn't known, but it appears to be in the neighborhood of two out of three MCTD patients, and is often the cause of an MCTD patient's death.

Raynaud's phenomenon. Raynaud's (pronounced ray-NOSE) condition involves super-sensitivity to cold, usually in digits (toes and fingers). Around 5 to 10 percent of the U.S. population has Raynaud's. Among us PH patients, 10 to 14 percent have it. The vast majority is female. In Raynaud's, the nerves that tell a blood vessel to open or close up don't send the right signals. There can also be problems in endothelial cells (as in PH). Spasms in the small arteries cut off the digits' blood supply and turn them white, blue, or blotchy red. Sometimes the spasms are triggered by emotional upset. (Raynaud's can also be caused by a narrowing of the small arteries, such as occurs in scleroderma or diabetes.) The spasms can last seconds or hours, and can be painless or cause throbbing or tingling.

People with Raynaud's are more likely than others to get migraine headaches, angina, and PH. Only a small percentage of people with Raynaud's develop a collagen vascular disease or PH. When Raynaud's occurs by itself with no other health problems it is called **Raynaud's disease**, rather than Raynaud's phenomenon, and is not usually a serious problem.

If you use a prostanoid or calcium channel blockers to treat your PH, you may find the drugs also help control Raynaud's. On the PubMed website you'll find papers discussing the iloprost form of prostacyclin as a treatment for Raynaud's. In PH patients with scleroderma, the iloprost form of prostacyclin given intravenously is perhaps more effective at relieving the symptoms of Raynaud's than the oral form of the drug. Alpha-adrenergic blockers or drugs to improve blood flow are also used (e.g., pentoxiphyline).

You can try to reduce Raynaud's symptoms by avoiding cold, wearing gloves, running warm water over your hands, or using hand warmers. Really warm socks can be often found at stores that sell hiking boots, winter sports gear, and Birkenstock-type sandals. REI sells a 2-pack of Grabber Mini Heater Handwarmers for $1.50, or you can get a big box of handwarmers at Costco for less. When exposed to air, a nontoxic chemical reaction starts that provides heat up to 7 hours inside a pocket or gloves. REI also has similar toe heaters. (www.rei.com) Reusable warmers are also available. Biofeedback helps some sufferers. Pampering your skin helps (avoid harsh cleaners, use moisturizers). Smoking decreases blood flow to your digits and can make Raynaud's worse.

1.3.2. Congenital Heart & Lung Disease

"Congenital" means something you're born with. Doctors think faulty genes interacting with things in the womb environment might cause congenital defects. The environmental factor often can't be identified. These problems can be complex, and it is important to get an exact diagnosis. The good news is that, along with standard PH treatment medicines, there are often surgical treatment options not available to other PH patients. Some congenital problems can now be corrected in infancy or even while the fetus is still in the uterus, which greatly reduces the chances of getting PH. A cardiac catheterization is often needed to find out what's going on; echocardiograms can also be useful. Many problems, like atrial septal defects, ventricular septal defects, and patent ductus arteriosis (all are explained below) can now be repaired during a catheterization, avoiding the need for open-chest surgery and going on a heart/lung machine.

The following are only some of the congenital heart and lung diseases that can lead to PH.

Atrial septal defect (ASD). An ASD is a hole in the wall (*septum*) dividing the two upper chambers of the heart (the *atria*). The theory is that the hole can cause excessive blood flow through the lungs (it *shunts* the blood away from its usual route—the pink blood goes to the blue blood side of the heart), and the excessive flow can damage the linings of pulmonary arteries. Three times as many girls as boys are born with an ASD. It's somewhat hard to pick up in a routine office exam, and symptoms (which include shortness of breath and an enlarged right heart) may not develop for years.

Doctors generally prefer to close up these holes when the patient is between 1 and 6 years old, although an ASD can sometimes be repaired when you're older. People who were once told it was too late for surgery are now being reevaluated, although this remains controversial. A 23-year-old with a huge ASD had it sewn up, with a nice resulting drop in pressures. If you already have PH when you have surgery, you may have to deal with the PH. Fortunately, it's treatable with epoprostenol.

There is disagreement over whether ASDs in adult patients actually cause PAH. Some doctors say perhaps 20 percent of adults with an uncorrected ASD will develop PH, but there are no good studies to support this. Other doctors think differently, and point to studies that compared medically treated vs. surgically treated adult ASD patients over long periods. Some of these studies found no significant difference in mortality or in the development of PAH. It's possible that ASD patients with PH really have IPAH, which they would have developed even if they didn't have an ASD. Therefore, surgery on adults to close an ASD should only be done if there is relatively little disease in the pulmonary arteries. This must be determined by expert cardiologists, because the subtleties that are involved may be complex.

Unfortunately, some people who do not have their ASD repaired before adulthood may die before age 50, of heart failure. But some people with a gaping hole live to be PH-free geezers and grannies.

Now here's a mystery: even if your ASD is caught and corrected in childhood, some doctors think you still have a greater-than-normal chance of developing PH in, say, 20 or 25 years. Therefore, if you have a corrected ASD, you might still want to get an echo once in a while and make sure it's not happening to you. A participant at PHA's 2002 conference developed PAH only 6 months after her ASD was corrected. She asked the docs if what she had was IPAH. Technically no, she was told, because the cause of the PH was known. (Maybe these doctors were wrong; maybe she really did develop IPAH, or maybe she had it all along.) But the symptoms and treatment are the same. If your PH was triggered by an ASD, your doctor will still look for other things that could be making it worse, such as sleep or thyroid problems.

Patent ductus arteriosus. Inside the womb, when Mom supplies our oxygen with her own lungs, we all have a little artery (the *ductus arteriosus*) that allows our fetal blood supply to bypass our lungs. The artery normally closes off soon after we give our first lusty howl. Sometimes, however, it remains open (*patent*), and blood can still from the aorta to the pulmonary artery. Because of this, too much blood flows to the lungs and can eventually damage the small pulmonary arteries. The heart works too hard and makes a loud swishy sound.

Patent ductus arteriosus is more common in babies born prematurely (the artery often gets around to closing itself off in these babies), in babies born at high altitudes, and in babies whose moms had German measles early in their pregnancy. If the little artery does not close itself off after a while, it is easily repaired.

Ventricular septal defect (VSD). In this condition (the most common heart malformation) there is a hole in the wall separating the two lower chambers of the heart. The hole allows too much blood to flow to the lungs, and this often causes PAH if the hole is not closed early in life. (Almost half of all VSDs are small and close by themselves within a few months of birth.) Depending on the size of the hole, PH can develop in early childhood or many years later; it usually appears early on and only rarely appears later in life. It is important to repair this defect surgically (when possible), before permanent PH changes develop. If uncorrected in infancy or childhood, PH is much more likely to develop than with an ASD. If PH has already developed, closing the hole may not help (although new thinking on this is more optimistic).

Atrial ventricular canal (AVC). An ASD + a VSD = an AVC. This condition is commonly seen in Down syndrome.

Eisenmenger's complex (a.k.a. Eisenmenger's reaction). This term is used when PH is found in connection with a VSD or other long-standing congenital heart shunt. Dr. Bruce Brundage said that when he was in med school, students were taught that Eisenmenger's was inoperable and there was nothing to do to help the patient. This attitude is outdated.

Mitral valve stenosis. A rare congenital problem, it is a narrowing of the mitral valve (between the upper and lower chambers on the left side of the heart), that restricts blood flow into the lower chamber and causes pressure to build in the upper chamber and back pressure to build in the lungs. This can cause PH. Fixing the valve usually reverses the PH. Back when rheumatic fever was common, many people—both children and adults—had mitral valve stenosis, which was caused by an autoimmune response to the germs that cause infection of the tonsils (streptococcus).

Pulmonary branch stenosis. If a woman gets German measles in the first trimester of pregnancy, intermediate-sized vessels in the lungs of the fetus can be constricted. This is rarely found today. It can be treated with angioplasty, but doing so is difficult.

Ebstein's anomaly. This rare condtion affects males and females equally. In some hearts, the little leaflets that form the tricuspid valve (between the upper and lower chambers on the right side of the heart) are displaced in the right ventricle and don't touch one another properly when they close. Because this is more a problem of the right ventricle than of the pulmonary arteries, you usually don't develop PH unless other problems also exist.

Cyanotic congenital heart disease patients. *Cyanosis* means blue skin (from lack of oxygen). It can be caused by structural abnormalities such as transposition of the great arteries (the aorta and the pulmonary artery) or truncus arteriosus (when the pulmonary arteries, the aorta, and the coronary arteries all originate in a single big artery). Surgery to help these conditions can often be done on infants or young babies.

1.3.3. Portopulmonary Hypertension

The liver is a wonderful machine—part sewage treatment plant, part factory—and it's practically maintenance free. Blood flows through the big portal vein that goes from your intestines to your liver. Inside the liver, poisons, other waste materials, and some drugs are removed, and yummy proteins are manufactured. But if liver disease causes obstructions in the liver, then the blood pressure in the portal vein rises. When this high pressure is found in association with PH, the syndrome is called *portopulmonary hypertension* (we'll call it "portoPH").

The lungs are downstream from the liver. In portoPH, blood that normally goes through the liver before going to the lungs ends up going directly to the lungs, injuring the pulmonary arteries. Even the experts are still baffled by exactly how liver disease, portal hypertension, and the pulmonary circulation relate to one another. So the material in this section of the *Survival Guide* is somewhat speculative.

Liver disease, usually cirrhosis, is the most common cause of portal hypertension and is therefore also the most common cause of portoPH. But you don't have to have liver disease (or cirrhosis) to develop portal hypertension or portoPH. Some patients with unusual circulatory plumbing can develop portoPH without having portal hypertension.

Liver disease can also cause something called the *hepatopulmonary syndrome*, which is the shunting of blood through the lungs and low oxygen levels in the blood. This condition is not often associated with PH. PH has appeared in such patients several years after a successful liver transplant, or because of certain surgical shunts used decades ago to relieve portoPH. It isn't known why one patient with liver disease gets PH, another gets hepatopulmonary syndrome, and another gets neither. In fact, the condition might change from hepatopulmonary syndrome to portoPH over some years. The extremely high cardiac outputs associated with hepatopulmonary syndrome may, by themselves, cause PH, but in contrast to IPAH/FPAH and portoPH, there is usually no abnormality of the pulmonary circulation itself.

Fortunately, considering the outbreak of hepatitis C in the U.S., only 4.7 percent of people with cirrhosis and portal hypertension develop PH. There does not seem to be a direct connection between the severity of the liver disease and the likelihood of PH. Because not everybody with liver problems gets PH, a genetic susceptibility is probably involved.

A different kind of problem occurs when IPAH/FPAH is so severe that it causes a back pressure and harms the liver (along with the kidneys, often).

Compared to IPAH/FPAH. If you put lung tissue under a microscope, IPAH, FPAH, and portoPH look alike. They also look alike on a chest x-ray. There are clinical differences, however. Most PH patients have platelet counts in the normal range; counts run much lower in portoPH. Cardiac output is usually low or normal in PH, but in hepatopulmonary syndrome it can be very, very high. In portoPH it is considerably lower than in hepatopulmonary syndrome, but generally higher than in PH.

Diagnosis. All new PH patients should be checked for portoPH. Your doctor will feel for your spleen and look for the little red "spiders" on your skin (they don't come and go, but are always there) that are associated with liver problems. Liver function tests reveal a lot. Other clues are a high INR in a patient who is not taking warfarin, low albumin levels in your blood (which suggests your liver isn't synthesizing protein well), a low platelet count, ascites, and a wasted look. These clues are enough reason to order a CAT scan of the liver, which can reveal scarring, shrinking, or enlargement. Echocardiograms with Doppler echo can suggest PH (especially when the systolic PAP is over 40 mm Hg, or a reversal of portal flow is seen). But when someone is really sick, the pressures found in an echo will not agree with those found when a (more reliable) catheterization is done. During a right-heart cath, your hepatic vein wedge pressure can be measured, telling if portal hypertension exists (this is not routinely done because docs can learn what they need to know from easier tests). A high cardiac output, which will also be found during a cath, is a red flag. In liver disease, your heart may pump 8 to 9 liters a minute instead of 3 to 5 liters. But

as liver disease progresses, your cardiac output falls, which is a bad sign because it means the right side of your heart is failing.

Cirrhosis. As already mentioned, a frequent cause of portal hypertension is liver cirrhosis, when healthy liver tissue is destroyed and replaced by scar tissue. Alcohol abuse, certain drugs and toxic chemicals, infections such as hepatitis B and C, and many other things can cause cirrhosis. In a survey done by the Cleveland Clinic, lung disease didn't appear until patients had had liver disease for about 6 years, and not everybody with PH had cirrhosis. Can you heal your liver by avoiding alcohol and making dietary changes? The liver can improve somewhat if there is not severe fibrosis, but advanced cirrhosis is not reversible. See Chapter 6 for information on liver transplants.

Other routes to PH. It might be that portal hypertension leads to PH because vasoconstrictors or toxins that the liver normally removes are left in the blood stream. Autoimmune problems might possibly lead to both liver and lung disease.

1.3.4. HIV Infection

If you are infected with the human immunodeficiency virus (HIV), you have an increased risk of developing PAH, even if you haven't developed AIDS. (In Paris, nearly a third of the HIV/PAH patients don't have symptoms of AIDS.) Still, only a very few people with an HIV infection ever develop PH; a genetic trait might influence which persons do.

By the year 2000, over 131 persons infected with HIV had been found who also had PH. Now that people with HIV are living longer, more are developing PH. The time between diagnosis of HIV infection and the diagnosis of PPH ranges from 0 to 9 years: a survey in 2000 found the mean interval to be 33 months. The median time from diagnosis to death was 6 months. Most deaths of HIV / PH patients are due to the PH. A look at the genes of 19 patients with HIV/PH found no germ cell mutations of the "PH gene" that might have made them vulnerable to the disease.

Scientists aren't sure why HIV infection triggers PH. Perhaps it does so indirectly, through recurrent respiratory disease. (This is an argument for the aggressive treatment of such opportunistic infections.) Or the HIV virus might cause higher levels of platelet-derived growth factor (a substance that can cause smooth muscle cells and fibroblasts to grow and migrate) or some other growth factor. It is also conceivable that the HIV virus itself acts directly on pulmonary endothelial or smooth muscle cells. (If this is so, might not other viruses trigger PH in some persons?) Or, because of weakened immune systems, HIV patients might be more likely to catch another virus (such as a herpesvirus or cytomegalovirus) that, in turn, injures the vessels and causes PH.

Herpesvirus 8 Infection

(A bonus section not in the WHO classification.)
Researchers at the University of Colorado Health Sciences Center published an article in the September 18, 2003, issue of *The New England Journal of Medicine* that suggests that the herpesvirus 8 (HHV-8) might be a triggering cause of much IPAH. DNA from the virus, and antibodies to it, were found in the lung tissue of 10 of 16 sporadic IPAH patients (62 percent), but not in lung tissue from 14 patients with PH secondary to another disease. (This article used the old slippery term PPH, but as a synonym for IPAH. Fenfluramine users and those infected by HIV were considered to have secondary PH.) Patients who had PAH running in their families were not included in this study. Two of the IPAH patients also had Castleman's

disease, a rare disorder where someone develops non-cancerous tumors in lymph node tissue. One form of Castleman's is associated with HHV-8.

HHV-8 is in the family of herpesviruses that cause chickenpox/shingles, Epstein-Barr (a cause of infectious mononucleosis), and herpes simplex 1 and 2 (oral and genital herpes). Like all herpesviruses, HHV-8 causes a primary infection followed by a latent phase that lasts the rest of the person's life, so it can sometimes be reactivated. When someone first catches HHV-8 they may have a fever that lasts from 2-14 days and a rash that lasts for 3-8 days. Then the patient feels better, but the virus is still lurking in the patient's body.

HHV-8 is already known to cause some blood cancers. The researchers found HHV-8 both inside the nasty plexiform lesions in PH patients' pulmonary arteries, as well as in other cells. This discovery, if borne out, could mean that PAH is viewed as a form of malignancy. The virus might promote endothelial cell growth by messing with molecules that control it.

AIDS patients are familiar with this virus, because it also causes a type of skin cancer, Kaposi's sarcoma, which usually appears as a purple blotch on the skin, but can also sometimes involve internal organs. Kaposi's sarcoma is seldom a cause of death in AIDS patients. Post-transplant patients who are on immunosuppressive therapies may also develop Kaposi's sarcoma.

The lesions produced by Kaposi's sarcoma and those produced in PH look and act very much alike. But neither DNA nor viral antigens to the HIV virus have been found in PH lesions.

It is not known how HHV-8 is transmitted between individuals. There is evidence that it can be sexually transmitted. Because the virus is found in children in Central Africa and the Mediterranean, it appears there must be a nonsexual method of transmission. Some evidence points to saliva. The virus is found only in humans.

HHV-8 is rare and mild in persons with normal immune systems who don't have IPAH. In the U.S., up to 3 percent of blood donors without HIV infection show evidence of HHV-8 infection, so it isn't a virus that gets around a lot. And very few of those 3 percent have IPAH. However, it might be that having IPAH makes it more likely that you will catch an HHV-8 infection (as is the case in HIV-infected individuals). And remember that even if HHV-8 does cause PAH, it would only do so in people with a genetic vulnerability to PAH.

If the Colorado researchers are correct, it will move many patients from the IPAH category into a new HHV-8 category of PAH. It may also suggest treatments aimed at stopping the proliferation of mutant blood vessel cells, which would be of enormous help to PH patients who aren't helped by vasodilator drugs. Maybe it could even lead to a vaccine. As Dr. Norbert Voelkel told a PH patient who e-mailed him (and who posted the doc's response on the PHA message board): "The point of our paper is that we must find anti-angioproliferative drugs for those patients not very much helped by the vasodilator drugs. An effective anti-angioproliferative treatment might amount to a cure—or make patients significantly better permanently."

1.3.5. Drugs & Toxins

At the 1998 WHO Evian World Symposium on PPH a consensus, of sorts, was reached on which drugs and toxins might be linked to the onset of PAH. Not all doctors and researchers agree on all of these. One noted researcher, for example, suspects a link between oral contraceptives and estrogen replacement therapy that she would like to see investigated more thoroughly. Here is a summary of the consensus:

Definite link to PAH: aminorex (European diet pills), fenfluramine, dexfenfluramine, toxic rapeseed oil. (Basis: at least one major controlled study or epidemic.)

Very likely link: amphetamines, a contamination of some L-tryptophan. (Basis: several large case series and studies not attributable to considered biases, or a general consensus among experts.) [A "case series" or "case control study" is a paper that describes several patients rather than just one, and that compares the PH patients to healthy controls who are otherwise similar to them.]

Possible link: methamphetamines, cocaine, and chemotherapeutic agents (mitomycin-C, carmustine, etoposide, and cyclophosphamide). (Basis: an association based on case control studies, registries, or expert opinions.)

Unlikely to be linked: anti-depressants, birth control pills, estrogen therapy, cigarette smoking. (Basis: risk factors that have been proposed but not yet found to have any association from controlled studies.) [While cigarette smoking is not directly linked to PH, it is indirectly linked because it causes emphysema and bronchitis that can, in turn, trigger PH.]

Contaminated rapeseed (canola) oil. In Spain in early 1981, the consumption of contaminated rapeseed oil made 20,688 people sick with a multisystemic disease. About 5 to 8 percent of them developed PH (only 2 percent had it after 8 years). When the oil was removed from the market, the number of new cases of PH dropped to normal.

Contaminated L-tryptophan. This amino acid "food supplement" was linked to an outbreak in 1989 of a disease called eosinophilia-myalgia syndrome (EMS). Eosinophils are a type of white blood cell, and in eosinophilia there are too many of them in the blood. EMS affects many systems in the body. Symptoms include muscle weakness and pain, swelling, and hardening of the extremities, especially the legs. About 20 percent of people with contaminated L-tryptophan-induced EMS developed PAH.

Crotalaria (a type of plant also known as a "canary bird bush") and crotalaria-fulva are linked to PH in humans and known to cause PH in rats. The seeds and leaves of these plants are used to make bush tea. Drinking the tea can cause pulmonary venous occlusion.

Substance abuse. At least one major PH treatment center sees more PAH caused by street drugs like methamphetamine (a.k.a. speed, meth, crank, ice, met), chalk, and crystal, than from diet pills, even during the diet pill epidemic. One PH doc calls meth "super fen-phen" because of its ability to cause PAH. Cocaine causes pulmonary blood vessels to constrict, which might lead to PAH, although the data on this is soft.

In an international study, a small increased risk of getting PAH was associated with the use of intravenous drugs or cocaine. The blood clots caused by intravenous drug use, and the associated liver disease and HIV infections make it hard to tell what is the direct cause of the PH. Young people who have sniffed a lot of glue (toluene) or smoked crack have also gotten PAH

Diet pills. Drugs that work by causing a loss of appetite (*anorectic agents*) include pills containing fenfluramine or dexfenfluramine

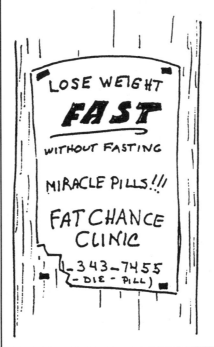

(such as Redux, Pondimin, and "fen-phen"). Such pills can trigger PAH. PAH caused by anoretic agents was traditionally called IPAH (they used the old term, PPH), because blood vessel abnormalities look just like those found in IPAH/FPAH, and the symptoms of the two groups of patients are also the same.

An association of PAH and heart-valve problems with the use of anorectic diet pills occurred in the U.S. shortly after dexfenflura-mine was approved for extended use by the FDA in April 1996. The makers of the pills yanked them from the market in September of 1997. The outbreak did not surprise PH specialists, because a sudden ten-fold increase in PAH in Europe between 1967 and 1973 was linked to a similar drug, aminorex. About 0.1 to 2 percent of people who took aminorex pills got PAH. Less than 0.02 percent of people who took fen-phen got PH, but this figure is higher than the figure for IPAH/FPAH (.0001 to .0002 percent).

In fact, PH specialists in the U.S. were so confident (given the introduction of the pills and the rising obesity rates in the U.S.) that there would be a rise in the number of PH cases diagnosed, that they set up a surveillance team at 12 PH centers soon after the FDA approved the pills. Their findings were reported in an article by Dr. Stuart Rich and others in the March 2002 issue of *Chest*. The 579 patients studied were divided into two groups: those that were diagnosed by their own PH doctor as having PH secondary to another disease ("SPH" patients), and those for whom no cause of their PH could be found ("PPH patients"). The first group served as a control group for the second. The researchers asked about the use antidepressants and amphetamines as well as diet pills.

Only the use of diet drugs containing fenfluramine or dexfenfluramine was found to have "a significant preferential association with PPH as compared with SPH." If somebody used a diet drug for longer than 6 months, he/she was found more likely to have developed PAH than somebody who used the drug for a shorter time.

An unexpectedly high number of SPH patients (11.4 percent) reported using the diet pills as well. It appears possible, therefore, that the diet drugs might have been a trigger (or an additional trigger) for some of these patients' PH.

Dr. Jane Morse has looked at the genes of anorectic pill users who developed PAH and found BMPR gene mutations only in about 15 percent. It has thus far not been possible to cause PAH in animals (other than humans) by giving them diet pills.

What are the odds of getting PH from the pills? Six million people took anorectic diet pills between September 1996 and December 1997. The vast majority of these people will not get PAH. The longer you used the pills, the greater your risk. If you used these diet pills for more than 3 months, your chance of getting PAH greatly increases. However, as little as 23 days of exposure has been known to trigger the disease. The background rate of IPAH in the U.S. population is about 2 in a million. Among those who took these diet pills for over 3 months, a well-done study found that 46 out of a million develop PAH. That is a 23-FOLD increase, not just a 23 percent increase (a 2,300 percent increase!). This is a *much* stronger association than smoking is to lung cancer.

If you took Redux or "fen-phen," and haven't already had a checkup, do so. Three federal agencies—the FDA, the NIH, and the CDC—recommend that anybody who took either type of pill get a medical checkup for possible heart damage, and that any pill user who has developed shortness of breath, a new heart murmur, or other heart problem, get an echocardiogram.

Sometimes the PAH seems to disappear, but according to some experts, it virtually always returns. PAH can appear quite a long time after someone stops taking the pills; in many people it might not become obvious until years later. When can pill takers "breathe easy" and stop worrying? Doctors have seen patients who didn't develop PH symptoms until 5 years after they ceased taking diet pills. One PH specialist says he wouldn't be surprised if, in a few people, 10 years pass before they notice PH symptoms. A study in France of people who took different anorexigenic pills there, well before the fen-phen madness in the U.S., looked at how much time passed from the time someone swallowed their first pill to the appearance of the first symptoms. The mean time was 4 years (the study followed users for 10 years). Because Redux and fen-phen were taken off the market in 1997, we are well past the 4-year mark now, and new cases seem to be dropping off.

An international study that looked at diet pill use and PAH also looked at other risk factors and did not find any correlation between obesity, smoking, recent pregnancy, the use of thyroid preparations, or other evaluated variables, and the likelihood of getting PAH. It is possible that a synergistic effect between diet drugs and living at a high altitude would make PAH more likely, although this has not been proven.

Why would these diet pills cause PAH?
Two hypotheses are the "potassium channel hypothesis" and the "serotonin hypothesis." Some scientists suspect the diet pills affect the potassium channels in the membranes around the smooth muscle layer of blood vessels, or their associated nerves, causing an influx of calcium and making it hard for vessels to relax. Dr. Rubin M. Tuder and his colleagues at the University of Colorado speculate that—in persons who already have a predisposition to develop PH—diet pills stimulate the overgrowth of endothelial cells. Fenfluramine inhibits the reuptake of serotonin, so more of it accumulates in the blood. (Serotonin is a vasoconstrictor and apparently stimulates the growth of smooth muscle cells. IPAH patients seem to have elevated levels of it.) Diet pill / PAH patients seem to have much more abnormal endothelium than do comparable sick PAH patients.

There are other theories, too. Some people have genetic reasons for metabolizing these types of drugs more slowly than other people. It appears that pill takers who develop PH are more likely to have the "slow" genes. Therefore the drugs hang around longer in their bodies and do more damage. Fenflura-mine might also alter the metabolism of a catecholamine (epinephrine or norepine-phrine). (The chemical formula for fenfluramine is very similar to that for epinephrine.) It is possible that the drug might overstimulate the adrenergic receptors in pulmonary arteries, causing constriction and the proliferation of muscle cells.

As you know from hundreds of media stories and lawyer's ads, Redux and fen-phen can also cause fibrotic changes in heart valves. Heart valve damage can cause PH, but the reverse is not true. Sometimes it's hard to sort out what's really going on. A postmortem study of one patient found both IPAH and PH secondary to valve damage.

What about other types of prescription diet pills? Phentermine, the second half of fen-phen, has not been proven to cause PAH when used alone (whether it really helps anyone lose weight is another question). Several cases have been reported of PAH patients who used phentermine alone, but it might not have been the drug that caused their PH. Phentermine is marketed under about a dozen different trade names.

Sibutramine (trade name Meridia), works a little differently from fenfluramine and Redux. The FDA approved this drug over the objections of its own scientific advisors, who called it too risky, in November 1997. The FDA says the new drug should be avoided by anyone with poorly controlled hypertension, heart disease, or irregular heartbeat, or who has survived a stroke. There is a long, long list of other persons who should not take this drug. In an ad run in July 2000, the Knoll Pharmaceutical Company, which makes this drug, says in some fine dense print that: "In clinical studies, no cases of PAH have been reported with Meridia. Because this disease is so rare, however, it is not known whether or not Meridia may cause this disease." The Health Research Group at Public Citizen (Washington, DC) says the FDA has received many reports of cardiac and cardiovascular adverse events and would like to see the drug banned.

Dexatrim was pulled from the market for other reasons. Dexatrim, an old diet drug, is an amphetamine. It *might* be linked to PH, because it constricts blood vessels. A drug that has been on the market some time, phenter-mine resin (Ionamin) Capsules C-IV is made by Medeva Pharmaceuticals. Medeva sent out letters addressed to "Dear Doctor or Health Care Professional." In these letters the company says: "Medeva is aware of only a few isolated case reports of PPH possibly associated with phentermine monotherapy over the last 38 years. Although present data do not support an association between PPH and phentermine monotherapy, the possibility cannot be ruled out."

When fenfluramines were withdrawn from the market, some doctors began prescribing, as a substitute, a combination of fluoxetine (Prozac) and phentermine. Like the old diet pills, fluoxetine raises the levels of serotonin in the bloodstream. A study by Dr. Ken Weirs' group (University of Minnesota, Veterans' Administration Hospital) suggests, however, that Prozac and venlafaxine (Effexor) present less risk than fen-phen of causing PAH (at least through their effect on potassium channels).

An anorectic diet drug that has been on the market for a long time, Tenuate (diethylpropion hydrochloride), can elevate blood pressure and is something those with PH should definitely avoid. Like any amphetamine-like drug it has the potential to cause PH. Likewise, stay away from herbal appetite suppressants containing ephedra leaf or bitter orange, other amphetamine-like compounds. (See Chapter 9.)

Orlistat, a newer diet drug, works by preventing up to 30 percent of fat from being absorbed in the intestine. It offers only modest weight losses and has side effects that include explosive diarrhea. Which brings us to the bottom line: talk to your PH specialist before trying any diet drug, be it prescribed or "natural."

Don't blame the victims. The author has encountered several PH patients who think diet pill users don't have "real" PH, and who sort of resent the monetary damages some of the diet pill users have received. One even said that a diet pill user probably really got her PH because she was obese and just sat around all the time. Three thoughts on this. First, as Dr. Stuart Rich said at the Irvine PHA conference: "Most of the Chicago Bears are overweight and they can run 100 yards much faster than I can, so I'm very reluctant to blame somebody's weight on their inability to do exercise, until I look further." Second, people took diet pills because they were seriously trying to lose weight. Third, even with treatment, it's possible that someone who got PAH from diet pills has a bleaker outlook than someone with IPAH (see Chapters 5 and 7). We're all in the same leaky boat and we need to paddle toward safety together.

Use of Indomethacin by pregnant women. It is thought that this nonsteroidal anti-inflammatory drug (NSAID) may cause an interruption in the supply of blood to a fetus, leading to pulmonary hypertension in a newborn. (See Chapter 8.)

1.3.6. Other (Thyroid Disorders, Glycogen Storage Disease, Gaucher's Disease, Hemorrhagic Telangiectasia, Hemoglobinopathies, Myeloproliferative Disorders, Splenectomy)

Sickle Cell Disease. (This condition might also be put under category 4.3, below—there really isn't a consensus yet.) Millions of people around the world, primarily those with roots in Africa, the Mediterranean, or India, suffer from this inherited disease. It is thought to affect 80,000 or so people in the U.S. The disease is characterized by sickle-shaped red blood cells. These cells are stiff and have jagged edges; they can't carry enough oxygen around and are more likely to stick to the inner walls of pulmonary arteries (as well as sticking to the insides of small blood vessels in the spleen, bones, etc.) where they block blood flow. To add insult to injury, excess free hemoglobin in the blood leads to too little nitric oxide, so blood vessels are more likely to constrict.

Symptoms of sickle cell disease include anemia, stomach, and bone pain, and nausea (in young persons). PH is only one way this painful disease can cut lives short (one study estimated that about 3 percent of sickle cell patients die of PH). New research, from the National Institutes of Health and the Howard University Center for Sickle Cell Disease, and reported in the February 26, 2004, issue of *The New England Journal of Medicine,* suggests that about 20 to 40 percent of sickle cell patients have moderate to severe PH. Many are unaware that they have the disease. A lead doctor in the study, Dr. Mark T. Gladwin, says that in sickle-cell patients, PH appears to be the number one predictor of sudden death syndrome in these patients. Dr. Gladwin believes that about 60,000 sickle cell disease patients in the U.S. should be regularly monitored for PH.

Sickle cell patients with PH are in real trouble: less than 2 years after being diagnosed with PH, up to 40 percent have died. PH / sickle cell patients might have mean PAPs that suggest only mild PH and still be in danger.

Until recently there was no known treatment for sickle cell/PH. The authors of the study mentioned above suggest that the first thing to do is to aggressively treat the sickle cell disease (with things like the drug hydroxyurea, blood transfusions, and inhaled nitric oxide gas). Inhaled nitric oxide has been shown to be of benefit for PH, as well. In 2003, researchers at Children's Hospital, Oakland, CA, reported that the supplement arginine, taken orally, resulted in a 15.2 percent reduction in systolic PAP after 5 days of treatment. Arginine (which the body needs to make nitric oxide) has few side effects. The study involved only 10 patients. Still, it's encouraging news.

Clinical trials are finally underway to learn more about PH secondary to sickle cell anemia. Some trials may not involve anything more dangerous or unpleasant than giving a blood sample. Other trials may try out certain PH drugs (such as prostanoids and CCBs) on sickle-cell patients. You can learn more at www.clinicaltrials.gov, or by calling the National Institute of Diabetes and Digestive Kidney Diseases, toll free phone: 1-800-411-1222; TTY: 1-866-411-1010. To learn about an INO Therapeutics inhaled pulsed nitric oxide trial call 1-908-238-6605. PH in African Americans is being missed as a diagnosis far too often, and much more research and awareness is needed. Remember, the squeaky wheel gets the grease.

Thyroid disorders. A retrospective record review of 41 "PPH" patients done by the Cleveland Clinic Foundation, Ohio, and published in 1999, found a much higher rate (22.5 percent) of hypothyroidism (when the thyroid gland produces too little hormone) than is found in the general population. An earlier study at the University of Colorado also found a higher rate of hypothyroidism among PH patients. It is not thought that either disease causes the other, but that some underlying mechanism, perhaps an autoimmune disorder or a genetic glitch, leads to a defect in cell signaling, which in turn encourages the development of both conditions. In experiments on animals, hypothyroidism raised levels of the vasoconstrictor endothelin-1. Hashimoto's thyroiditis (an autoimmune form of an inflamed thyroid where there is an enlarged thyroid and hypothyroidism) also seems more common among PH patients. *Hyper*thyroidism might also be more common among PH patients, although there is not as strong an association as with hypothyroidism

Myelofibrosis. It is not known what causes this disease, in which blood cells in the bone marrow are replaced with fibrous tissue. Oddly shaped red blood cells, anemia, and enlarged spleens result. A small study by G.

Garc'a-Manero and others (see Bibliography) at the Thomas Jefferson University in Philadelphia looked at six myelofibrosis patients who also had PH. All six had an unusually high number of platelets in their blood. The researchers speculate at possible links between the two diseases. They think that the increased tendency of these patients' blood to clot, or the possibility that their red blood cell production process infiltrated essential working parts of their lungs, or their left ventricular failure might partly account for their development of PH. The authors recommend that patients with myelofibrosis and shortness of breath be screened for PH.

Gaucher's Disease. People with this disease have difficulties metabolizing fat, and products of fat metabolism called gluco-cerebrosides accumulate in tissues. It's most common in Eastern European Jews, and leads to an enlarged liver and spleen and bone abnormalities.

Hereditary Hemorrhagic Telangiectasia. Also called Rendu-Osler-Weber disease, malformed blood vessels are really fragile and prone to leaking. When vessels under the skin on the face break, bruise-like discolorations occur. It might be that the structure of the air sacs if affected, causing some interstitial lung disease (if this proves to be the case, this condition really belongs in category 3, below, which covers PH triggered by hypoxemia).

Splenectomy. A German study found that persons who had had their spleens removed were more likely than others to develop IPAH. Some speculate that this might be due to the loss of the spleen's role in filtering out old platelets; patients with very high platelet counts have an increased risk of PH.

1.4. Associated with Significant Venous or Capillary Involvement

1.4.1. Pulmonary Veno-Occlusive Disease (Clogging of Pulmonary Veins)

Sometimes the pulmonary veins get clogged from the inside by fibrous material. This is called *veno-occlusive disease (PVOD)*. The cause is unknown. PVOD is about 10 times less frequent than IPAH/FPAH, which makes it a really rare disease. A lung biopsy is the best way to find out if you have it, but such biopsies are dangerous for PH patients and may delay the only presently known remedy, lung transplantation. A biopsy might possibly be necessary to distinguish PVOD from interstitial lung disease, for which there are treatments other than transplant. Clubbing of fingers might be present in PVOD.

Although tumors usually create problems by pressing on pulmonary veins, sometimes they invade the veins as well (lung cancer is usually involved), and this can lead to PH.

1.4.2. Pulmonary Capillary Hemangiomatosis

Many benign vascular tumors can form on pulmonary capillaries, blocking the blood flow and causing pressures to rise in pulmonary arteries. This type of PH is rare. Researchers in Barcelona, Spain, scanned the literature and identified 35 cases. Chest x-rays and CAT scans will usually show signs of these blockages, but they look a lot like veno-occlusive disease/PH. This is one of those rare situations where a pulmonary biopsy might be needed to find out what's really going on, but such biopsies are dangerous for PH patients, and might unnecessarily delay lung trans-plantation. There is not yet an accepted drug treatment for this type of PH (prostanoids are not helpful; interferon has been tried, but still lacks a promising track record).

1.5. Persistent Pulmonary Hypertension of the Newborn (PPHN)

See Chapter 8, Children and PH.

Category 2: Pulmonary Venous Hypertension

Hypertension in the *veins* of the lungs—after the blood has passed by the air sacs.

2.1 Left-Sided Atrial or Ventricular Heart Disease

Various left-heart problems that develop after birth can dam up blood flow and cause back pressure in the lungs, triggering mild increases in the thickness of pulmonary veins (although the veins themselves are passive in this process). This is the sequence of events: left ventricular diastolic pressure (and/or left atrial pressure) increases, which leads to an increase in pulmonary vein pressure, which leads to an increase in pulmonary artery pressure. If this causes the tiny arteries to constrict, pulmonary artery pressure goes way up (as does right ventricular pressure, which reflects the **PAP**).

When a left-heart problem can be corrected, it usually resolves the **PH**.

Left-heart problems come in many forms. Maybe the heart has been damaged by a heart attack, or maybe there is longstanding hypertension, which eventually weakens the left ventricle. The veins of the lungs may not drain well because of a tumor or growth in the left atrium, or the patient's left ventricle may be giving out from a variety of causes. If the left side of the heart is stiff and doesn't relax quickly enough to accept blood from the pulmonary veins (*left ventricular diastolic dysfunction*), the blood can back up and cause PH.

In PH it's right-heart failure we have to deal with, when our right ventricles poop out. But in the general population more people have left-heart failure. When the left ventricle gives out, pressure in the pulmonary artery increases, because of the backup phenomenon, and this can cause PH. You can end up with biventricular congestive heart failure.

2.2 Left-Sided Valvular Heart Disease

Heart valves, particularly the mitral valve, may not work well. For example, *mitral stenosis*, a narrowing of the mitral valve, is common in patients who had rheumatic fever. Here is how it can lead to PH: blood cannot get through the mitral valve from the left atrium into the left ventricle, so pressure in the left atrium is too high. This high pressure backs up into the pulmonary veins (which drain into the left atrium). The pulmonary veins are, in turn, fed by the pulmonary venules (small veins). The backup keeps on going—from the pulmonary venules back to the pulmonary capillaries and into the pulmonary arterioles, where the PH vascular changes get underway.

Category 3: PH Associated with Hypoxemia

3.1. Airway Disease

Diseases that block the airways of the lungs include chronic bronchitis, emphysema, and asthma. You can have more than one of these diseases at the same time. Many people who have one or more of these diseases are said to have COPD. Over 16 million people in the U.S. have COPD, and in some of them it will lead to hypoxemia (see below) and to PH. Long-term cigarette smoking (and age) account for 85 percent of the risk of getting COPD. Roughly 15 percent of smokers develop COPD and a very small percentage of those go on to develop PH. Air pollution may also contribute, as can environmental irritants in the workplace.

Not surprisingly, genetic factors may help determine which people with COPD get PH. Researchers in France and the U.K. looked for subtle variations in gene sequences (gene polymorphisms) in 103 patients with COPD, and 98 control subjects who didn't have COPD. They learned that a polymorphism in the serotonin transporter (5-HTT) gene, which plays a role in the overgrowth of smooth muscle in pulmonary arterioles, appears to determine the severity of PH in hypoxemic patients with COPD. It was the LL genotype polymorphism that was to blame.

For bronchitis to be considered "chronic" and fit into this category, you must be coughing up icky stuff for at least 3 months in each of 2 successive years.

Emphysema sufferers have difficulty breathing because of abnormally big air spaces in their lungs, and a loss of elasticity in the walls of the spaces. (The walls of the little air spaces in their lungs break down to form big non-functioning air spaces.)

People with asthma have attacks during which they wheeze and have great difficulty breathing because their bronchial airways spasm and are narrow. The airways' linings are also inflamed and secrete mucus. This happens because people with asthma have lungs that are hypersensitive to something (it might be pollen, dust mites, cold, exercise, etc.—things that wouldn't bother normal airways). If the airflow obstruction can be completely unblocked, asthma sufferers are not said to have COPD.

Organic dusts can cause what is called *occupational asthma.* There are a zillion possible allergens that fall into this category including dust from castor beans, grains, red cedar wood, formalin, teas, epoxy resins, several antibiotics, and enzymes used in making beer and leather.

Cystic fibrosis is an inherited disease that occurs most often (but not exclusively) in white people. It affects several body systems and can manifest itself as COPD, bronchiectasis (see below), bronchitis, respiratory failure, etc. PH develops in a significant portion of cystic fibrosis patients who have too little oxygen in their blood, but it is usually mild.

3.2. Interstitial Lung Disease

"Interstitial" refers to the spaces between the individual air sacs *(alveoli)* in the lungs. This is a sprawling family of roughly 180 types of disease caused by breathing in various substances. They all involve an inflammation of the walls of the lower respiratory tract and problems with the walls of the air spaces in the lungs. (Sometimes these diseases are lumped in with COPD.) Interstitial lung diseases are chronic, noninfectious, and nonmalignant. Patients with these diseases are short of breath and might sometimes develop PH. Sometimes the cause of the interstitial lung disease isn't known, so it's called *idiopathic pulmonary fibrosis.*

Often it is possible to trace the illness to the patient's breathing something harmful from the environment, like certain mineral or organic dusts (*pneumoconiosis*). Miners and stonecutters often breathe in mineral dusts like silica, coal, asbestos, and beryllium. Each substance has its own disease label: anthracosis (coal), silicosis (quartz), asbestosis (asbestos), and berylliosis (also called beryllium poisoning or beryllium granulomatosis).

Another organic dust problem, byssinosis, is caused by inhaling little bits of cotton, flax, or hemp. Sometimes interstitial lung disease stems from drugs, radiation, or another illness.

In bronchiectasis part or all of the passages leading from the trachea (windpipe) to the lungs are chronically dilated and parts of the lungs are infected. The disease can be inherited, congenital, or secondary to TB, whooping cough, chronic bronchitis, and other conditions. Breathing particles of silica, talc, or Bakelite, or inhaling injurious gases can cause it, as can immunologic deficiencies. Bronchiectasis actually overlaps into several categories of PH.

3.3. Sleep Disordered Breathing

About 12 million Americans have *sleep apnea:* they stop breathing several or many times an hour while they sleep. This disease wasn't well known until recently, and most people who have it are unaware that they do. There is much more to be learned about sleep apnea. Sufferers are drowsy during the day and are said to be more dangerous on the road than drunk drivers!

To be classified as having sleep apnea you generally have to stop breathing for at least 10 seconds at least 30 times in a 7-hour period (and often over 100 times in an hour!). The condition is found most frequently in very heavy middle-aged men who snore, but it is certainly not limited to them. A clue, in obese

patients with IPAH, is the swelling of both legs. If present, it might make a doc wonder about whether the patient has obstructive sleep apnea.

If you don't breathe often enough, you don't maintain enough oxygen in your blood (the saturation falls below 90 percent for a significant time). This lack of oxygen can cause pulmonary vasoconstriction (see the discussion of hypoxemia, below), and a resulting rise in PAPs.

Those who have the most common kind of sleep apnea, obstructive sleep apnea, keep trying to breathe but can't pull in enough air because of a blockage in the upper airway. (Rarely, sleep apnea is caused by a problem in the brain stem.) PAH is moderately prevalent, but mild, in obstructive sleep apnea patients. On the other hand, the incidence of sleep apnea among PAH patients is probably low, but this isn't known for certain. It appears more often when other risk factors for PH are present, such as obstructed airways and obesity with hypoxemia. As Americans increase in size, more develop sleep apnea. If we get too heavy, we might breathe shallowly at night and not get enough oxygen during the day, either. This is called *obesity hypoventilation syndrome.* Someone with the syndrome might not huff and puff, because a lot of fat seems to reset some people's brains so they don't signal the need for more oxygen!

Dr. Brian Mulhall of Walter Reed Army Medical Center has another idea on what might contribute to sleep apnea: acid reflux. If larger studies confirm the preliminary findings of his group, treating your acid reflux might decrease or cure your sleep apnea.

A few sketchy studies suggest that sleep apnea alone might cause PAH, but most studies point to daytime hypoxemia (due to other pulmonary problems) as the cause of

PAH in sleep apnea patients. Industrial

strength, permanent PAH is probably not caused by sleep apnea alone, although apnea could worsen it.

When the hypoxemia that sleep apnea causes is prevented, the changes in the pulmonary vessels appear to be reversible. Sleep apnea is a rare situation where it is possible that supplemental oxygen might actually "cure" PAH; at least one woman's PAP returned to normal when she began oxygen therapy.

Continuous positive airway pressure (CPAP) is the remedy usually tried first. It involves a breadbox-sized machine attached to an "interface" with tubing. A mask and headgear are the most common interface. Because of its intrusive nature, many users do not warmly embrace CPAP. A doctor's prescription is needed. You can rent a machine for $30-40 a month and see if it helps. Unfortunately, the longer you use CPAP, the more problems you are likely to have with it.At a recent PHA conference, two sleep apnea patients (one of them PH specialist Dr. Michael Krowka of the Mayo Clinic, Rochester, Minnesota) complained that CPAP forced air out of their tear ducts! Some might find this unsettling. A full-face mask might help. On the other hand, the wife of a sleep apnea patient says a CPAP machine saved her marriage by allowing *her* to get some sleep.

After being set up and watched for a while by technicians trained to do this, you breath oxygen while sleeping. It's not the same as just slapping on an oxygen mask and dozing off, because the pressures must be set for you individually and there is a danger of heart rhythm problems. If it's not adjusted well for both comfort and effectiveness, you may get unnecessarily discouraged.

Because there is evidence that treatment with CPAP lowers PAPs, some PH docs like to use *polysomnography* (continuous measurement of things related to your breathing while you sleep) or 4-channel cardiopulmonary sleep studies to find if their patients have problems. These studies are usually done overnight at a sleep center. It's also possible to borrow an oximeter and do some testing yourself, at home. You can learn more about these tests, CPAP, and how to work with your insurance company to get CPAP coverage, from the American Sleep Apnea Association (www.sleepapnea.org; telephone 202-293-3650).

If your PH doctor doesn't ask you if you snore, raise the subject yourself. Is your snoring so loud it can be heard outside your room (be honest)? Are there pauses followed by a loud snort? This usually indicates you stopped breathing for a bit. Are you sleepy during the day? (Some patients have no daytime symptoms.)

When the patient is obese, weight loss is recommended. There are other remedies, including surgery, that help in some cases.

Don't confuse sleep apnea with *insomnia*, which is trouble falling asleep or staying asleep (although sleep apnea might keep waking you up, too). PH patients have more sleep complaints than most people. This is because nearly all congestive heart failure patients have sleep problems, and many of us have congestive heart failure. Being attached to a tube or waking up at night in a state of fear because we sense an unusual heartbeat can make it hard to sleep. We tend (with some reason) to be more anxious about unusual things going on in our bodies, and anxiety is a prime cause of insomnia. Symptoms seem more threatening at night, which is why emergency rooms are so crowded as the clock hands point upward.

3.4. Alveolar Hypoventilation Disorders & Hypoxemia

Alveolar hypoventilation happens when there is not enough air exchange in the small lung sacs. This is usually due to mechanical or neurological problems involving muscles, nerves, or the brain. For example, musculoskeletal problems can prevent the lungs from fully expanding. Even if there is nothing wrong with the lungs, hypoventilation might be caused by the obesity/hypoventilation syndrome, sleep apnea, or drug overdose.

When there is not enough fresh air in the lungs, too little oxygen is available to be taken into the blood, and *hypoxemia* results. Sensing this lack of oxygen, the pulmonary arteries tighten up in their effort to direct blood to other places, where there might be more oxygen. Hypoxemia is a potent vasoconstrictor; vasoconstriction might eventually lead to PH.

Symptoms of hypoxemia include the symptoms of hypoxia (see the next section) plus fatigue, memory troubles, more shortness of breath with exercise, depression, and waking up a lot at night. Hypoxemia is not only present in alveolar hypoventilation disorders, but is also found in connection with some of the other lung diseases discussed earlier, and with living at a high altitude (see the next section).

3.5 Living Too High: Altitude & PH

A lack of oxygen in the air you are breathing (*hypoxia*) can also cause hypoxemia. As is the case with alveolar hypotension, your pulmonary arteries tighten up in their effort to direct blood to places where there might be oxygen. Living at a high altitude is one reason for hypoxia.

Three highs that can make you low: elevation, temperature, and humidity. As you climb above sea level, the air pressure drops as the air thins, resulting in less available oxygen for your lungs to absorb. The higher the elevation, the more likely you are to get hypoxic vasoconstriction. Healthy people can function pretty well up to around 10,000 feet. Up to about 5,200 feet (the altitude of mile-high Denver), lung pressures usually get only slightly higher. Many PH patients do okay in high-altitude cities. But some who do fine at sea level will need supplemental oxygen if they visit high places like Salt Lake City or Denver. Sometimes, PH patients are advised to move to a lower altitude; it's an individual thing and there is no general rule about what altitude is safe.

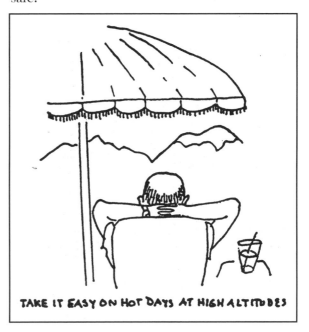

TAKE IT EASY ON HOT DAYS AT HIGH ALTITUDES

High temperatures and high humidity also thin out the air. Airplanes require longer runways to take off at high altitudes, and also when the air is hot and moist. You, too, might have to put more effort into getting up and off on hot, humid days, or when you are visiting friends in Leadville, Colorado (elevation 10,200 feet). (Please don't really go to Leadville. It's so high that they say cats can't even give birth to live kittens.) Of the three (altitude, temperature, and humidity),

humidity is the least important to us. Really *dry* air can also be hard on lungs.

Symptoms of hypoxia include impairment of vision, euphoria, lightheadedness, breathlessness, hot and cold flashes, reasoning difficulties (like repetitive thought patterns), headache, slowed motor responses, tingling fingers and toes, increased perspiration, nausea, vomiting, and finally unconsciousness.

Be alert for such symptoms (okay, it's hard to be alert for unconsciousness, but pay attention to the others) when you are flying on commercial airliners, which are engineered to provide a cabin pressure of at least the equivalent of 8,000 feet above sea level (in practice, airlines usually do better than that, and pressurize to the equivalent of 5,000 to 7,000 feet).

The low-pressure situation on airplanes is made worse by pollutants and high levels of carbon dioxide in recirculated cabin air. Airplanes that fly at high altitudes always carry emergency supplemental oxygen; ask for it if you need it. (For how to get oxygen on airplanes, see Chapter 10.)

Category 4:
PH Due to Chronic Thrombotic and / or Embolic Disease

The PH in this category is caused by clots and other obstructions in the lungs.

An *embolus* is a clump of something (even air bubbles), that has plugged up a blood vessel. An *embolism* is the blockage of a vessel by an embolus. In our case, it's usually a blood clot that has formed somewhere else and traveled to the lungs. A *thrombus* is a fibrinous blood clot that obstructs a blood vessel. Both emboli and thrombi can be thought of as clots. Clots probably cause around 10 percent of all cases of PH.

Nearly always, blood clots dissolve on their own, and if you survive the original event, you need not worry about PH. If clots do not dissolve, but persist for years and cause PH, and if they are big enough and lodged in the larger vessels, they can often be removed by a procedure called a pulmonary thrombo-endarterectomy (see Chapter 6), so it can be good news to learn that this is your problem.

4.1. Thromboembolic Obstruction of Proximal Pulmonary Arteries

This category deals with clots that generally are found in medium to small-sized arteries, but that can occur in other arteries as well.

Clots usually form in a leg vein and travel to the lungs, where they sometimes become wedged. Each year, about 500 to 2,500 patients in the U.S. who previously survived an acute pulmonary embolism event, but have a clot still in their lungs, go on to develop chronic thromboembolic PH (CTEPH). Although a big majority of PH patients are female, slightly more men than women develop CTEPH. (It used to be thought that tiny, tiny clots formed in the legs and then traveled in the bloodstream to the lungs where they wedged together in small pulmonary arteries to cause PH, but this theory now lacks credibility.)

Because it's possible to have a pulmonary embolism without knowing it, or without knowing that a clot has remained, the clots often work in secret until the PH process is well underway. After a clot lodges in the lungs and grows into the wall of a vessel, there may be a honeymoon period that lasts months or even decades before PH symptoms appear and you are diagnosed. Dutch researchers recently found that a surprising 3.8 percent of people who survive pulmonary embolisms have PH 2 years later.

When birth control pills contained higher doses of hormones (until the mid -1980s), doctors saw more such clots. They can also form when you are sick in bed for a long time and are not taking an anticoagulant, or if you sit in one position for a long time, like when you're traveling by air, car, or bus.

Why do only a few people have clots that don't dissolve, and why does PH develop in only some people who get clots? A minority of CTEPH patients have inherited factors in their blood that make it more prone to clotting. For example, elevated amounts of clotting factor VIII and high-level cardiolipin autoantibodies (lupus anticoagulant) are found more often in CTEPH patients than in the general population or in persons with PH that does not involve chronic thromboembolisms.

Surgeons who operate to remove these clots used to think that if you take out the clot, you cure the patient. Now they know it's often more complicated. When PH develops, something is going on in the smaller vessels farther out from the central clots (*distal* vessels). You would think that a vessel downstream from a clot would be protected, at least from higher pressures. But like vessels in the unobstructed parts of the lungs, they also show some remodeling typical of PH (although somewhat less than vessels not sheltered behind a block). In other words, the degree of vessel obstruction does not always correlate with the development of PH. Possible factors are the amounts of vasoconstrictors circulating in your blood, a genetic predisposition to PH, how your right ventricle adapts to the increased pressure, etc.

The symptoms are much like they are for all PH: first breathlessness when you move about, and then swollen ankles, chest pain, dizziness, etc. In 30 percent of patients doctors can hear unusual high-pitched blowing sounds over the lungs. Such sounds can be caused by other diseases, but are not heard in IPAH / FPAH. Misdiagnoses are common: patients are told they are just out of shape, getting old, have asthma or another lung or heart condition, or that they have psychological problems.

The gold standard for finding out about clots in your lungs and whether they are operable is pulmonary angiography and an ultrafast CT scan. In the near future, new magnetic resonance techniques may replace angiography and CT scans in many patients.

4.2. Thromboembolic Obstruction of Distal Pulmonary Arteries

Sometimes very tiny clots form right in place (*in situ*) inside the tiny arteries (the "twigs," using the above analogy) in the lungs. This occurs in patients who already have severe PH. Not much is known about whether tiny clots do or do not tend to dissolve on their own. They cannot be removed by surgery, so we take anticoagulants to prevent them from forming. The data is still murky, but researchers believe that PH gets worse over time even if no tiny clots are involved, and that in situ clots don't play a starring role in the progression of PH.

4.3. Non-Thrombotic Pulmonary Embolism (Tumor, Parasites, Foreign Material)

Even small amounts of cancer can cause clots. Tumors arising from glandular organs are particularly likely to cause clots. Small fragments of tumors can also break off, travel, and block blood vessels in the lungs. Or lung cancer can directly affect the small vessels.

Schistosomiasis. Hundreds of millions of people, especially in Asia, Africa, and South America, suffer from this parasitic disease caused by blood flukes living in the blood vessels of internal organs. Although this disease is seldom seen in the U.S., on a worldwide basis, it is one of the most common causes of PH. It can cause PH either by causing portal hypertension (which, in turn, leads to PH), or by fluke eggs blocking blood vessels in the lungs and causing fibrosis.

Behçet's Disease. Behçet's disease is found mostly (but far from exclusively) in the Turkish population. It attacks the small vessels that provide the walls of larger vessels with blood. Nearly every organ can be involved. In the lung vessels of these patients, thrombotic and "inflammatory" changes lead to PH. (Symptoms of Behçet's include recurrent canker sore-like ulcers in the mouth and on the genitals, and eye inflammation. Behçet's can involve any organ and can affect the central nervous system. Skin lesions, arthritis, bowel inflammation, meningitis, and cranial nerve palsies are other possible symptoms.)

Category 5: Miscellaneous

As in Category 4 this category involves some things that cause PH by directly blocking the flow of blood through pulmonary vessels. Pressures build up behind the blockage and this can lead to PH. Schistosomiasis and sarcoidosis also involve inflammation.

Another cause of venous PH is —take a deep breath—**lymphangioleiomyomatosis (LAM)**. This is a very rare disease in which smooth muscle cells can grow in places they don't belong in the lymph system.

Diseases involving granulomas. Granulomas are growths that result when macrophages attempt to destroy foreign bodies or mycobacteria. (Macrophages are a type of white blood cell that has left the circulation and settled in a tissue. They can identify and clean up "garbage" in the form of foreign antigens.) Granulomas occur in diseases like leprosy, yaws, syphilis, and leishmaniasis, which are all diseases caused by known infectious agents.

The cause of the chronic disease called sarcoidosis is unknown, but it also involves the formation of granulomas as well as other infection-fighting cells. Sarcoidosis may affect almost any organ system, but especially the lungs. For some reason, white blood cells travel to the lungs even when there are no known triggers, inflaming the lungs and swelling lymph nodes. People from Scandinavia seem more prone to the disorder, which might explain its higher incidence in Northeast Wisconsin. Or it might be that exposure to beryllium (found in some soils and used in building aircraft), or working with certain ceramics can trigger sarcoidosis. African Americans are also more likely to have sarcoidosis.

Histiocytosis X, a.k.a. Langerhans' cell granulomatosis, includes a group of diseases where scarring is caused (often in the lungs and bones) by the overgrowth of cells that scavenge for foreign material (histiocytes) and cells involved in allergic reactions (eosinophils). Pulmonary histiocytosis X happens only in smokers, and is rare. The lungs are made stiff by scarring. Common symptoms are coughing, shortness of breath, fever, chest pain, and weight loss.

Squeezing of central pulmonary veins. An inflammation of the tissue separating the right and left lungs can cause scar-like tissue to form (*fibrosing mediastinitis*). If enough of the fibrous tissue forms that it squeezes central pulmonary veins, it can lead to PH. If lymph nodes or tumors compress these veins it can also cause PH.

PH Treatments: the Basics

Today there are treatments to help most PH patients, and additional therapies are peeking over the horizon. Although PH has various causes, many treatments can focus on the common final disease pathways.

It isn't possible in the *Survival Guide* to tell all you need to know about treating PH. Your PH medical team can give you more information on options, risks, side effects, drug interactions, dosages, etc. A good doctor welcomes questions. Be sure that you are diagnosed (or have your diagnosis confirmed), and your treatment begun, only at a PH specialty treatment center. Because PH has many causes, *treatments that might save one PH patient's life could easily harm another.* Specialists at PH centers might also be participating in clinical trails that are evaluating potential new therapies that may be of interest to you. You can learn about them on PHA's website (www.PHAssociation.org), in the "Research Corner" of *Pathlight,* or by signing up for *PHA News,* which will send you bi-weekly
e-mail reports. *PHA News* is free; you don't have to join PHA to receive it. If you are a PHA member, you still have to ask for it (sign up on PHA's website).

Our discussion of treatments is divided into three chapters: an overview in this Chapter 4 (which includes a look at basic treatments that tinker with PH more than control it); PH Drugs (Chapter 5); and Surgical Solutions (Chapter 6).

How Do Doctors Decide on a Treatment?

Nearly all PH patients receive at least some "conventional therapy": oral anticoagulants, diuretics, oxygen, and digoxin.

If a patient does not have really severe PH, and if he or she responds well and quickly to vasodilators, doctors usually begin treatment by trying to lower lung pressures with calcium channel blockers (Norvasc, Procardia, Aldalat, etc.). The calcium channel blockers come in pill form, are easy to administer, and cost much less than alternative treatments. Unfortunately, few patients respond to this treatment (see Chapter 5).

If calcium channel blockers don't work well, and the patient is in Class III (see Chapter 1), endothelin receptor antagonists (Tracleer, etc.), some form of prostanoid therapy (Flolan, Remodulin, iloprost, etc.), and/or phosphodiesterase inhibitors (Viagra, etc.) will be considered. If these don't do the trick, or the patient is in Class IV, chronic intravenous epoprostenol (Flolan), perhaps in combination with other drugs, is usually preferred. If this fails, lung transplantation is an option in selected patients. At any stage, investigational therapies can also be considered. Certain patients might go straight to surgical treatments.

The above are not cookbook rules, only rough guidelines. There are types of PH for which particular therapies are not appropriate. A specialist's decision is also influenced by factors such as the age of the patient (quality of life may be more important than longevity to an 85-year-old), whether a patient has rapidly advancing HIV disease (it can take months to benefit from epoprostenol), the patient's ability to comply with a particular therapy, etc.

As new drugs become available, shifts are seen in the percentages of patients on each type of treatment. An interesting (but unscientific) poll on PHCentral's website, taken in April of 2003, showed a drop from 27 to 11 percent over the preceding several years in the use of calcium channel blockers, a drop and from 35 percent to 27 percent in the use of epoprostenol (Flolan), and a large increase in the use of an endothelin receptor blocker (Tracleer). See www.phcentral.org.

What about Treating "Mild" PH?

Dr. Ron Oudiz (Harbor-UCLA, Torrance, CA) polled his fellow PH specialists on this topic in 2000. The poll confirmed what most PH docs already knew: a big gap in our knowledge is how those with little or mild PH should be treated.

What is "mild" PH? There's no exact definition, but it might be someone with a systolic PAP around 40 when diagnosed, and with few or no symptoms. Mild symptoms do not necessarily mean you have only mildly elevated PAP; symptoms and pressures do not always go together. It isn't even known for sure if "mild" patients will continue to get worse, as do patients with more severe disease, and if so how fast they will worsen. It is possible that prostanoids or other PH drugs would prevent such patients from getting worse; doctors just don't know.

Dr. Oudiz's informal survey found that for Class I patients with only moderate systolic PAPs (say 60 mm Hg), all the doctors who replied would prescribe warfarin, half would

use digoxin, and all would use calcium channel blockers if the patient was a responder to an acute vasodilator. Epoprostenol (Flolan) would probably not be used. Treprostinil (Remodulin) might be used, however, if the patient was a nonresponder to calcium channel blockers. For Class II patients, more doctors would use treprostinil or an investigational drug if it was oral, but very few would consider epoprostenol. Many experts would not add specific therapy aimed at the treatment of PH, because there is no information showing that the treatment of Class I patients stops disease progression or improves survival. This survey was done before the FDA had approved endothelin antagonists, and before the increased use of phosphodiesterase inhibitors to treat PH. These options might well be considered now for treating mild PH. Hopefully, new clinical trials will address these and other related questions.

Secondary PH: Treatment of Underlying Disease

As long as an underlying disease exists, it will continue to cause PH. For example, if you suffer from a chronic obstructive lung disease (like bronchitis) that has led to your PH, this obstructive lung disease needs to be treated (maybe with bronchodilators) in addition to your PH. Pneumonia or acute bronchitis usually need to be treated with antibiotics. Schistosomiasis can be treated with the anti-parasite drug praziquantel (unfortunately, anti-parasite drugs are toxic and not always very effective). Those with Gaucher disease can now be treated with glucocerebrosidase enzyme replacement therapy. Researchers at Tokyo Women's Medical University, Japan, have found that in their systemic lupus erythematosus/PH patients, treating them with immunosuppressive agents shortly after their PH appears improves their prognosis. These are just a few examples.

Once you have PH, especially if you have had it for some time, curing the disease that caused it may not make the PH go away, so the PH itself will need separate treatment. Remember, once PH gets started it will often continue to worsen over time. Sometimes, however, curing the underlying problem does cure the PH. Repairing or replacing a leaky or narrowed mitral valve, for example, often cures the patient's PH. Having a thrombo-endarterectomy to remove big clots in your lungs is another treatment of an under-lying condition that can sometimes cure PH.

Substance Abuse: It's Hard, But Essential, To Quit

The head of a PH treatment center in a large city estimates that a third of the PH patients that come to that center are hooked on street drugs, especially cocaine and methamphetamine. That center has seen more patients who developed PH from the use of street drugs than from diet pills. The street drugs linked to PH are addictive. Even when a patient knows that his/her drug abuse caused PH, that the abuse makes effective treatment impossible, and that the abuse will probably lead to death, the patient might be unable to stop.

Some patients even use the epoprostenol IV access catheter to inject a street drug, with dire results. If they survive, they tell a dozen different lies about what happened to their catheter. When a doctor, physician's assistant, or nurse has struggled to keep a patient alive and give him/her a chance at a good life, it is heartbreaking to learn the patient could not resist the siren's call, and has died.

The bottom line is this: you've got to help yourself survive by getting appropriate treatment and joining a support group, by sticking with a program or therapy, and by

finding other things to make life exciting and rewarding. Yes, this is a big order, considering the changes inside the brain caused by addiction. But many others have quit, and so can you.

Treating the Symptoms and Slowing the Progress

Before turning, in the next two chapters, to the more advanced treatments touched on above—treatments that can halt or even reverse progression of PH—here are some widely used basic treatments that may make you feel better or slow the progress of the disease just a bit. With the exceptions mentioned, and although oxygen has been shown to help patients with PH due to emphysema, the author is unaware of any scientific trials that have been done to prove that these drugs truly improve PH patients' lives or life spans. But common sense supports their use, where appropriate.

Anticoagulants

Anticoagulants make blood less likely to clot. Sometimes called "blood thinners," they don't make you feel better, but might lengthen your life. Although the blood itself in most PH patients is no more prone to clotting than the average Joe's blood, the damaged blood vessels in the lungs of PH patients are less resistant to clotting. These clots (*thrombi*) in the small lung vessels can worsen PH. Microscopic layers of clots may form inside the vessels. Some researchers think that the vessels in the lungs of PH patients do not break down fibrin (a substance that helps form blood clots) as well as normal lungs do, because a lot of thrombotic lesions are found in the small pulmonary arteries of many patients with PH.

Some PH patients form fairly big clots in their veins (typically their leg veins) that eventually break loose and travel to the lung vessels (pulmonary arteries), where they block blood flow. The tendency to clot is sometimes hereditary in this group of patients. A study sponsored by the National Heart, Lung, and Blood Institute, and carried out at Brigham and Women's Hospital and Harvard Medical School, found that after treating such clots with full-dose warfarin for a few months, thereafter *low* doses of warfarin went a long way toward preventing future clots and reducing the danger of bleeding. (See the section in Chapter 6 on thromboendarterectomy, a "cure" for this type of PH.)

Now back to "typical" PAH patients: three studies *suggest* that PAH patients who use anticoagulants live longer than those who do not use them. The first study was the largest. It was a retrospective study done by Dr. V. Fuster (Mayo Clinic) and others, and was published in *Circulation* in October 1984. Another retrospective study looked at "PPH" patients who had taken aminorex (a diet drug used in Europe in the 1960s). It found that warfarin (the most commonly prescribed anticoagulant pill) increased long-term survival and significantly improved the quality of life of "PPH" patients, especially those who had taken the diet pills. A small, prospective, but nonrandomized study by Dr. Stuart Rich and his colleagues found that 91 percent of PH patients taking Coumadin (a brand of warfarin) were alive at the end of a year, versus only 67 percent of those not using the drug. The benefits of

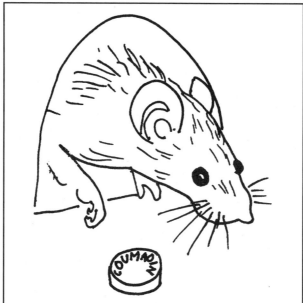

warfarin were particularly apparent in patients who did not appear to benefit from calcium channel blockers (see below). (Don't be scared by these numbers; the study was published in 1992, before epoprostenol and other new drug treatments were available.) Dr. Rich cautions that the study was not designed to test the influence of anticoagulants, and that the researchers might have been unconsciously biased in the selection of patients given Coumadin. (See the graph in Chapter 7.) Dr. Bruce Brundage also cautions that a long-term, randomized, placebo-controlled study is needed to find out if warfarin really helps PH patients.

Warfarin. Yes, warfarin is the chemical used in rat poison, but the pills intended for humans are more carefully manu-factured and government-regulated. Doctors might prescribe the Coumadin brand of warfarin, made by DuPont Pharma-ceuticals. The patent on Coumadin has expired, however, so other companies are now making warfarin. Generic warfarin works just fine and is a lot cheaper. If you switch to a generic form, get your INR checked soon afterwards, because the right dose may be a little different than with Coumadin. And don't jump around from one generic version to another: each time you switch manufacturers, your INR needs rechecking. Open the little bottle before leaving the drug store counter and make sure your new pills look just like your last ones.

Doctors may decide not to use anti-coagulants if your PH is mild, if you tend to fall down, play contact or extreme sports, or have a history of significant bleeding (i.e., from a peptic ulcer or leaky blood vessel in your brain).

Aspirin. Aspirin has some properties that prevent clotting and is inexpensive. So why not use it instead of warfarin? Because aspirin acts on the *platelets* in the blood, and warfarin acts on little fiber-like agents. Many researchers think that it's the fiber-like agents that are more likely to contribute to PH. Aspirin, unlike warfarin, has not been tested on PH. Some researchers think it possible that the right amount of aspirin would improve the production of prostacyclin and decrease the production of thromboxane—substances our bodies make that have been implicated in the development of PH. However, what the right amount might be for PH patients is unknown. Because aspirin can't be patented (thus no maker of aspirin has a financial interest in studying it in PAH), and because there are so many drugs that urgently need clinical trials, there might never be a study of aspirin's effects on PH (although inside sources suggest a trial is being considered). In the meantime, doctors just have to use their best judgment with the knowledge available. It would be dangerous to experiment on your own. Unless your doctor tells you to, don't take both warfarin and aspirin: aspirin can cause stomach irritation or ulcers, and warfarin could make you bleed more severely if you develop an ulcer. Sometimes doctors may use both low-dose aspirin and warfarin (usually in people with artificial heart valves), with careful monitoring.

Ximelagatran (Exanta® or Exarta®, H 376/95) was initially investigated as an anticoagulant that would eventually replace warfarin (Coumadin). In 2006, its manufacturer AstraZeneca announced that it would not market the medication in the US after reports of liver damage. It also discontinued its distribution in other countries where the drug had been approved. Fortunately, other companies are working on similar drugs which will hopefully fare better than Exanta and pave the way for blood thinners that don't require blood test monitoring.

Thrombolytics. These drugs don't just keep clots from forming, but actually break them up—a little like Drano unclogging a drain. Today they are mostly used in patients with heart attacks or certain types of strokes, and in those with a new, massive, acute pulmonary embolism who are likely to die if treated only with conventional blood thinners. Otherwise, there is no role for thrombolytics in chronic PH.

How to Use Warfarin

It is important not to be over- or under-anticoagulated. Unfortunately, a zillion foods, meds, and other things (e.g., how your body metabolizes the drug) affect how well warfarin works. The list of foods and drugs that interact with warfarin is too long to include here, but you should be able to get such information from the place that monitors your clotting time.

INR (International Normalized Range) checks. The INR is a measure of exactly how much your blood has been anticoagulated. "INR" is sometimes used interchangeably with "pro-time" ("PT"). Although these two are not exactly the same (the INR is more accurate), they are both used as indicators of how "thin" your blood is. The INR was developed as a universal standard measurement so that test results from different laboratories can be compared.

To keep your warfarin dosage right, you need regular INR checks to measure the time it takes for your blood to clot. Most patients prefer a finger-stick to a blood draw, because they can learn the results in under 2 minutes. Checks are typically done about once a month; how often you're tested depends on how stable your INR is.

One of the most annoying things about using warfarin is the need for frequent trips to the clinic or lab for these checks. The technician has to ask intrusive questions about your personal life: How many margaritas did you drink on the cruise? Exactly what drugs do you take? Umm hum. Is that a new antidepressant for you? Have you managed to lose weight? Lord knows how long they keep those files, but it's not hard to imagine an insurance company subpoenaing them and saying, "Ah ha! You have started going to the gym and are using weights! Are you *really* disabled?"

PH doctors disagree as to exactly what INR to aim for in PH patients; generally they seek a number between 1.5 and 2.0, although some like it higher. There can also be clinical reasons for a higher or lower dose. Just because you take more warfarin than someone else does not mean you are sicker or that your INR is necessarily higher. Your liver might just metabolize the drug more efficiently, your diet might be different, or your other medications may be different.

Home testing. The FDA has approved several home testing systems, available only by prescription, that allow you to check your INR more conveniently. See "INR home testing kits" under Nongovernmental Resources in Chapter 14.

Forgot to take a dose? The general rule seems to be that if it's still the same day, only later than the time you usually take your warfarin, go ahead and take it. But don't take two doses in the same day without your doc's okay.

Pre-surgery precautions. If you plan an operation or serious dental surgery, it will often be necessary to stop taking warfarin for about 5 to 10 days before the procedure. This is because warfarin takes a while to clear from your system, and its effects cannot easily be reversed in an emergency (in a pinch, some doctors may use shots of vitamin K to try to drop your INR). For most PH patients, the risk of stopping warfarin for 5 to 10 days is negligible. As a substitute for the warfarin, your doctor may prescribe **heparin**, another anticoagulant that inhibits the formation of fibrin. It's always given by injection, often into the fat on your tummy. The advantage of heparin is that it has a much shorter half-life and its effects are more easily reversed.

Side effects to report to your doctor. There are potentially serious side effects to anticoagulant therapy. You'll want to take particular care to avoid cuts and to protect your head and body from injury. Tell your doctor if you experience:

- Blue or purplish toes or fingers, if they weren't this color before you started taking warfarin. Call your doctor at once!
- A head injury. Call your doctor at once!
- Prolonged or unusual bleeding, including increased menstrual flow, red or dark brown urine, red or tarry-black stools, coughing up blood or vomiting stuff that looks like coffee grounds, bleeding gums when you brush your teeth, hard-to-stop nosebleeds or prolonged bleeding from cuts. Call your doctor at once!
- Unusual bruising for unknown reasons.
- Fevers, diarrhea, vomiting.
- Signs of internal bleeding like a swollen or painful abdomen, back pain, dizziness, joint pain, stiffness, and a severe or long-lasting headache.
- Coumadin contains a bit of lactose: if you are lactose intolerant, and notice diarrhea,

bloating, or cramps after taking Coumadin, talk to your PH doctor.

Be cautious when changing your diet and meds. Let the person who monitors your INR know if you go on a diet and lose a significant amount of weight, because losing weight can also affect your INR. So can a change in how physically active you are. Also report changes (adding, discontinuing, or changing a dosage) in your use of prescription drugs, nonprescription drugs, and vitamins. Even flu shots have reportedly increased INR (this is not, however, a reason to avoid getting your annual flu shot).

Common drugs that interact with warfarin. Hundreds of drugs mess with your INR levels. You can often take these drugs, but might need to adjust your dose of warfarin. We all react differently, so don't try to make an adjustment on your own.

To help prevent dangerous bleeding, do not use aspirin (acetylsalicylic acid), or aspirin-containing drugs like Excedrin, unless your doctor tells you to. As mentioned earlier, aspirin can cause bleeding in the lining of the stomach. It can also increase the effect of the warfarin. The salicylate in Pepto-Bismol can increase bleeding. Avoid, too, ibuprofen-containing drugs like Excedrin IB, Motrin, Advil, Nuprin, Voltaren, diclofenac, and Naprosyn. Acetaminophen (Tylenol) may possibly increase INR, but it's generally okay to take it for pain relief if you don't take more than four extra-strength tablets per day for a week.

Antibiotics (including erythromycin, tetracycline, Bactrim, Cotrim, Septra, SMZ-TMP, Sulfatrim, Uroplus, Flagyl, and Protostat) can change the effect of warfarin, so use them only with your doctor's informed consent.

Barbiturates, thyroid hormones, gout medicines, antifungal agents, heartburn meds, cholesterol meds, seizure meds, and binge drinking can all affect your INR.

Women on warfarin need to consult with their doctor before taking Monistat or other vaginal creams and suppositories that contain the antifungal drug miconazole. It can interact with warfarin to cause nosebleeds, bleeding gums, and bruising.

Ways your diet interacts with warfarin: Vitamin K (phylloquinone) increases the synthesis of four clotting factors, and therefore makes warfarin less effective. It is found in large amounts mostly in leafy green vegetables, but also in fish, fish oils, canola oil and soybean oil. Veggies and fish are good for you, so don't stop eating them. But do not suddenly change your diet to eat a lot more things high in vitamin K, without getting your warfarin dose adjusted. Nobody really knows exactly how much vitamin K you will find in a given vegetable, because the outer leaves (or peels) have more of the vitamin than the pale inner leaves (or fleshy parts). Where and when the plant was grown also affects the amount of vitamin K. Cooking, freezing, or drying a food does not seem to affect the vitamin K content, but not much is known about this.

Here are some common foods that are REALLY high in vitamin K, so approach them with caution if you don't regularly eat them. If you are just using a few sprigs of an herb, don't worry. But if you eat a cup of cooked parsley, it might promote clotting.

Mint	Swiss chard
Parsley	Cucumber peel
Spinach	Kale
Green tea leaves	Brussels sprouts

In the baby food category, creamed, strained spinach is high in vitamin K.

Common foods high in vitamin K, but not as high as the above:

Broccoli	Green scallions
Cabbage	Liver
Collards	Endive
Watercress	Tofu

Other foods to watch out for: these less common foods are loaded with vitamin K – amaranth, ashitaba, bell tree dahlia, chrysanthemum garland, coriander leaf, mituba, nightshade, perilla, purslane, roctish, samat, toumyao (Chinese), purple laver algae, hijiki algae.

A big dose of vitamin E, on the other hand, *boosts* the effect of warfarin. A double-blind trial found no effect on anticoagulation of daily vitamin E supplements of 400 IU or lower. So let the person who monitors your INR know if you take over 400 IU, or change your dose.

Important dos and don'ts if you use warfarin:

♦ Do not use oral anticoagulants during pregnancy; they can cause birth defects.

♦ Get your INR checked on a regular basis; keeping your INR within the range set by your doctor can help you avoid some nasty side effects.

♦ Protect your head: use your shoulder harness or seat belt, and if a sport or activity calls for a helmet, wear one. Avoid contact sports and activities likely to result in serious thumps or cuts.

♦ Wear a MedicAlert bracelet or necklace, or carry a wallet card, to let emergency medical technicians know you take warfarin (see Chapter 14 for how to order).

♦ Let all your health care providers and your dentist know you take warfarin.

♦ Use alcohol only in moderation and let your doctor know if you change your drinking habits. (Alcohol can either increase or decrease your INR. Go figure.)

♦ Be meticulous about taking the exact dose your doctor prescribes, and take it at the same time each day. A pillbox with a space for each day of the week is helpful.

Digoxin (Lanoxin)

This drug appears to help a weak or failing right ventricle to squeeze better, and is prescribed for some PH patients, although its use remains controversial. There is no solid research supporting the chronic use of digoxin to treat PH, or showing that it helps PH patients to live longer. A small study of 17 patients with right ventricular dysfunction because of "PPH" found that intravenous digoxin modestly, but significantly, improved their cardiac output, although pulmonary artery pressure increased as well. Digoxin can be used with calcium channel blockers.

Digoxin interactions. An overdose of digoxin could kill you. Its effect can be increased by some drugs used to treat PH, such as nifedipine (Procardia), or diltiazem (Cardizem, Dilacor XR). Potassium-depleting diuretics can also increase its effect. If you use digoxin, your doctor will want to monitor your potassium levels, because if your blood levels of potassium are too low or high, your heart's electrical system can be seriously affected: skipped beats (even stopping), extra beats, very fast or very slow heart rates, etc., can occur. (See Diuretics, below, for a list of potassium-rich foods.)

Digoxin interacts with lots of other drugs, as well, including antacids, laxatives, certain antibiotics, stomach ulcer medicines, and anti-anxiety medicines. Large amounts of fiber can decrease the absorption of digoxin. You don't have to give up oatmeal or oat bran, just be fairly consistent about how much roughage you eat.

Symptoms of too much digoxin include nausea, loss of appetite, abdominal pain, diarrhea, anorexia, headache, confusion and hallucinations, depression, disturbed vision (such as a yellow-green vision), nightmares, and disrupted heart rhythms.

Diuretics

Fluid retention and swelling (*edema*), especially in the legs and belly, afflicts many PH patients. (Blood clots are another, less common, cause of edema in the legs.) When less blood is pumped to the kidneys, they "think" you're losing blood from an injury and stop secreting fluid. Fluid then leaks out of the blood stream and into spongy body tissue. Fluid retention leads to weight gain. By weighing yourself at the same time each morning you can catch early signs of a build-up of fluids.

Avoiding salt in your diet can help a lot to reduce fluid retention. Cutting down on salt has other benefits. It can help prevent systemic hypertension (the kind measured by a cuff on your arm), and may reduce the risk of osteoporosis and kidney stones. All PH patients should try to limit their salt intake, whether or not they also use diuretics.

If cutting back on salt doesn't help enough (and it usually doesn't), your doctor can prescribe a diuretic (a "water pill") to help your kidneys eliminate water. Two commonly used diuretics are furosemide (Lasix) and spironolactone (Aldactone). Aldactone isn't really much of a diuretic; it's used to spare potassium. (Doctors sometimes prescribe Aldactone for its potassium-sparing effect when a patient is on a potent diuretic like furosemide.) Other diuretics are bumetanide (Bumex), torsemide (Demadex), ethacrynic acid (Edecrin), hydrochlorothiazide (HydroDIURIL, etc.), indapamide (Lozol), tri-amterene combined with hydrochlorothiazide (Maxzide), and metolazone (Zaroxolyn). Like Aldactone, Maxzide spares potassium. More than one diuretic may be prescribed for the same patient. Diuretics reduce swelling in the legs and abdomen and can substantially improve overall functioning.

It isn't known why diuretics make you breathe and feel better, but they do. There is a trend to use them earlier and more often to treat PH patients, but they are a "maintenance" drug, and do little, if anything, to halt the progression of PH.

Different diuretics have different side effects. Common side effects include dehydration and resulting low systemic blood pressure (too much water is lost), and low levels of potassium and/or magnesium (leading to heart rhythm problems). Dehydration can be very dangerous for a PH patient. At high doses, some diuretics can make your ears ring or, less commonly, affect the ear's sense of balance.

For severe fluid retention, diuretics can be given intravenously, to remove the fluid more quickly. If ascites (fluid in the abdomen) is present, the fluid can be removed through a needle temporarily inserted into your abdomen (a *paracentesis*). This is done in the hospital.

Keep an eye on potassium levels and watch out for licorice! When using most diuretics (except the potassium-sparing ones), more of the mineral potassium is excreted than usual, so be careful to keep up your potassium levels by eating potassium-rich foods like bananas, cantaloupe, honeydew melon, potatoes, and orange juice. Do not eat a lot of licorice, which can cause potassium depletion (by the way, it can also impede sexual performance in men). In the U.S., black "licorice" candy is actually flavored with anise, not licorice, so eat it if you must. But avoid the supplement licorice root. Because potassium is important to the electrical stability of your heart (it helps your heart keep up its regular beat) some docs order blood work on some patients every few months to check potassium levels.

Salt substitutes and potassium pills. Just as

too little potassium is dangerous, too *much* potassium can cause the heart to stop (*cardiac arrest*). For this reason, PH patients should avoid potassium pills unless a doctor prescribes them. If you take a lot of diuretics, your doctor may recommend potassium pills and follow you closely with regular lab work. Otherwise, it's easy to get enough potassium from the right foods, and you can't overdose from them. Spironolactone (Aldactone) is a potassium-sparing diuretic, so potassium pills are unlikely to be needed in the rare instance where it is the sole diuretic taken. Be cautious about using salt substitutes, because if one of their ingredients is potassium chloride, they can contain too much potassium for those patients who have kidney problems or are taking certain blood pressure or heart medications.

Mind your magnesium, too. Your doctor may want you to keep up your levels of magnesium, which can also be depleted by diuretics. Most Americans don't get enough magnesium in their diets, because we don't eat enough of the right foods. A magnesium deficiency can cause irregular heart rhythms and muscle weakness. Magnesium-rich foods include bananas, beans, whole grains, nuts (especially almonds, cashews, and peanuts), green veggies, grains, and milk.

Oxygen

A lack of oxygen can cause PH, but PH itself sometimes causes reduced oxygen in the bloodstream. Low levels of bloodstream oxygen make PH worse and increase the heart's workload. Most PH patients have an adequate amount of oxygen in their blood. But many patients, at one time or another during the course of their treatment, need supplemental oxygen. Some PH patients need continuous use. Others may only need supplemental oxygen when moving around, or sleeping, or visiting a place high above sea level, or when traveling in an airplane. It depends on the individual.

Oxygen saturations above about 92 percent when you are sitting and around 88 to 90 percent with exercise are generally considered tolerable. If you repeatedly go lower than that for sustained periods, you may find that oxygen therapy improves your mental and physical functioning. If you have irregular breathing while you sleep (a condition unrelated to sleep apnea), and your oxygen saturation falls too low, this can be improved or prevented by using oxygen through a nasal cannula at night. This type of irregular breathing occurs more often in patients with severe PH.

Checking your oxygen saturation level. You can generally rely on a pulse oximeter (which gives a range and measures trends) to learn if oxygen therapy will help you, but in some cases you may need to have a blood draw from an artery. Because it is hard for a doctor to predict whether you will need supplemental oxygen when you fly to Tibet to visit Aunt Lulu at her ashram, you may want to do a test run on a shorter airplane flight. Also, check out PHA's Consensus Committee's recommendations on travel on PHA's website. The Pulmonary Vascular Disease Program at the University of Washington has a beeper-sized mountain climber's oximeter from REI that it loans to patients going on trips. Abigail borrowed it and learned she could forgo buying expensive supplemental oxygen on some short airplane trips. (See Chapter 12.) You can also borrow (or buy—again see Chapter 12) such an oximeter and drive up a mountain, and see what happens to your oxygenation as you climb. Abigail drops below 90 percent at around 3,000 feet.

Equipment options. Oxygen comes in several forms: liquid, compressed, and concentrated out of ambient air. Each form

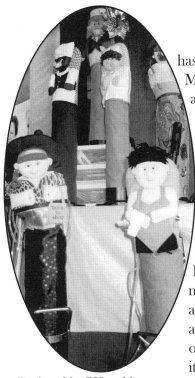

Designed by PH and heart patients, many styles of upbeat liquid oxygen tank and Flolan pump covers are available from Able Bodied Works. Phone: (504) 393-9891. www.ablebodied works.com.

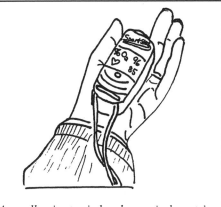

A small oximeter is handy on airplane trips or when exercising.

has pros and cons. Medicare covers them all.

Liquid oxygen can be delivered to your house in waist-high thermos tanks, in which it is stored at a temperature of about minus 300 degrees Fahrenheit. A flow meter and regulator are attached so you can adjust the flow of oxygen, which warms as it leaves the tank and becomes a gas. You can use a big "mother" tank to refill smaller, portable tanks. You have to be careful to keep liquid oxygen tanks upright. It evaporates slowly from the small tanks. If you're traveling, you need a vehicle big enough to haul the "mother" tank along. Liquid oxygen is silent when in use. It weighs much less than compressed oxygen— you get more oxygen (hours) per pound of weight. The mother tank must be refilled once a month or so, and you have to be home when it's delivered.

Compressed oxygen also comes in a tank with a flow meter and regulator. You have to handle this kind of tank carefully, too, because it's under pressure (a broken valve can turn it into a missile). Unlike liquid oxygen, it doesn't evaporate. So if you don't use it at night, it will all still be there in the morning. The tanks are heavier than liquid oxygen tanks, however, and they don't last as long. If you don't need supplemental oxygen all the time, this can be a good choice.

The most convenient form when you're away from the house is a **portable oxygen-conserving unit** (such as the Oxylite, Helios, or Escort) that has a much smaller, lighter container than a regular liquid oxygen tank. The units save oxygen by delivering it in tiny pulses only when you inhale. They are used with a nasal cannula. Such systems can provide up to 2 liters/minute for 10 hours and weigh as little as 3.5 pounds when filled. Not all systems are available in all countries. If you need a flow rate of over 6 liters/minute, you can't use a pulse system.

Concentrators. You can rent an oxygen concentrator, a rather noisy machine about the size of a large suitcase that sucks oxygen right out of room air. (Actually, it takes out the nitrogen, leaving you with oxygen that's about 87 to 95 percent pure.) Many home oxygen users have

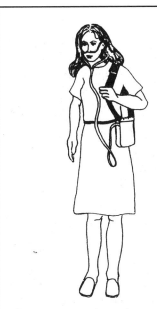

Oxygen conserving units are light weight, easily portable, and provide oxygen for up to 24 hours.

Illustration by Andrea Rich.

such a machine. Some devices really put a spin on your electric meter (one user says it costs him about a dollar a day), and some generate heat, which can be a negative if you live in a warm climate. And because a concentrator doesn't store oxygen and there is always the possibility of a power outage, you should have another source of oxygen available. The part of the machine that humidifies the oxygen must be cleaned frequently so you don't breathe germs or mold. It would be nice to be able to stick it in a closet so you couldn't hear the noise, but the machine has to be placed where there is a good supply of fresh air. You can often put it in another room and use a long tube. A retractable oxygen-tubing reel is available from Colvin Designs & Distribution, 1-888-870-5266. A concentrator cannot be used to fill portable tanks.

If you have an RV or camper, ask for a **transportable concentrator**. It will be too heavy to carry and still needs to be plugged in, but has wheels and a handle. Some can run off a car's battery if you use an inverter, or off an RV's auxiliary generator.

A new device is the **truly portable concentrator**, such as the LifeStyle made by AirSep. It weighs less than 10 pounds and has a battery that can run it for almost an hour. It might be particularly handy for trips to the doctor (run it off his/her electricity for a while). It stores no oxygen, so you can carry it aboard an airplane and put it in an overhead compartment. PHA and other groups are lobbying hard to get the FAA to order airlines to allow you to plug a little concentrator into an outlet aboard an airplane and use it in your seat. A little concentrator has AC and DC adaptors. Between fights, in airports, you can fight with laptop users for scarce electrical outlets. (To find an outlet, look for a laptop user. Often there's a free socket.) The disadvantages are that some of us would need a cart to carry 10 pounds, and it is expensive and might not be covered by insurance.

On your face. Except for the oxygen-conserving unit, which requires a cannula, oxygen can be inhaled through either a facemask or a cannula (nasal prongs). Outside of a hospital, nearly everybody uses the latter. Cannulas make it easier to talk and eat. Special prongs are available for people with sensitive noses. To help prevent respiratory infections, clean your cannula regularly. If you are a high-flow user who needs 6 liters per minute or more, cannulas aren't recommended.

Safety concerns. Because oxygen supports combustion—it makes things burn faster and hotter—be very careful if you use it while cooking, especially if you have a gas stove (ask your oxygen supplier if cooking over gas is a task you should delegate). Keep yourself, your tank, and your tubing a safe distance from any open flame or lit cigarette. Your oxygen company will provide an "Oxygen in Use" sign to post on your door and more guidance on safety.

The FDA has received reports of oxygen cylinders with aluminum regulators burning or exploding. Most aluminum regulators were Life Support Products and Allied Healthcare Products. If you still have one of these old aluminum regulators on your equipment, ask that they be replaced with brass regulators.

Too much oxygen is not a good thing. Once you are adequately oxygenated, extra oxygen does no good. If you increase the level too high it can cause carbon dioxide to build up in your blood and body, and this can be dangerous (this is much less likely to happen with a cannula than with a facemask). Too high a flow also dries out your mucous membranes.

Information on the web. While researching for this book, the author found a good website, www.portableoxygen.org, which is run by a retired guy who uses oxygen, who claims to have no financial links to its sale, and who appears to be obsessive about ferreting out facts. There is much more information on his site than could be included here.

Patient reports. Jessica, who uses oxygen, went to a graduation rehearsal and saw people she hadn't seen for years and *not a single person* mentioned her oxygen! She found it very strange how something so obvious "can just be taken out of a conversation when it is sitting there the whole time sticking out of your nose." Abigail wore her oxygen, in a backpack, to an art exhibit opening. The gallery had been freshly painted. Another art patron asked her, "Where did you get that oxygen? I need some, too. The smell of the paint is making me dizzy." It's not those of us who use oxygen who are strange, it's the others.

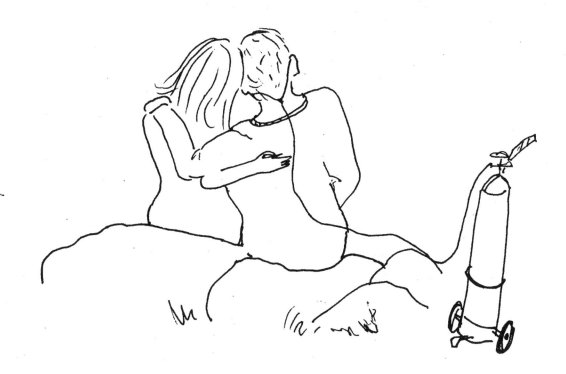

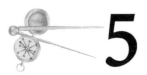

PH Drugs

Revised for the March 2008 reprint by
Glenna Traiger, RN, MSN & Juliana Liu, RN, MSN, ANP

This chapter is about treatments that may slow, stop, or even undo some of the damage PH has caused in your lungs. Nearly all PH patients need to take at least one of these drugs (in addition to one or more of the general treatments covered in Chapter 4). Because there are now so many PH drugs, it can get confusing. To help you keep them straight, Cathy Anderson-Severson, an RN, BSN at the Mayo Clinic, has prepared a summary in chart form (pages 74-75). The drugs are listed in alphabetical order. This chapter will review all the PH specific therapies, some experimental therapies and a separate section on combination therapy.

At first, PH doctors were hesitant to use more than one heavy-duty drug at a time on a PH patient. If there's a bad reaction it's hard to tell which drug is to blame. Now, however, many PH patients are using more than one of these drugs. For instance, a controlled trial on drug combinations has been published (BREATHE-2); however the study was too small to draw conclusions on safety and effectiveness. Therefore, combinations are still approached on tiptoes. Because PH is really a cluster of diseases, therapies will become more individualized as new drugs are added to the mix. Someday, your drugs may be matched to your genetic makeup as well as to your symptoms. Using combinations of drugs can sometimes allow lower doses of drugs that have bad side effects; when a dose is lowered, side effects tend to lessen or even disappear.

PH drugs are outrageously expensive. That's partly because manufacturers charge what the market will bear, and also because relatively few patients are using meds that cost millions to bring to market (see below). When people must take a medicine daily to stay alive, they will pay whatever it takes, even if it means impoverishing their families. To quote one PH patient, who uses treprostinil and sildenafil, "It feels as if they are living off me." Other costs must be added to that of the medicine itself: the cost of supplies; required blood tests; hospitalizations for central line placement, infections, or adverse events; medicine to treat site pain and other side effects; and specialist visits for medication adjustments. Patients worry that they might well hit the "lifetime caps" of their insurance coverage, and this adds significantly to their stress.

But there's a Catch 22 in the drug price issue. We are a small market that would ordinarily be ignored by drug companies. It's only because the companies can charge so much that they work on developing drugs to keep us alive. To be fair, drug companies sometimes provide drugs free or at a steep discount to the already poor. And, as a group, we are far better off today than we were a decade ago, thanks new Cadillac drugs. Another reason PH drugs cost so much is the small number of prescriptions for them written by doctors worldwide. Although few people use the drugs, the cost of developing, making, and marketing them is high (easily over $800 million), so a drug company must charge a lot per dose.

		Type of PH It Shows Promise For WHO Class	Who Should Not Use It	Evidence	Form
Arginine		Sickle cell/PH, but trials still underway		Case reports; A food supplement not regulated by FDA Clinical trials underway	oral
Calcium Channel Blockers	amlodipine besylate (Norvasc) nifedipine (Procardia XL - Adalat [Canada]) diltiazem (Cardizem, Tiazac)	IPAH, if patient responds really well to an acute vasodilator challenge, and is not in right-heart failure.	Most other PH patients	Clinical trial (nifedipine and diltiazem), but not perfect design	pill
Endothelin Antagonists	ambrisentan (Letairis)	PAH patients in Class II-IV		Clinical trials	pill
	bosentan (Tracleer)	PAH patients in Class III-IV (US) and Class III (EU)		Clinical trials	pill
	sitaxsentan (Thelin)	PAH patients in Class II-IV		Clinical trials	pill
Nitric Oxide (NO)		Newborns with persistent PH and older PH patients with other lung disease, too, such as some patients with scleroderma, sarcoidosis, sickle cell disease, portopulmonary hypertension.		Clinical trials (for full-term PPHN infants) For older patients, used in acute vasodilator trials and chronically in a few cases	inhaled gas
Phosphodiesterase Inhibitors	sildenafil (Viagra, Revatio)	PAH	Patients taking nitro-glycerine, other nitrates	Clinical trials	pill
	vardenafil (Levitra)	Probably similar to sildenafil	Patients taking nitro-glycerine, other nitrates		pill
	tadalafil (Cialis)	Probably similar to sildenafil	Patients taking nitro-glycerine, other nitrates	Phase III trial concluded enrollment. Results expected at the end of 2007.	pill
Prostanoids	beraprost sodium (Domar -[Europe], Beradrak, Procyclin)	Classes II-III	Class IV patients	Uncontrolled, retrospective trial in Japan with gen. favorable results; No active trials in US	pill
	epoprostenol (Flolan)	FDA approved for IPAH, PAH associated with scleroderma spectrum of diseases. Medicare will also cover it for PH associated with thromboembolic disease, HIV, cirrhosis, diet pills, and congential left-to-right shunt in heart; Classes III-IV	Pulmonary venous hypertension, PH due to congestive heart failure or severe left ventricular systolic function	Clinical trials	IV & pump
	iloprost (Ventavis)	PAH Class III/IV WHO Group 1		Clinical trials	inhaled aerosol; IV (outside US)
	treprostinil (Remodulin)	FDA approved for PAH, connective tissue/PH, maybe portopulmonary hypertension/II-IV		Clinical trials	Under-the-skin catheter and IV

Side Effects	Sometimes Used Along With	Where * Available	Manufacturer/Comments	
			Our bodies need arginine to make NO.	Arginine
Edema, headache, dizziness, fatigue, hypotension, constipation, nausea, bradycardia, flushing	True responders might not need any other PH drug, but occ. used with most other PH drugs	Essentially worldwide		Calcium Channel Blockers
Teratogenic, increased liver enzymes, headache, edema, flushing, nasal congestion, abdominal pain, constipation		US	Gilead. Has orphan drug designation in EU. Marketing application underway. No drug interaction with sildenafil.	Endothelin Antagonists
Increased liver enzymes, teratogenic, headache, edema, flushing, hypotension, dyspnea, nausea/vomiting, abdominal pain, influenza, dizziness	Combination study with iloprost. Often used in combination with other prostanoids and sildenafil.	US, EU, Aust., Can., Brazil, Iceland, Israel, Nor., Switz., China, Japan, Korea, Taiwan	Drug interaction exists with sildenafil.	
Edema, headache, dizziness, nasal congestion, increased prothrombin time/INR		Europe, Australia, and Canada	Encysive Pharmaceuticals (company to be acquired by Pfizer in 2008) STRIDE III study in the US terminated. FDA requiring further data to approve drug.	
Sometimes severe rebound after discontinuation, fainting when temporarily stop use	Always used along with oxygen	Only in hospitals or as participant in study	NO is not an FDA-regulated drug, but a commercial product.	Nitric Oxide (NO)
Headaches, flushing, upset stomach, visual disturbances, nasal congestion, diarrhea, insomnia, nosebleeds	Bosentan, prostanoids	Essentially worldwide		Phosphodiesterase Inhibitors
When used for erectile dysfunction: headaches, flushing, indigestion, nasal congestion, mild color vision disturbance		Essentially worldwide	Bayer	
When used for erectile dysfunction: headache, indigestion, back pain, muscle ache, nasal congestion, flushing, skin rash, and possible color vision disturbance		Essentially worldwide	Lilly ICOS. PHIRST (Phase III) trial closed enrollment in US and Europe. Official results pending.	
Jaw pain, headache, flushing, nausea, diarrhea, vomiting, heel pain		Japan, Europe, Kuwait, Korea, Philippines	Toray Industries (United Therapeutics license in US); Trials stopped early in US as patients did better at 3 and 6 months but benefits later disappeared. Has orphan drug designation in EU.	Prostanoids
Jaw pain, headache, flushing, nausea, diarrhea, vomiting, pain in calves and feet, risk of infection	Bosentan, sildenafil	US, EU, Canada, Chile, Columbia, Israel, Japan, Syria, Taiwan	GlaxoSmith Kline; No controlled studies yet on whether it's useful for PH secondary to HIV infection, portopulmonary hypertension, or congenital heart disease/PH; Must be mixed shortly before use and kept cold; Half life measured in minutes; Available in US only through Accredo Therapeutics.	
Cough, flushing, headache, jaw pain, nausea, palpitations, insomnia, dizziness	Bosentan, sildenafil	EU, US, Argentina, Australia, Chile, China, Columbia, Finland, Norway, Taiwan, Thailand	Schering (US license: Actelion); An oral form of iloprost for PH/scleroderma is in trial. Can also be used intravenously (UK and Germany)	
Site pain, jaw pain, headache, nausea, diarrhea, flushing, heel pain	Sildenafil, CCBs, bosentan	EU, US, Aregentina, Can., Israel, Norway, Taiwan, Venezuela	United Tx; Inhaled version under clinical trial. Premixed, refrigeration not needed; 2-3 hour half life. When used subcutaneously, less potent than Flolan; Avail. in US only through Accredo, Caremark, and Curascript.	

* For up-to-date information about the availability of treatments around the world, see our World wide Therapies Distribution List at www.phassociation.org/wwtherapies/.

In most discussions of each drug you will find estimates of their cost. The cost of oral therapies is easier to determine than the various inhaled, subcutaneous or intravenous therapies because this category of drugs involves pumps or devices and their dosage is very variable: the higher the dose, the higher the costs. In addition to the cost of the drug itself, you must also consider the cost of treating side effects and complications, the cost of starting therapy if it involves hospitalization and many other factors. Although it is a consideration, when your doctor discusses which PH treatment you will start or add to your regimen, cost is not their primary concern. Drug effectiveness, side effects, lifestyle impact and quality of life are all important considerations.

CCBs: Nifedipine (Procardia, Adalat), Amlodipine Besylate (Norvasc), Diltiazem Hydrochloride (Cardizem, Cartia XT)

If you had a positive response to an acute vasodilator challenge, your doctor will probably start a monitored trial of a calcium channel blocker (CCB). For patients who tolerate CCBs, they can be very effective long term (but should be closely monitored), they come in pill form, and they cost much less than all of the alternatives. From the early 1980s to the mid-1990s, CCBs were the only PH drug therapy available. (A few dozen patients were in Phase I and Phase II Flolan trials in the early 1990s, but it wasn't FDA approved until 1995.)

How they work. The smooth muscle cells in arteries cannot constrict without cellular calcium. CCBs slow the influx of calcium ions into muscle cells, so the cells (and arteries) stay relaxed. This lowers blood pressure. In persons without PH, these drugs are used to lower systemic blood pressure and to treat chest pain.

In PH patients, the goal is to lower the pressure inside our lungs; lowering our systemic pressure is more of a problem than a good thing. When the blockers work, the change is usually immediate and dramatic. Patients who respond well to these pills see an improvement in symptoms, a reduction in mean PAP, and a cardiac output that stays the same or improves.

How long will they work? There is no known time limit. A tiny handful of patients respond well for a very brief time and then stop responding. The patients in a study by Dr. Stuart Rich (*The New England Journal of Medicine*; July 9, 1992) were still doing well when he checked on them over 10 years later. Some patients have been on blockers for 20 years. For those with a *dramatic* reduction in pulmonary artery pressure and pulmonary vascular resistance, the benefits appear to be life-long. Dr. Rich says these fortunate few see progressive improvements year after year.

Who will benefit? The most recent information from Dr. Olivér Sitbon (Hôpital Antoine Beclere, Assistance Publique-Hôpitaux de Paris, Université Paris-Sud, Clamart, France) and others suggests that less than 10 percent of PAH patients benefit, the vast majority of whom have IPAH (i.e., vasoreactivity is very rare in associated PAH (APAH); see below). A positive vasoreactive response is BOTH a fall in mean PAP of more than or equal to 10 mm Hg and a resulting mean PAP of less than or equal to 40 mm Hg. The cardiac output (the amount of blood the heart can pump in 1 minute) must stay the same or increase. Patients that Dr. Sitbon studied who met these criteria did very well on CCBs after one year, and were called "long term responders". CCBs are contraindicated (should not be given) when patients are in right heart failure (typically Class III or IV, and low cardiac output, and high pressure in the right atrium) because they decrease the contractility or squeezing ability of the heart muscle (this is called a *negative* *inotropic effect)*. If someone is already in heart failure, a drug that can decrease contractility would make matters worse. Dr. Michael McGoon (Mayo Clinic, Rochester, Minn.) suggests that PH patients with a mean right atrial pressure of over 15, or cardiac output of less than 2.0 liters, should not be tested or treated with CCBs, because it might cause their right hearts to fail. Vasoreactivity testing might still be done in patients in heart failure because the response might help your doctor determine how advanced your PH is. But regardless of the result of the vasoreactivity testing, a CCB should not be prescribed if your doctor thinks you are in heart failure.

CCBs are less likely to help patients with PH triggered by another disease (associated PAH). A doctor at a major PH center says he has not personally seen CCBs make a significant difference in such patients. Scleroderma patients, for example, are much less likely to respond to vasodilators. Portopulmonary hypertension patients can't use CCBs because the swelling in their lower extremities becomes worse. Diet pill/PH patients can use CCBs if they are responders.

A common mistake doctors make is to use CCBs in patients who aren't responding well to them. If you are taking CCBs and have not seen a dramatic improvement, ask your PH specialist about other options. In most patients, unfortunately, CCBs have little effect and can often make the disease worse. One doctor quotes a nursery rhyme: "When they are good, they are very, very good, and when they are bad, they are horrid." Adverse effects include dangerously low systemic blood pressure, pulmonary edema, right ventricular failure, and death.

Without an acute vasodilator trial there is no way to be absolutely certain who the lucky responders will be. But research by Dr. Melvyn Rubenfire's group (University of Michigan) discovered that when echocardiography finds signs of really bad PH (such as a smaller-than-usual left ventricle or a bowing into that ventricle of the wall that divides the two chambers), the patient does not benefit from CCBs. Partly because of the danger of severe systemic hypotension and the long-lasting effect of CCBs, it is unwise to use CCBs when doing the diagnostic workup of such patients, or to give the patients a "trial run" on CCBs.

Many PH patients also have essential hypertension, or plain old high blood pressure. CCBs may be used for high blood pressure in standard doses in these patients. When used for PAH, the dose is usually much higher.

Which CCB will my doctor use? The most commonly used drugs are nifedipine (Procardia or Procardia XL, called Adalat XL in Canada and the U.K.) and amlodipine besylate (Norvasc). Diltiazem hydrochloride (Cardizem, Cartia XT) is also sometimes used. Nifedipine is nearly always given in its extended-release form, except for children unable to swallow these bigger pills. The CCB verapamil should not be used to treat PAH.

You might respond differently to different CCBs. Amlodipine is favored by at least one PH center because they find it has fewer side effects. CCBs reduce the heart's vigor of contraction by just a little; newer forms of the drugs (like amlodipine) do this slightly less. Your doctor might experiment with several drugs, or combinations of them, to find what works for you. Experimentation is best done under close medical supervision that includes closely monitoring your hemodynamics. After 3 months of therapy, if the patient has not improved to Class I or II, usually another PAH drug is added, with or without the CCB.

Dosage and cost. Dosage is a very individual thing. If your dose is higher than your PH pen pal's, it doesn't necessarily mean you're sicker. For PH patients, doctors usually prescribe much higher doses than are used for other medical conditions (your pharmacist may question the dose on the prescription). A few of us are helped with standard doses. Most doctors do a heart catheterization to determine the most effective dose. The author's Procardia XL costs her around $5.30, U.S., a day, for two 60 mg tablets (at Costco). Generic nifedipine costs less, but look for an extended release form. Two 60 mg tables of generic time-release diltiazem can be had for about $1.65, U.S., from Canada. A typical dose of Norvasc is 10-30 mg/day. (In the U.S., Norvasc is only recommended for use up to 10 mg/day because it wasn't approved with PH in mind. But some US doctors still use higher doses in spite of this) The Canadian price for a hundred 10 mg pills of Norvasc is around $193, U.S.

Side effects. CCBs relax all the blood vessels in your body- not just the ones in your lungs-so the side effects can include swollen feet, ankles, and lower legs. Your blood pressure might even drop to the point you feel dizzy. These side effects are also symptoms associated with worsening PH, however, so it's sometimes hard to tell what's causing them. In general, if the medications have made you feel much better and less short of breath, the swelling of your feet and legs is probably just a side effect that can be controlled with diuretics. If your feet swell and your breathing has not improved, or even worsened, the swelling should be immediately called to your doctor's attention. Headaches are another common side effect, but they tend to go away as you adapt to the drug. A few patients report thickening of the gums, and need to get their teeth cleaned three to four times a year. Heartburn is another possible side effect, because CCBs may relax the esophageal sphincter, allowing stomach acid to rise into the esophagus. Bloating, nausea, blurred vision, sweating, and sleep disturbance are also possible. Infrequently, patients say their muscles don't seem to contract quite as well or that they get muscle cramps. There are scattered reports of joint pain, brief mental confusion, and an inability to sit down because of anxiety and

muscular quivering (acathisia).

Diltiazem is more likely to cause a slow heartbeat, and nifedipine more likely to cause a too-rapid heartbeat or palpitations, headache or flushing, and diarrhea.

Allergies to CCBs are rare, but would include rash, itching, facial swelling, and trouble breathing. Call your doctor about these or other odd effects.

The matrix that contains the timed-release form of nifedipine might irritate some tummies. A pharmacist at the University of Washington says they have many complaints of nausea, abdominal cramps, discomfort, and occasional vomiting from patients taking Procardia XL. When patients have such problems, the pharmacist suggests they take the drug right after a full meal, and divide the dosage into smaller pills taken after breakfast and after dinner.

Precautions for CCB users. Never suddenly stop taking CCBs. Going off them should be done only under a doctor's close supervision. Sudden withdrawals have resulted in death. Do not chew or divide a timed-release tablet, because that will destroy the matrix (the built-in structure that delivers the drug at a constant rate over a 24-hour period).

A big glass of **grapefruit juice** can mess up your dosage of a CCB by making it more powerful. How much it will affect you depends on how much of a certain enzyme you have in the wall of your small intestine. If you have a lot of this intestinal enzyme, grapefruit and grapefruit juice can really affect your reaction. The enzyme breaks down CCBs (and some other common drugs, like Seldane and cyclosporine). A chemical in grapefruit juice latches onto the enzyme like "The Club" onto a car wheel, so the enzyme can't work. This leaves more medicine to be absorbed into your bloodstream over a longer time. The effect lasts a day or more. Grapefruit can also affect the digoxin you might take along with your CCB. Furthermore, it interacts with most of the "statin" cholesterol-lowering drugs, some anti-anxiety drugs (benzodiazepines such as Halcion or Valium), several HIV drugs, and some immunosuppressants and antihistamines. Whole grapefruit messes with the drugs, too, as do sour oranges, limes, and tangelos. Sweet oranges and lemons are okay.

The popular herb **St. John's wort** (hypericum, known as y fendigedig in Welsh) is suspected of having an effect similar to that of grapefruit. Do not take this (or any herbal) without asking your PH doctor.

There is no evidence that taking CCBs leads to osteoporosis and it is okay to take calcium supplements while on the blockers.

Combined with other PH drugs. Some patients thrive on a combination of CCBs and prostacyclin. Liz is one of them. A practicing lawyer, she runs 2 miles a day. Now that there are six FDA approved medications specific for PAH more PAH patients will likely be treated with a combination of drugs, which may, in some cases, include CCBs. Dr. Vallerie McLaughlin (University of Michigan) cautions, however, that a true responder to CCBs will already be Class I or II and have an excellent prognosis. So why risk drug interactions, drug reactions, and run up big medical bills?

Endothelin Receptor Antagonists: Ambrisentan (Letairis), Bosentan (Tracleer), Sitaxsentan (Thelin)

Endothelin (ET) is present in blood. IPAH/FPAH patients and those with PH triggered by other diseases tend to have higher-than-normal levels of it. Endothelin is secreted by the cells that form the endothelium, the innermost layer of all blood vessels. It binds to - and activates - two types of receptors in the layer of smooth muscle cells that surround it: endothelin-A and endothelin-B (ETA and ETB) receptors. Once it binds, it causes vasoconstriction and the growth and development of new smooth muscle cells. It may also increase fibrous tissue formation.

Designer molecules made in laboratories can keep endothelin from binding to receptors. These drugs are called endothelin receptor antagonists. A great advantage of these drugs is that they come in pill form (woohoo!).

Endothelin receptor antagonists prevent endothelin from activating endothelin receptors. By doing so they vasodilate and seem to inhibit unwanted growth and proliferation of cells. Patients using them may not see immediate improvement. It may take a month or more for noticeable benefits to show up. Eventually, most patients plateau; others keep improving for a long time.

ETA receptors are thought to be mostly responsible for the vasoconstriction and increased cell growth. ETB receptors appear to have other roles, including possibly promoting scarring inside the blood vessels that is seen in PH. Results from the STRIDE -1 trial show that exercise improvements with ETA antagonists are in a similar range to improvements with dual (ETA and ETB) antagonists. Moreover, ET binding to ETB receptors may have some beneficial effects, so, at present, it isn't known for sure if selective or dual antagonists are better or whether differences are even detectable at a clinical level.

Bosentan (Tracleer)

Bosentan (BO-sen-tan) was the first endothelin receptor antagonist to be approved and marketed. Tracleer (Truh-CLEAR) is its trade name. Bosentan is a dual endothelin receptor antagonist. It received FDA approval in the U.S. in late 2001 for use in Class III or IV PAH patients. In Europe, Tracleer is approved only for PAH class III patients. Tracleer is also available in Australia, Canada, China, Brazil, the European Union, Iceland, Israel, Japan, Korea, Norway, Switzerland, and Taiwan. For updates, go to the Actelion (the manufacturer) website.

An early study. In November 2000, Dr. Lewis Rubin (principal investigator, University of California at San Diego) reported on the results of a double-blind, placebo-controlled clinical trial, sponsored by Actelion, and involving 32 patients. (The first author on the subsequent paper in Lancet in 2001 was Dr. Richard Channick, also with UCSD.) Some of the patients had "PPH," some had scleroderma/PH. They were all Class III or IV. After 12 weeks on bosentan, they had significant improvements in both their exercise ability and hemodynamics (pulmonary artery pressure, cardiac output, etc.). Patients getting the real drug walked 70 meters farther in 6 minutes than they had at the start of the trial. Those getting a placebo walked 6 meters less. Dr. Rubin said, "The improvements were significant enough that 43 percent of the patients (9 of 21) receiving Tracleer were reclassified as 'moderate' from their previous 'severe' status, as compared to only 9 percent of patients (1 of 11) receiving placebo."

A follow-up of these patients concluded that longer-term treatment (for over a year) was safe and was associated with better hemodynamics, functional class, and exercise capacity.

BREATHE-1. Dr. Rubin was also the principal investigator of a large, international, randomized, placebo-controlled, double-blind, Phase III study (BREATHE-1) involving over 213 PAH patients ("PPH" or PH associated with connective-tissue disease). The results were reported in the March 21, 2002, issue of The New England Journal of Medicine. The researchers concluded that oral bosentan is an effective therapy for PAH patients and is well-tolerated at a dose of 125 mg twice daily.

At the end of 4 months, when compared to the group of patients receiving placebo, patients taking bosentan significantly improved their walking distance (by 36 meters), had less breathlessness, increased the time to clinical worsening, and improved their WHO functional class status. Those getting a placebo decreased their walking distance by 8 meters.

BREATHE-1 patients receiving bosentan were further divided into two groups: those getting 125 mg twice a day, and those getting 250 mg twice a day. Except for liver function problems (see below), which were greater in the higher-dose group, the drug seemed to be equally well tolerated at both doses. Potential liver problems are why the researchers recommend the lower dose.

A sub-study of BREATHE-1 undertaken by researchers at the University of Bologna, Italy, found that for a subset of patients in BREATHE-1, bosentan was good for the heart: it reduced the size of the right ventricle, improved its functioning, and increased the size of the left ventricle while improving its function, too. (This study used echocardiograms to follow the patients). The study was not designed to see if bosentan increased the lifespan of PAH patients, or if the drug's effectiveness continues over a long period.

BREATHE-5. This study examined the use of bosentan in patients with congenital heart disease and PH. Investigators tested 54 patients with atrial septal defect, ventricular septal defect, or both. 17 of the patients received placebo and 37 had 4 weeks of 62.5 mg twice daily bosentan, and 12 weeks of the 125 mg twice daily dose. The results showed that treated patients walked on average 43 meters more in their 6 minute walk tests. The placebo group walked 10 meters less. The oxygen saturation of treated patients improved on average 1.5%. Worsening disease will cause these patients' blood to shunt more and thereby result in worse oxygen saturation. The pulmonary vascular resistance (or the amount of resistance found in the pulmonary vessels as measured by cardiac catheterization) also improved somewhat in the treatment group.

Side effects. Bosentan appears to be well tolerated. Increased swelling of legs and ankles has turned out to be a greater problem than

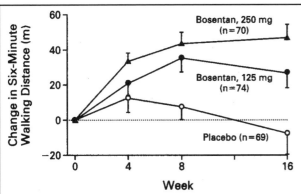

Mean (±SE) Change in Six-Minute Walking Distance from Base Line to Week 16 in the Placebo and Bosentan Groups. P<0.01 for the comparison between the 125-mg dose of bosentan and placebo, and P<0.001 for the comparison between the 250-mg dose and placebo by the Mann-Whitney U test. There was no significant difference between the two bosentan groups (P=0.18 by the Mann-Whitney U test.

This figure is reprinted with permission from an article by Lewis Rubin et al., "Bosentan Therapy for Pulmonary Arterial Hypertension," The New England Journal of Medicine, 346: 896-903 (Mar. 21, 2002). Copyright © 2002 New England Journal of Medicine.

appreciated during clinical trials: if you have such swelling, you may need to increase your dosage of diuretics. Other side effects (often not severe or long-lasting) include headache, flushing, inflammation of nose and throat passages, low blood pressure, dizziness, and (at higher doses) nausea. The biggest problem is liver toxicity (see the discussion below).

It is possible that all endothelin antagonists may affect male fertility, because in very high doses bosentan has affected fertility in animals. Scientists don't know if human males will be similarly affected, but it is being studied.

At least one case has been reported where bosentan seemed to significantly decrease the anticoagulant properties of warfarin. It is thus smart to get an INR check after you start taking bosentan.

Liver toxicity. About 13 percent of BREATHE-1 patients getting bosentan developed significant liver problems. Actelion literature says about 11 percent of patients develop elevated liver enzymes and that, to date, these elevations have been reversible by reducing the dose or discontinuing the drug.

Symptoms of liver toxicity include nausea, vomiting, fever, abdominal pain, unusual tiredness, and jaundice (yellowish skin or a yellow tint to the whites of your eyes). But most patients with liver problems initially have no

symptoms. Ninety percent of liver toxicity shows up in the first several months, although it can appear later. Call your doctor right away if you develop any symptoms.

Because of possible liver toxicity, everyone taking bosentan must get blood draws at least once a month to check their levels of the liver aminotransferases (ALT and AST, also called SGPT and SGOT). If your levels are up, notify your PH specialist and get rechecked in a few days; don't wait a month. Some experts recommend checking bilirubin and alkaline phosphatase as well as the usual liver function tests; a change may show up first in some patients' alkaline phosphatase. Your specialist may want to decrease or stop your dose depending on how high the ALT and AST are. Right-heart failure can also cause liver enzymes to increase-if this is your problem, it may not be necessary to change your bosentan dosage. In any case, you absolutely have to stop taking the drug if you have an elevation greater than eight times the upper limit of normal values for ALT and AST. To avoid irreversible damage, thereafter, the drug should not be retried.

Which PH patients should (and should not) consider bosentan. As noted above, BREATHE-1 included "PPH" and connective tissue/PH patients, and the drug is FDA-approved for such patients who are Class III or IV. A recent placebo-controlled study by Dr. Carol Black (Royal Free Medical School, London) and colleagues involved 122 scleroderma patients without PAH. Those getting the real bosentan developed significantly fewer ulcers on their fingers and toes. This study may be of interest to scleroderma/PH patients who are troubled by such ulcers.

None of the patients in BREATHE-1 had portal hypertension or were infected with the HIV virus, or had PH secondary to a disease other than a connective tissue disease. A study using no placebos found that bosentan helped HIV/PH patients walk farther and improved their hemodynamics and quality of life. And researchers at Mount Sinai School of Medicine in New York tried bosentan on two patients with chronic thromboembolic disease/PH, nine with pulmonary fibrosis/PH, three with obstructive lung disease/PH, three with corrected left heart disease/PH, and one with Gaucher's disease/PH. All improved significantly. Bosentan is not for women who are, or who may become pregnant, because of the danger of birth defects. If you are a sexually active, fertile woman, you'll need a test to prove you aren't pregnant before you start taking the drug, and you should have a pregnancy test monthly while using bosentan. It's not enough to be "on the pill;" bosentan may alter the metabolism of birth control drugs and reduce their effectiveness. Of course, patients with PH are advised not to become pregnant anyway.

If you are using glybenclamide (also called glyburide, a pill for diabetes) or cyclosporine you should not use bosentan.

Bosentan combined with other PH drugs. Bosentan may be the only PH medicine some PAH patients need. In other (perhaps most) patients, it may prove helpful when used in combination with other drugs. Thus far, it appears safe when used with intravenous epoprostenol, subcutaneous treprostinil, nebulized iloprost, and oral beraprost, but the jury is still out on combination therapy.

There is, however, a known interaction with bosentan and sildenafil. Specifically, when taken together, it will increase the amount of bosentan and decrease the amount of sildenafil available in your body. It is not fully known if this interaction has a significant clinical affect, but those on this combination should discuss the potential risks and benefits with their PH doctor. In 2006, Actelion began the large Compass 2 double-blind placebo-controlled clinical trial to investigate the benefits of bosentan in combination with sildenafil. The study is scheduled to be completed at the end of 2009. Meanwhile there have been several small studies that have looked at the usage of both bosentan and sildenafil together. While the results of these studies indicate some additional efficacy by using this combination therapy, given the small size of the studies, the efficacy of this combination therapy for a broad based group of PH-ers is still not conclusive.

In severely ill PAH patients, the addition of bosentan to intravenous epoprostenol may be of benefit. Dose adjustments of prostacyclin might be needed to avoid an increase in flushing and a drop in blood pressure. A multi-center study, BREATHE-2, tested a combination of intravenous epoprostenol and bosentan (or placebo) in severely ill PAH patients requiring intravenous epoprostenol. They were tested for 4 months, and started taking bosentan (or a placebo) at the same time they started on epoprostenol. The combination appeared safe, was well tolerated, and the patients taking bosentan did a bit better on their walk tests and hemodynamics than those taking a placebo, but most of their improvements weren't statistically significant. Therefore, insurance companies might balk at paying for both drugs.

Dr. Richard Channick and other researchers at UCSD report successfully weaning patients from intravenous epoprostenol or subcutaneous treprostinil by adding bosentan to their meds. All patients were able to significantly reduce the amount of prostanoid they took without making their PH worse; a few patients were able to completely stop taking a prostanoid after about 7 months (some later had to return to a prostanoid). This study involved 36 epoprostenol patients and 8 treprostinil patients. Researchers at Baylor College of Medicine in Houston report similar results.

In the STEP trial, patients already treated with bosentan had inhaled iloprost added. This trial proved that combination of bosentan with inhaled iloprost was safe, and some benefit was observed.

Ongoing blood tests. In addition to the

pregnancy tests and liver tests mentioned above, a blood test will need to be done at 1 month, 3 months, and every 3 months thereafter to count your red blood cells.

Tracleer providers. Tracleer is only available through specialty pharmacy distributors: Accredo Therapeutics, Caremark, CuraScript, and PharmaCare Specialty Pharmacy. If your PH doctor would like to start you on Tracleer, they need to send a referral to PAH Pathways (formerly known as Tracleer Access Program or TAP) who will verify benefits and pass on the referral to one of these distributors. PAH Pathways can be reached at 1-866-228-3546.

Cost. In the U.S. treatment with bosentan runs in the neighborhood of $3500 to $4000 per month, whether you use the 62.5 mg pills or the 125 mg pills. Tracleer is generally covered by insurance companies and HMOs for approved indications (although some have been slow to pay), and by all state Medicaid programs. It is covered by Medicare under its part D prescription drug program. However, some part D plans categorize not only bosentan, but many of the PH drugs as a "specialty" or Tier 4 drug. If this is true for the plan you have, you are asked to pay a significant portion of the cost of the drug. Unfortunately, many of the patients cannot afford the medication and are forced to go onto non oral drugs because of this scenario. Actelion has a patient assistance program for those who do not have prescription drug coverage. It also works with non-profit organizations such as Caring Voices Coalition to help patients with high co-pays. If you are running into such situations, contact PAH Pathways for more information.

Ambrisentan (Letairis)

Ambrisentan (trade name Letairis) is the most recently approved oral drug for the use in PH. It was approved by the FDA for commercial use in the U.S. on June 15, 2007. It was approved for PH patients with functional class II or III symptoms. Like bosentan, the first oral drug approved for use in PH, it is an endothelin antagonist. Unlike bosentan, it only blocks the ETA receptor. In fact, it has a 4000 times stronger affinity to the ETA receptor than the ETB receptor.

The FDA approved the medication based on the study results from the ARIES I and II studies. A total of 393 patients with PH were tested in these two multi-center trials. The study lasted 12 weeks, and both compared the efficacy of the drug against placebo. ARIES I compared the once daily dose of 5 and 10 mg doses in North America. ARIES II compared the once daily 2.5 or 5mg doses outside of North America. In both studies, patients combined ambrisentan to conventional PH therapies such as blood thinners, diuretics, CCBs, or digoxin, but not to any other specific PH therapies. No hemodynamic measurements (cardiac catheterizations) were done on these patients; change in 6 minute walk test distance was the main indication of the efficacy of the medicine. Investigators also took into consideration whether patients' functional class or subjective rating of breathlessness got worse. Though all classes of PH patients were included, most were functional class II (38%) or III (55%). IPAH, PH patients with connective tissue disease, HIV, and diet pill use were included. There were no patients with congenital heart disease in the study. In both studies, treatment with ambrisentan compared to placebo showed an improvement in the 6 minute walk test. It also appeared the improvement increased with dose. In ARIES I, patients on ambrisentan on average walked 31 and 51 meters more than placebo on the 5mg and 10 mg dose respectively. The placebo patients walked 8 meters less than their baseline. In ARIES II, patients on ambrisentan walked on average 32 and 59 meters more than placebo on the 2.5 mg and 5 mg dose respectively. Placebo patients walked on average 10 meters less than their baseline.

The studies also kept track of any events indicative of clinical worsening as defined by hospitalization, death, transplantation, or atrial septostomy. In ARIES I there were 4 clinical worsening events (3%) as opposed to seven (10%) in the placebo group. In ARIES II, there were 8 events (6%) versus 13 (22%) in the placebo group. On the extension trial of ambrisentan, 95% of the patients were alive on ambrisentan therapy after 1 year of treatment. Of that group, 94% were on ambrisentan alone without the addition of any other PH specific therapies such as sildenafil or prostacyclin therapy.

Side effects. Some of the common side effects of ambrisentan include mild swelling of the legs, nasal congestion, sinus congestion, flushing, palpitations, abdominal cramping, and constipation. Like bosentan, it can cause severe birth defects. Patients need proof they are not pregnant before and throughout the use of ambrisentan.

Liver toxicity. Even though in their 12 week clinical trial, no patient experienced elevation in their liver enzymes, monthly liver function tests are still mandatory since 2.8% of the patients on the extension trial experienced an increase in liver enzymes. In a separate study, among 36 patients who had previously had to stop bosentan or sitaxsentan because of elevated liver enzymes, none developed a clinically important increase of enzymes when treated with ambrisentan for a year.

Ambrisentan combined with other PH drugs. No studies have been done to test the combination of ambrisentan with other PH drugs. However, unlike bosentan, ambrisentan does not interact with sildenafil. Because many patients are on sildenafil already, this may end up being a favorable characteristic of ambrisentan. It is not known if this lack of interaction will result in better clinical outcomes for PH patients on both ambrisentan and sildenafil. Ambrisentan also does not interact with warfarin.

Ongoing blood tests. Because of the potential for liver injury, patients must have a liver function test every month. Pregnancy testing is needed if you are a female of child bearing age. A drop in the hemoglobin (blood count) has been observed, so it is also a good idea to check that before, at 1 month and periodically thereafter while you are on the medication.

Ambrisentan providers. Like most PH drugs, ambrisentan is available through specialty drug providers. Your PH doctor needs to send a referral form to the Letairis Education and Access Program (LEAP) who will verify your medical coverage and send the referral to one of the following pharmacies: Accredo, Aetna Specialty Pharmacy, Caremark, Cigna Tel Drug, CuraScript, Fairview, Walgreens Specialty Pharmacy, or Precision Rx Specialty Solutions. For questions about the LEAP program, call 1-866-664-5327.

Sitaxsentan (Thelin)

Another selective endothelin antagonist was developed by Encysive Pharmaceuticals (as of February 2008, Encysive is to be acquired by Pfizer). Like ambrisentan, sitaxsentan targets only the ETA receptor and shows an ability to reduce pulmonary pressures with no bad effect on systemic pressures or a patient's heart rate. The STRIDE-1 and STRIDE-2 studies examined the effect of sitaxsentan on patients with PAH. Although some benefit was observed, the FDA still believes that it did not adequately show evidence of effectiveness needed for approval. *Thus, the drug is not currently available in the U.S. In response to this, Encysive plans to conduct another Phase III trial called STRIDE-5. This trial will use 6 minute walk tests as an indicator for improvement in exercise capacity. It is unknown presently when this medication will be made available in the U.S. Currently, the medication is approved in Australia, Canada and the European Union. For up-to-date information see PHA's "Therapies around the World" list at* www.PHAssociation.org/wwtherapies.

STRIDE-1 & STRIDE-2 trials. In the first STRIDE trial, undertaken by Dr. Robyn Barst (New York's Columbia- Presbyterian Pulmonary Hypertension Center) and colleagues, and reported on in the February 15, 2004, issue of the American Journal of Respiratory and Critical Care Medicine, 178 PAH patients in NYHA Class II, III, or IV participated in a 12-week double-blind, placebo-controlled trial to assess the safety and usefulness of sitaxsentan. Those not receiving a placebo got either a 100 mg or a 300 mg dose of the drug once a day. Dr. Barst says that patients receiving either dose showed equal and significant improvement in 6-minute walk tests, in their functional classifications, and in their heart and lung hemodynamics. (The patients improved their walk distance by about 35 meters, or 9 percent.) In an attempt to compare patients in the sitaxsentan trial with patients in previous PAH trials, the researchers identified a subset of patients in STRIDE-1 who fit the patient characteristics of the patients included in bosentan or epoprostenol trials (generally sicker patients who couldn't walk very far before being treated). Within this subset of patients in the sitaxsentan trial, a 65-meter increase was seen (as compared to patients taking a placebo). Doctors caution comparing results in one trial to those of another trial, so the significance of this 65 meters is unclear. Only the higher dose showed an improvement in predicted peak VO2 (peak amount of oxygen delivered by the heart to the body; which was to be the key thing looked at in this study, although the walk test is the usual standard). The STRIDE-2 trial was a 248-patient, 18-week study, which included Class II-IV patients. Patients with either "PPH" or PAH due to connective tissue disease or certain congenital heart defects were included. Patients were given a placebo, 50 mg, or 100 mg of sitaxsentan or bosentan. The trial included a randomized test against bosentan. This was the only study to date which compared one PH drug directly against another. The study examined how patients in the various groups did in their 6-minute walk tests and looked for changes in functional class, breathlessness, and the occurrence of problems requiring a trip to a PH doctor. All treatment groups improved in their 6 minute walk distance. Once adjusted for the placebo, they improved by 24 and 31 meters for the sitaxsentan 50 and 100 mg groups respectively, and 29 meters in the bosentan group. 1% of the patients who received 100 mg of sitaxsentan experienced worsening in functional class as opposed to 23% of the placebo group. The percentage of patients who experienced a worsening in functional class did not differ significantly between the 50 mg sitaxsentan, bosentan, and placebo groups.

At the American College of Chest Physicians' meeting in October of 2007, Canadian researchers reported the findings of an open label (meaning there was no placebo used in the trial) 1 year study of PH patients on 100mg of sitaxsentan. Patients improved an average of 22 meters on their 6 minute walk tests. 24% stopped the medication due to liver function test abnormalities, patient choice or non-compliance, 3 died and 8 worsened. Overall 62% remained on the therapy for one year. Although the medication is not yet available in the U.S., this Canadian report suggests that this medication may be beneficial for PH patients for a longer duration.

It should be noted that even though there are not many long-term studies where a placebo was used, PH docs still believe that the above drugs continue to work over the long haul. Unfortunately, because PAH is rare, it is very time consuming and costly, not to mention next to impossible to follow enough patients long enough in a placebo-controlled trial, we may never have definitive "proof" that these medications work for more than a few months.

It is also considered unethical to expose PH patients to a placebo for long periods of time.

Side effects. The most frequent side effects, aside from liver problems, were headache, peripheral edema, nasal congestion, and dizziness. An increase was seen in some patients' INR, which measures the effect of warfarin; sitaxsentan interacts with a liver enzyme that metabolizes warfarin, so *patients need to reduce their dose of warfarin to avoid the risk of bleeding.*

Nitric Oxide & Arginine

Nitric Oxide

Nitric oxide (NO) is approved by the FDA for treating newborns with persistent pulmonary hypertension of the newborn (PPHN). Its use in PH is "off label" (used for a non-FDA approved purpose). At PHA's International Conferences, it has not been uncommon to meet PH patients who are breathing a mixture of nitric oxide (NO) and oxygen. A few PH patients have been successfully treated with NO for many years. The neat thing about NO is that because the gas is inhaled, it selectively dilates only the *pulmonary* arteries. This eliminates most side effects. NO (not the same thing as *nitrous* oxide, the laughing gas dentists use) is one of the most potent vasodilators known. NO is also, by the way, a key component of air pollution. Dr. Richard Channick says that, "On a smoggy day in L.A. you probably have therapeutic levels of NO." Of course, smog also carries harmful pollutants.

NO works by causing the blood vessels to make more of a substance that dilates the pulmonary blood vessels. This substance is called cyclic GMP (cGMP). Interestingly, cGMP is degraded in the blood by an enzyme known as phosphodiesteras-5 (PDE-5). Sildenafil blocks the breakdown of PDE-5 which makes cGMP stay around longer, enhancing the effects of NO. (See Chapter 4 for more on this).

The last decade has seen an explosion of medical uses for this gas. When certain medical problems arise suddenly and are of short duration, the use of NO is widely accepted. In hospitals it's used for acute vasodilator testing, to judge the likelihood of success of some heart repairs, to treat PPHN, to treat postoperative PH in congestive heart failure, etc. NO may be used during and right after any major surgery to stabilize PH patients, in addition to their usual PH drugs. The gas can be given through a ventilator (breathing machine) or by nasal cannula. The gas is gradually weaned off as the PH patient undergoing surgery stabilizes.

Doctors working with continuous inhaled NO therapy to treat PH in persons other than the newly born are careful to emphasize that the research is at an early stage and the sample of patients is still too small to draw conclusions. There has not been a large, placebo-controlled study.

What it does. The creation and use of NO in our lungs is exceedingly complicated. NO is formed by the endothelial cells lining our blood vessels; the cells send it as a messenger to adjacent smooth muscle cells, telling them to relax. As a chemical formed naturally in our bodies, NO dilates vessels everywhere in our bodies. Inside our lungs, it not only relaxes vessels, but also prevents platelets from sticking

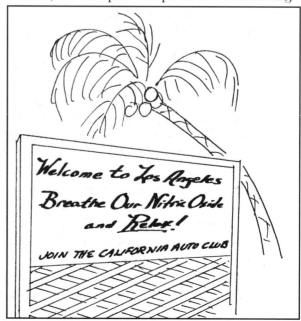

together and keeps smooth muscle cells from proliferating and clogging vessels. When used for a long period, some researchers think it might reverse some of the vessel thickening that PH causes. So far, there is only anecdotal evidence of this.

Getting tanked. The NO used in inhalation therapy has a half-life of about 15 seconds, so it must be breathed continuously. When used as continuous, outpatient therapy, it is delivered from a portable tank. A device senses when you are starting to draw in a breath and releases a little spurt of NO into tubing attached to a nasal cannula. This conserves NO and prevents overdoses. A second tank and tube deliver oxygen, which enhances the vasodilative effect of the NO, so the patient gets both gases with each breath. Instead of using the pulsing method, the gasses can be "T'ed" together into a cannula. The gases can't be premixed in one tank because of the possibility they will form toxic metabolites.

One patient wears a backpack holding an NO tank, an oxygen tank, and epoprostenol. Imagine the fun when he tries to board a commercial airliner! Pat, the fourth patient in the country to go on the gas chronically, said it gave her back a very good quality of life. She was Class IV when she started and improved to Class I or II. Lynn takes her little D cylinder with her everywhere-even when she's riding horses or body-building.

Doctors are looking for ways to make NO's effect last longer, perhaps with sildenafil or other drugs.

Who is most likely to benefit? Inhaled NO therapy is an option that patients who are not helped by other therapies might want to consider. It may be as, or more, expensive than some other approved PH therapies. Researchers at Duke University have found that NO dilates the pulmonary vessels of PAH patients. They anticipate that in some PH patients, inhaled NO will prove to be the best therapy. NO might turn out to be most effective in PH patients who also have lung disease, such

as scleroderma patients or patients with sickle cell anemia. Epoprostenol makes some of these patients worse; this is because a "mismatch" may happen if newly dilated vessels carry blood to places in the lungs that aren't getting oxygen (because air sacs are not working). Inhaled NO goes only to places with air, so there's no mismatch. A small study at the Mayo Clinic found that inhaled NO could successfully reduce the PAPs of persons with portopulmonary hypertension (these PH patients aren't supposed to use bosentan because of its risk of liver damage, but the truth is that some are already taking it, and some have had no liver problems). Inhaled NO has also helped PH patients with acute chest syndrome in sickle cell disease. It has been used on a compassionate-use basis in end-stage PH. Sarcoidosis/PH patients might also benefit.

A short-term pilot study (by Dr. Michael Landzberg and others at Children's Hospital and Brigham and Women's Hospital in Boston) with very small groups of "PPH" patients and patients with PH secondary to other diseases had results pretty similar to short-term trials of epoprostenol. (But epoprostenol seems to have more beneficial effects on the heart than NO.) There were more events of fainting or near-fainting than expected. Most fainting occurred when patients had removed their cannulas or were changing tanks. For patients that have been using NO for some time, they may be able to go without the gas for short periods, to run to the store, for example. Pat went without her NO for 12 hours because it was delivered to the wrong hotel (she was in Dallas for the PHA Conference). Another patient went off NO long enough to get married. Of course, some patients might rapidly get worse when their NO is interrupted, so stopping it for any length of time could be very dangerous (see *Side effects,* below).

Dosage and use as combination drug. The most commonly used concentrations are 10-40 parts per million. (Concentrations up to 1,000 parts per million are found in cigarette smoke.) Optimum dosages aren't known, nor whether NO would be more effective if combined with other drug therapy. NO is being tried in combination with drugs like epoprostenol, bosentan, and sildenafil. Patients have had a mixed response to the combination of inhaled NO and bosentan-in some, it made their side effects worse.

Side effects. There is concern about the sometimes-severe rebound effect after discontinuation of NO therapy. When NO is used acutely at Children's Hospital in Boston, doctors have avoided the fainting problem by either taking the children off NO slowly, over several days, or by giving them sildenafil. Aside from fainting when you discontinue or temporarily stop breathing the gas, no significant side effects of NO therapy have been described using concentrations up to 40 to 80 parts per million. Long-term side effects are unknown.

It's possible that the commercial NO doctors use outside of hospitals might carry contaminants. So far they have seen no toxic build-up, but there is a theoretical possibility that NO might lead to the creation of free radicals, those nasty little cell-aging and cancer-causing chemicals you read about in face cream and supplement ads. Another concern is that NO may be mutagenic (capable of being damaging to your DNA).

Arginine-NO from a Pill?

Arginine is one of the things our bodies use to make nitric oxide. Researchers have been taking a closer look at its possible helpfulness in reducing the symptoms of PH.

Arginine is an essential amino acid. "Essential" means our bodies can't make their own arginine, so we need to get it from the foods we eat. A normal endothelium makes enough NO to control pulmonary artery pressure, but the endothelium in a PH patient is damaged and might not be up to the task. We

can't get therapeutic doses by just changing our diets; we have to use pure L-arginine sold as a food supplement. (When arginine is manufactured from a nonfood source it is called L-arginine, the label used on bottles of supplements. For our purposes, arginine and L-arginine are the same thing.)

An average person probably has borderline levels of arginine. Pregnancy, aging, and stress can further lower levels. Adding arginine to your diet *may possibly* improve your levels of NO. It isn't yet known if adding an arginine supplement to your daily diet will help your lungs heal. It seems to help in rats that have PH. One doctor points out that PH patients tend to be short on the enzyme that converts arginine to NO, so it might be that no matter how much arginine we consume, it won't make a big difference.

Small studies have reached inconsistent results. A 2001 study by Dr. Noritoshi Nagaya (National Cardiovascular Center, and Osaka Seamen's Insurance Hospital, Osaka, Japan) and others found that giving PH patients 0.5-grams of L-arginine per 10 kilograms of body weight 3 times a day improved the patients' hemodynamics and exercise capacity. It was a small study that lasted only a week. Mean PAPs declined from 53 to 48, there was a 16 percent decrease in pulmonary vascular resistance, and cardiac output improved. There were no bad side effects, except some short-lived gastric discomfort in one patient. Although the L-arginine lowered the subjects' mean systemic blood pressures as well as their PAPs, it did not do so significantly. Of the 19 patients involved in this study, 11 had "PPH." 7 had chronic thromboembolic PH, and one had residual PH after surgical correction of an opening between the two top chambers of the heart. The patients were randomized to receive oral L-arginine or a placebo, and the study was double-blind so neither patients nor doctors knew who was getting placeboes. However, patients with PH so severe they couldn't tolerate the exercise were excluded from the study.

Other researchers tried using the HeartBar, which is loaded with L-arginine. PAH patients were pulled from the study early, because they showed no improvement in walking distance when compared to patients taking a placebo. But some researchers think that walking distance might not have been the best measurement to use as a test.

A long-term, larger study on the effects of arginine is badly needed.

A word of caution: Some researchers investigated the use of L-arginine in patients who suffered a myocardial infarction (heart attack). 153 patients were randomized to take L-arginine for a target dose of 3 grams 3 times a day versus placebo. They looked at whether or not the stiffness of blood vessels or ejection fraction (how strong the left side of the heart was pumping) changed over a 6 month period. They found that there were no significant differences between the L-arginine group versus the placebo group. However, during the course of the study, 6 patients in the L-arginine group (or 8.6%) died versus none in the placebo group. Because this study seems to show that deaths occurred more in the treatment group, great caution needs to be exercised when taking L-arginine supplementation. Always consult your PH specialist before considering L-arginine.

Side effects. If you want to experiment with arginine, talk it over with your doctor first. Arginine and its effects on the body, including its long-term effects, are not well understood. Remember that the U.S. government does not test supplements for purity, safety, or effectiveness. Arginine may lower your systemic blood pressure, so if your blood pressure as measured by a cuff on your arm is already low (either naturally or because of your PH meds), that could be a problem. At doses above 10 grams, arginine can cause nausea, cramps, and diarrhea. If this happens, start with a half dose and slowly increase.

Those who have herpes simplex should avoid arginine because it can spur the growth of the virus. In fact, a low-arginine diet is sometimes used to decrease herpes outbreaks. What about the possibility that some IPAH might be triggered by herpesvirus 8? To be *super* cautious, if you are concerned that you might have herpesvirus 8, don't take arginine supplements until scientists learn more.

Things to consider if you use arginine. PH patient and nutrition writer Maureen Keane contributed a lot to this section on arginine. The next few paragraphs are straight from her. But first, a word of caution: a doctor reviewing this chapter asked us to let you know that if you take arginine, you may be excluded from many clinical trials of PH drugs that are likely to help you more.

How much oral arginine is needed to increase NO production in the pulmonary arteries is not known. The amount used in the Japanese study was about 11 grams for a 150-pound person. Other studies have used 12 grams per day to lower systemic blood pressure and to dilate the arteries in the penis to treat erectile dysfunction. This amount is best taken in two doses of 5-6 grams. (It's conceivable that there is a minimum dose below which arginine isn't effective, which is why breaking your supplement into two--rather than three--doses is sometimes recommended.)

All amino acids, including arginine, should be taken on an empty stomach. This means no food (especially protein) for 3 hours before and at least 30 minutes after you swallow the supplement. (Arginine shares its "transporter protein" with other amino acids; there are only so many seats on the transporter bus, and the arginine and protein end up competing for those seats and both lose.) On the other hand, carbonation and a little carbohydrate might enhance arginine absorption, so you might want to take your arginine with a dash of fruit juice in Perrier.

Arginine supplements (usually labeled L-arginine) are available in health food stores, some grocery stores, drugstores, by mail order, and on the Internet. It comes in capsules, tablets, powder (good for those who have trouble swallowing capsules), and in HeartBars. When deciding what size capsules or tablets to buy, remember that they come in milligrams, not grams, and think about how many you'll have to swallow to add up to at least 10 grams. Don't buy a supplement with additional ingredients; they add nothing, cost more, and can dangerously interact with your PH or PH medicines.

Arginine looks promising in sickle-cell anemia patients. Levels of arginine drop too low in patients experiencing a sickle cell crisis, which may lead to low levels of nitric oxide. A team of researchers that included Dr. Claudia Morris of Children's Hospital, Oakland, California, thinks that because of limited treatment options and a high mortality rate, arginine therapy is a promising new approach for these patients. They used oral arginine for 5 days in 10 patients, and found a 15.2 percent reduction in estimated PAP. Check www.clinicaltrials.gov to find studies recruiting sickle cell disease/PH patients.

Phosphodiesterase Inhibitors
(Cialis, Revatio, Viagra)

Viagra may do more than star in strange TV ads: it may help control PH. Sildenafil citrate (the chemical name) is a selective phosphodiesterase inhibitor (see below) used to treat erectile dysfunction (ED) in men. But just as it expands blood vessels in the penis, sildenafil (and its competitor Cialis) expand vessels in the lungs-and they do so fairly selectively. That means your systemic blood pressure doesn't drop too far, causing dizziness, etc. (*hypotension*). And unlike nitric oxide gas or inhaled iloprost, the effect can last for hours. Sildenafil has garnered a lot of interest due to its availability in pill form and its relative lower price. PH doctors started prescribing Viagra "off label" several years ago. Sildenafil was approved

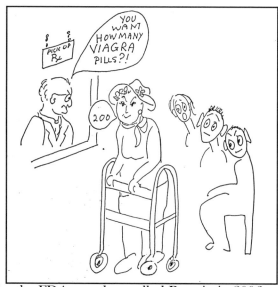

by the FDA as a drug called Revatio in 2006.

Almost as soon as Viagra came on the market, in 1998, it was tried at Boston Children's Hospital on children who were extremely ill with PH. The drug helped wean the children from inhaled nitric oxide so they could breathe on their own. The first paper on the use of Viagra in children, by Dr. David Wessel of Children's, and Dr. Andrew Atz, now with the Medical University of South Carolina, was published in 1999. To give the little blue pill to little children, it had to be crushed and diluted in water.

In 2001 reports began to appear of a few PH patients being helped by sildenafil. By 2003, the trickle was a torrent. Researchers worldwide (Australia, Canada, England, Germany, India, Japan, Spain, and the U.S.) were trying this drug on various types of PH patients who weren't doing well on other therapies.

Researchers often liked what they found, and called for larger, multi-center, longer-term studies. One such study, by the Mayo Clinic Pulmonary Hypertension Group, added sildenafil to the other vasodilating drugs being taken by 13 PAH patients. The sildenafil quickly caused them to be even more vasodilated, but the long-term effects on right-heart function and functional class were ambiguous.

The European Commission granted orphan drug status to sildenafil for use in PAH and chronic thromboembolic PH. (Orphan drug status in the EU means the drug is expected to be used in fewer than 5 in 10,000 people with a life-threatening illness and the drug appears to provide significant benefit over what's already available. Drug companies like to get such status for one of their products because they get a 10-year market exclusivity period during which other similar drugs won't get approved.)

An early study by Dr. B.K.S. Sastry at the CARE Hospital in Hyderabad, India included 22 patients with "PPH," and PAH related to connective tissue disease or corrected congenital heart disease. Patients got either a sugar pill or a weight-adjusted dose of sildenafil (20 mg, 40 mg, or 80 mg) three times a day for 6 weeks. Then they switched to the other treatment for 6 weeks. During sildenafil treatment, patients' exercise time on a treadmill increased by 44 percent compared to the period of time achieved while taking a placebo. This was a wonderful response, but remember that the study was small and short, and results varied greatly from patient to patient.

A double-blind, placebo controlled study of 278 patients with PAH (idiopathic or associated with connective tissue disease or repaired congenital shunts) was done using 20, 40 or 80 mg 3 times-a-day for 12 weeks. Patients receiving sildenafil increased their 6-minute walk distance by 45, 46 and 50 meters respectively compared to placebo. All doses reduced the mean PAP, and improved functional class although clinical worsening was no better than placebo. The hemodynamic improvements were most pronounced in the 80 mg group. Because there was not a statistically significant difference in 6-minute walk distance between the 3 groups the FDA only approved the 20 mg dose (called Revatio).

At the end of the 12 week study, patients could enroll in a long term open label trial where all patients received 80 mg 3 times-a-day. This trial has ended, but at this time the results are not available. An important note is that there will be no long term data on the 20 mg FDA approved dose, and so we may never know whether 20 mg 3 times-a-day is enough after taking it for 12 weeks.

A study of sildenafil added to chronic epoprostenol is still underway in the open label phase. In this study also, virtually all patients in the open label phase are on 80 mg 3 times-a-day.

Because of these issues, the optimal dose of sildenafil is controversial; some physicians only use 20 mg, others routinely use 80-100 mg 3 times-a-day, or more. The fact that the FDA approved only 20 mg has created insurance nightmares for patients and doctors who want to use more than 20 mg 3 times-a-day.

To make matters worse, a law went into effect January 1, 2007 stating that no CMS money (Medicare Part D or Medicaid) could be used to pay for Viagra or other drugs FDA approved for ED. The reason this law was passed was because Congress discovered that some sex offenders had their ED drugs paid for by Medicare or Medicaid. PH patients who had been on Viagra since 2003 or earlier, were suddenly denied coverage for Viagra and told they had to reduce their dose of 25 mg 3 times-a-day or more to Revatio 20 mg 3 times-a-day. Physicians often have to fight long and hard with the insurance companies to keep patients on 80 or 100 mg 3 times-a-day and to increase the dose beyond 20 mg if it is not enough. The cost of all the pills is the same, whether its Revatio 20 mg or Viagra 25, 50 or 100 mg. Therefore, getting 100 mg 3 times-a-day using Revatio costs 5 times as much as using Viagra 100 mg pills, but the insurance companies don't seem to care.

How they work. These drugs work by selectively inhibiting cyclic guanosine monophosphate-specific phosphodiesterase type-5 (PDE-5, for short). PDE-5 is an enzyme found mostly in lung and penile blood vessels. We have other types of PDE in our bodies-including one involved in making our hearts pump-so it's important for an inhibitor to be selective.

In case you were wondering, this is the chain of events:

1. You swallow a sildenafil pill, which enhances the effect of our old friend nitric oxide (NO).
2. NO relaxes vessel walls, allowing more blood to flow, and
3. both NO and sildenafil cause a substance called cyclic guanosine monophosphate (cGMP) to build up.
4. cGMP gets to work relaxing vessels even more.
5. PDE-5 clocks in, doing its work of breaking down cGMP, but it is slowed down a lot by a PDE-5 inhibitor like sildenafil, and so more cGMP can hang around in your blood for a longer time!

Doesn't look at all like the chain of events in ED ads, does it? Yet it is.

New PDE-5 option. Tadalafil (Cialis) (see-AL-iss),made by Eli Lilly, is a long acting PDE-5 inhibitor that is effective for a whopping 36 hours with just one dose (Viagra works for 4 to 5 hours for ED problems). Sildenafil and tadalafil are approved in Australia, Britain, France, Germany and many other countries. In 2003, tadalafil was being sold in at least 45 countries.

Multicenter clinical trials of tadalafil (Cialis) are ongoing. A randomized, double-blind, placebo controlled study of 2.5, 10, 20 or 40 mg daily was completed. This study enrolled patients with IPAH and PAH associated with collagen vascular disease and some types of congenital heart disease in any functional class (I-IV). Patients taking bosentan were allowed in the study, but no patients on any prostanoid could be enrolled. The primary endpoint of the study was 6-minute walk distance, secondary endpoints were functional class, Borg dyspnea score (a patient's subjective rating of how short of breath they felt), time to clinical worsening

(how long it took before PAH worsening occurred), hemodynamics and quality of life measures. Data is expected to be available in 2008. Currently, these patients are in a continuation study of either 20 or 40 mg for 1 year, thereafter the dose will be 40 mg daily.

ED options to opt out of. Another ED drug, Uprima, is a totally different sort of chemical and is not of interest to us as PH patients. Early studies used dipyridamole, but it lacked potency and selectivity. There is also no data or experience with Levitra (vardenafil) in PH.

Warning: do not try any of these drugs without first talking it over with your PH specialist. Although it's easy to get PDE-5 pills over the net without a prescription, please do the smart thing and discuss PDE-5 inhibitor therapy with your doctor first. PDE-5 inhibitors can interact with other PH drugs in unpleasant (as well as pleasant) ways. Sure, millions of men have taken sildenafil for years and lived to talk (or not talk) about it. But PH patients are unusually vulnerable to many drugs, and must balance combinations of drugs exceedingly carefully.

If you use any drugs containing nitrates (isosorbide, or Isordil, Ismo, etc), you shouldn't use these PDE-5 inhibitors. If you are taking PDE-5 inhibitors and need to go to an emergency room, especially for chest pain, tell the ER staff you are taking one of these drugs. Nitroglycerin (NTG) is one of the first drugs given to patients with chest pain and the combination of NTG with PDE-5 inhibitors may cause dangerously low blood pressure.

Recently, Pfizer (the manufacturer of Viagra) changed the package insert of the medication to include a warning about reported cases of sudden hearing loss for patients on Viagra. Although the direct connection from the hearing loss to the use of Viagra is not firmly proven, this action was taken as a safety precaution to warn patients taking this medication.

There have also been rare reports of patients taking Viagra experiencing blindness due to a rare condition called non-arteritic anterior ischemic optic neuropathy or NAION. This loss of vision is due to insufficient blood supply to the optic nerve. However, the incidence of NAION is higher in patients with diabetes, regular (systemic) hypertension, and increased cholesterol levels. The patients taking Viagra for ED may already have these risk factors. Therefore, the incidence of NAION associated with Viagra use may not be any higher than the incidence of NAION in the general population. No incidence of NAION has been reported with patients on Revatio. Talk about these issues with your PH doctor if you have further concerns.

Side effects in the general population.

Okay, this is what you really want to know: no, these drugs won't make you walk around in a state of arousal. Nor will they solve all your love life problems, in part because most of us are tired and on other meds that might blunt our enthusiasm. Nor are pumps and oxygen tanks aphrodisiacs, although there are PH patients using both who don't let the equipment get in their way. A female PH patient reported a day or two of "great discomfort," but it passed. Women's sex organs are not as affected as men's by sildenafil. In women, arousal is not a synonym for desire. Women with increased blood flow "down there" often say they don't even feel it. It seems that the vagina has four layers, and PDE-5 is present only in one layer.

Side effects for all these drugs are usually minimal.

For sildenafil (Viagra), the known side effects are heartburn, nasal congestion, diarrhea, flushing, headache, urinary tract infection, a transient inability to distinguish blue and green, increased sensitivity to light, and blurred vision.

Tadalafil (Cialis) side effects include heartburn, headache, indigestion, back pain, muscle aches, nasal congestion, flushing. Allergic reactions (skin rashes) may occur. Some men say it turns their vision blue; some

complain it doesn't work after a meal. In addition to not using nitrates, you should be wary if you have angina, hypertension, or hypotension.

Will tolerance develop? Doctors disagree on this. For ED, sildenafil is taken only sporadically, which is quite different from taking a drug every day, or taking a drug that lasts an entire weekend. Your body might compensate for the sudden surge of medicine by reducing the number of receptors for it.

What does sildenafil cost? Canadian researchers say that a monthly cost of $492 Canadian (roughly $492 U.S., as of February, 2008) might be safe and effective. Lucky Canadians-American prices are much higher, closer to $900 U.S. per month). As mentioned above, all doses of Viagra and Revatio 20 mg all cost the same, about $10 per pill. A Google search of "Viagra" turned up 15 million hits, and many of them appeared to be outlets of questionable reputation offering discount prices on what may or may not be Viagra equivalents. Ask your doctor for ideas on how to get the drug more cheaply. Ask if it makes sense, economically and medically, to buy a larger-dose pill and break it into halves or quarters (but make sure you can break each pill evenly). Some insurance companies refuse to pay for sildenafil for PH patients. Some have balked at paying for more than the normal, say, eight to ten pills a month. Others pay without any prodding. With the approval of Revatio, this is not as much of a problem, but the dosing issue has been troublesome (see above). PH patients do report getting strange looks when they ask a pharmacist to fill a prescription for 100 pills. Husbands have been known to get a prescription and then give the pills to their PH patient wife to try out (after talking it over with her PH doc). Tsk, tsk.

Patients' reports. Louise, a one-time climber of famous mountain peaks, and more recently a computer science teacher, writer, volunteer, and grandmother, lives in Maryland and has had PH for a long time. Recently, she went through a really bad spell. She had been taking bosentan and was going downhill faster than an Olympic skier. For 7 weeks she was hospitalized and a referral to a hospice was gently suggested. Her doctor then adjusted her drugs. She now takes 125 mg of bosentan twice a day and 50 mg of sildenafil 3 times a day. Of sildenafil, she says, "It's like a miracle drug for me. My condition has improved to between Class I and Class II."

The usual reminder: each of us is unique. Like most of us, Louise is also coping with other medical problems, and taking meds unrelated to her PH. The lesson is that little adjustments in our medications can make a world of difference.

Diane Adkins' story made *The New York Times* (April 10, 2004). Diane is vice-president of a floor-covering company and used to take epoprostenol. Sildenafil will cost her around $10,000 a year, which is about a tenth of the cost of epoprostenol. But her insurance company refused to pay for it (even though they paid for the more expensive epoprostenol) because she was not a male over the age of 18! Diane has hired a lawyer. She jokes that if her insurance company doesn't pay up, she'll get a sex-change operation-something the insurance company does cover.

Prostanoids: Beraprost (Dorner, Beradrak, Procylin); Epoprostenol (Prostacyclin, Flolan); Iloprost (Ventavis); & Treprostinil (Remodulin)

Prostacyclin is man-made, but acts like a substance (prostaglandin I2, a.k.a. PGI2) that occurs naturally in our bodies. (The guy who discovered it in 1976, Sir John Vane, was rewarded with a Nobel Prize. It's that big a deal.) Research suggests that those of us with PAH don't make enough of this important substance. So, just as diabetics are given insulin therapy, it makes sense to give us prostacyclin or prostacyclin-like substances. This group of medicines includes beraprost (Dorner, Beradrak, Procylin); epoprostenol (Flolan); iloprost (Ventavis); and treprostinil (Remodulin). Technically, epoprostenol is a synthesized form of the PGI2 that occurs naturally in our bodies. The others (beraprost, iloprost, treprostinil, etc.) are derivatives of PGI2. This book will just refer to them all as *prostanoids*.

Why does prostacyclin help PH patients? Prostacyclin does several things: it dilates blood vessels (but seldom enough so that lung pressures return to normal), reduces clotting by keeping platelets from clumping together, improves cardiac output, and slows the growth of smooth muscle cells. Pulmonary artery pressure and right atrial pressure fall, and oxygen saturation climbs. Symptoms decrease or even almost disappear. This change usually takes from a few weeks to a few months. In many patients, epoprostenol (an intravenous form of prostacyclin) appears to actually reverse the course of the disease.

How prostacyclin does all this isn't understood. But researchers know it does a lot more than just act as a vasodilator, because patients who do not respond to it initially often slowly get better over time. This is why those who don't respond well during an acute vasodilator challenge are often started on prostanoid therapy anyway. In an editorial in the January 29, 1998, issue of *The New England Journal of Medicine*, Dr. Alfred P. Fishman (professor emeritus, University of Pennsylvania, Philadelphia) put it this way: "Whether prostacyclin's mechanism of action involves the inhibition of coagulation as a result of the drug's anti-platelet-aggregation effects is speculative. However, it is quite likely that the response to the drug is related to its effects on vascular growth and remodeling, which are as yet poorly understood." A study published in 1999 by Dr. David Langleben (Jewish General Hospital,

Montreal) and others found that after 88 days of treatment with prostacyclin, patients' levels of endothelin-1 (a blood vessel constrictor) were closer to normal.

Prostanoids are chemically very similar to one another (they are *analogs*). Although they are all in the same class of drugs, they are not identical, and their toxicity, side effects, and effectiveness may differ.

Which PH patients will prostanoids help? Nearly all PH patients show at least some positive response to prostanoids. Some get just a little better; others return to a normal life style. As one doctor put it at PHA's Conference in 2000, "We don't know how prostacyclin works, but it successfully treats a disease we don't understand."

The following sections cover the pros and cons of each type of prostanoid. To avoid favoritism, they are listed in alphabetical order by their chemical names: beraprost, epoprostenol, iloprost, and treprostinil. The section on "Lines and Pumps" applies to epoprostenol and treprostinil when given intravenously (directly into the bloodstream by vein).

Beraprost

(Dorner, Procylin, Beradrak)

Toray Industries of Japan developed this chemically stable pill form of prostacyclin. In Japan and the Philippines, beraprost is an approved PH therapy. LungRx, an independent division of United Therapeutics owns the rights to it in the U.S., and new trials of a modified version of beraprost may soon be started in the U.S. Beraprost is under evaluation by the European Agency for the Evaluation of Medicinal Product (EMEA). It is also being tried in Australia.

Studies and trials. Beraprost has been used in Japan since 1995. Dr. Noritoshi Nagaya and others followed 59 patients consecutively, through the 1980s and 1990s. Although the data were uncontrolled and retrospective, the results were generally favorable: patients receiving beraprost, as opposed to conventional therapy, lived longer.

Beraprost vasodilates, discourages platelets from sticking together, discourages smooth muscle cells from proliferating, and inhibits inflammatory cytokines.

There have been two randomized, double-blind, placebo-controlled trials on PAH patients. One study, in Europe, led by Dr. Nazzareno Galiè (Instituto di Bologna, Italy) and others, involved 130 patients with "PPH" and PAH associated with connective tissue disease, congenital heart disease, portal hypertension, and HIV infection. The patients were functional Class II or III and got as much beraprost as they could tolerate for 12 weeks. In the group that got the real drug, the improvement in the 6-minute walk distance of the "PPH" patients was 45 meters; the others didn't walk any farther than they had at the start of the trial. Cardiopulmonary hemodynamics did not improve significantly.

The second study, in the U.S., by Dr. Robyn Barst and others, is fascinating. It looked at the effects of the drug on 116 Class II or III patients for a full year. The results of this study were a textbook illustration of why long-term studies are essential. At 6 months, the patients getting the real beraprost had less disease progression and improved their 6-minute walks by 31 meters. Sounds good, right? But this improvement disappeared: at 9 months and 12 months the patients getting the beraprost were doing no better than they had at the start of the study. So it might be possible that beraprost does some good for a while, but then its effects wear off.

A big gulp. The drug is absorbed fast after being swallowed, reaching a peak concentration in about half an hour, and then is eliminated over the next 35-40 minutes. Because beraprost has a short half-life, patients take up to 120 mcg 4 times a day (the pills are 20 mcg, so this adds up to a lot of pills). Some patients notice their symptoms returning between doses as the drug wears off, but all are able to go overnight without having to get up to swallow pills. An extended release form of the pill is being talked about.

Side effects. Side effects include nausea, flushing, headache, jaw pain, leg pain, and swollen feet. If you take the pills with meals, side effects lessen. There is little danger of overdose, because the pill form of prostacyclin can't reach blood level concentrations as high as can be obtained with epoprostenol.

Just to thoroughly confuse you as to your possible prostacyclin options, researchers in Japan have been testing an *inhaled* form of beraprost on rats.

Epoprostenol (Flolan, prostacyclin)

Members of PHA rejoiced when, in September 1995, the FDA approved the marketing of epoprostenol sodium for the long-term treatment of "PPH." Dr. Barst and many of her PH colleagues around the country did a randomized trial that showed that Flolan improved survival in addition to making the "PPH" patients feel better, walk further and have better pulmonary pressures, cardiac output and pulmonary resistance after only 12 weeks. Flolan remains the only drug we have for PAH that has been shown in a randomized study to improve survival in "PPH". Although it was known that the market would be small, the drug company, Burroughs Wellcome (which has now merged into GlaxoSmithKline), invested heavily in this drug, which it calls Flolan. In the U.S., Flolan is now marketed by Gilead. Epoprostenol is said to be available in Germany and Japan, but at great cost. It is available in the U.K., where patients call it prostacyclin, in Israel, and in some other places as well. Refer to the PH Drug Chart for further information.

Epoprostenol is still considered the "gold standard" for PH treatment for very sick, Class IV patients. Dr. Vallerie McLaughlin reports

that after a year of therapy pressures typically drop by about 20 percent, cardiac output is up by 60 percent and pulmonary vascular resistance (PVR) is cut about in half. People walk farther and feel better. Some can wave goodbye to their oxygen tanks. If you improve over the first year (say to Class II), you tend to do well for a long, long time. The lung pressures of patients using epoprostenol (or any other therapy) seldom return to normal, although there are cases where this happens, especially in children.

Epoprostenol delivery. Epoprostenol has a short half-life of only a few minutes, so it cannot be given in the form of a pill. Epoprostenol is continuously delivered, intravenously, usually through a central line right into the heart (it can also be administered temporarily through an IV (for example placed in the arm) while patients are waiting for a central line to be placed or while their central line is being changed because of an infection). See the section "Lines and Pumps" for discussion of catheters and pumps used for epoprostenol and other therapies.

It's heartbreaking to get a call on the PHA hotline from a man or woman who is so breathless they can hardly be heard on the phone above the wheeze of supplemental oxygen, someone who tells us they haven't gotten treatment because, "I could never stand

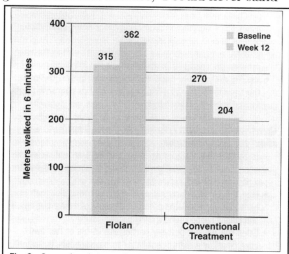

Fig. 2—Comparison between 6-minute walk distances at baseline and 12-week follow-up in patients with PAH treated with epoprostenol vs conventional therapy ($P < .002$).[2]

From Advances in Pulmonary Hypertension, *Vol. 1, No. 3.*

wearing a pump around." Before you decide that epoprostenol or another pump therapy is not for you, even if you are dying, please, please go to a support group meeting and talk to some folks using it, or at least call PHA's 800 number (see Chapter 14) and say you want to talk with a patient using epoprostenol or another prostacyclin-like drug. At PHA's first International Conference (1994 in Stone Mountain, Georgia), we watched one of our members, a beautiful girl, do an athletic dance routine that included flips, while wearing her pump. Most viewers couldn't tell where she had concealed her pump under her leotard. At the 1998 Conference (in Dallas), dozens of Flolaners line-danced to the country music. After meeting people of all ages, from infants to seniors, who live good lives because of epoprostenol, the nuisance and side effects seem much more bearable. Many epoprostenol users go to school, travel, and continue to work at their jobs.

Who benefits from infused epoprostenol.

When Dr. Bruce Brundage was at Harbor/UCLA, he found that over the long term (about 3 years) 70 to 80 percent of his patients responded well. In other words, although people with PAH may have initially gotten sick for very different reasons, when given epoprostenol nearly all found that their pulmonary pressures fell, pulmonary vascular resistance fell, and their cardiac output rose.

As mentioned, Flolan was first approved by the FDA for the treatment of "PPH" for patients in classes III and IV. Flolan is now also approved for the treatment of PAH secondary to the scleroderma spectrum of diseases (connective tissue diseases). Medicare will cover Flolan if a patient has "PPH" or PH secondary to one of the following conditions: connective tissue disease, thromboembolic disease of the pulmonary arteries, human immunodeficiency virus (HIV) infection, cirrhosis, PH due to diet drugs, congenital left-to-right shunts, etc. (There are additional criteria to be met; see Chapter

13.) Dr. David Badesch (University of Colorado) and a gaggle of some of the finest PH doctor/researchers at 17 PH specialty centers did a randomized, controlled, open-label study involving 111 patients with moderate to severe PAH secondary to scleroderma-type diseases, and concluded that the patients who got epoprostenol walked farther and had improved hemodynamics after using the drug 12 weeks. Their Raynaud's was less severe, they had fewer ulcers on their fingers and toes, and they suffered less breathlessness. Side effects were the usual for prostacyclin and included jaw pain, nausea, and anorexia. There were infection problems related to the entry site, plus cellulitis at the entry site (both problems also occur with IPAH/FPAH patients).

Some patients whose hands are badly affected by scleroderma may have trouble mixing epoprostenol and handling the pump.

Joyce has scleroderma/PAH, and had a soaring PAP when she was first diagnosed with PH in 2000. Most of her doctors (with the exception of her PH specialist) were not optimistic about her survival. But epoprostenol and later bosentan (when her PAP dropped way down she was weaned from epoprostenol) have done wonders for her. Joyce says, "Unlike what most rheumatologists have led patients to believe in recent decades, PAH is not the last stop on the stage headed for the cemetery. I have been fighting the various ugly heads of scleroderma for just over 4 decades and I'm living proof that PAH can be controlled. Neither Flolan nor Tracleer healed my scleroderma, but at least my PAH is under great control!"

There have not yet been any controlled studies on whether infused epoprostenol will work for patients with PAH associated with HIV infection, portopulmonary hypertension, or congenital heart disease. However, in a study by Hilario Nunes and others (Hôpital Antoine Beclere, Assistance Publique-Hôpitaux de Paris, Université Paris-Sud, Clamart, France), continuous epoprostenol infusion helped patients with severe HIV / PAH to survive longer. And Dr. Robyn Barst has found it helpful in treating patients with PH and congenital heart disease (Eisenmenger). Flolan has also been used in many children; and despite the pump, the children's growth and development only improve with no interference due to the pump. Other doctors have successfully used it for Gaucher's disease.

A small study by Dr. Stuart Rich (then at Rush Heart Institute, Chicago) and others found a higher mortality among patients with PAH triggered by diet pills. They were not responding as well as others to epoprostenol (their PAPs were not falling as much), although they did see an improvement in cardiac output and functional status. The study has not been replicated. A doctor in France says his diet pill/PAH patients seem to respond much like other PAH patients.

Pulmonary artery pressures (PAPs) have been successfully reduced in people with portopulmonary hypertension by treating them with infused epoprostenol. Dr. Michael Krowka (Mayo Clinic, Rochester, MN) reported on 15 portopulmonary hypertension patients using epoprostenol. They saw a nice reduction of PVR as measured in the cath lab, as well as a drop in mean PAPs, and improved cardiac outputs. There is still much to be learned about the impact of continuous epoprostenol infusion on people with portopulmonary hypertension. If epoprostenol causes a patient's cardiac output to go too high, it can worsen the portopulmonary hypertension and cause fluid to accumulate in the lungs. Ascites (fluid in the abdomen) may be made worse. Enlarged spleens have been reported, as have abnormally low numbers of platelets and white corpuscles in the blood. Spleen troubles may be the cause of the decrease in platelets and white blood cells. This is called hypersplenism, and may be unrelated to epoprostenol use. (If the PH is caught early

enough, treprostinil, beraprost, bosentan, and inhaled nitric oxide might also be of use for portopulmonary hypertension patients. And a liver transplant is sometimes an option if the PH can be well controlled with medical treatments for PH.)

Epoprostenol is often used to help patients get well enough to undergo a lung transplant, and its use is sometimes continued for some time after the operation.

Who should not use infused epoprostenol. In pulmonary venous hypertension patients, epoprostenol has not shown any benefits and might make the disease worse. GlaxoSmithKline warns that epoprostenol is not for those with congestive heart failure due to severe left ventricular systolic dysfunction. If you got your PH because of veno-occlusive disease, epoprostenol may not help and may even be harmful.

Don't suddenly stop taking epoprostenol! Once epoprostenol therapy has begun, it should never be abruptly stopped, nor should the dose be drastically reduced in one big step (unless your PH specialist says it is necessary). If you have severe PH and are highly dependent on your epoprostenol, you can clinically deteriorate ("crash") within just 5 minutes (although it usually takes somewhat longer) after you suddenly stop taking the drug. You must go to the closest hospital if your Flolan stops (and it is not due to your pump not working) to get it restarted. *Even such a brief interruption of medication could result in death.*

Will I have to take this stuff forever? Maybe not. Patients have been "weaned" from epoprostenol if they are doing quite well. However, many doctors are reluctant to do this even if a patient's pressures are low, because of the other pluses of epoprostenol (to repeat: it discourages platelets from clumping together, improves cardiac output, and slows down the growth of smooth muscle cells). "Weaning" usually means switching to another prostanoid, an oral PH drug or combination. A couple of cases have been reported where the weaned patient takes no medicine. This would only be considered if your pressures have returned to normal, and you would be very carefully monitored. (Just as systemic blood pressures [the blood pressure that your doctor measures on your arm] stay down only as long as a patient takes her medicine, so it nearly always is with PAH.) As with so many other PAH treatment decisions, a mistake could be life-threatening.

Common side effects. Prostanoids, as a group, have very similar side effects. As far as doctors know, nobody is allergic to epoprostenol. Most side effects are easily treated or at least bearable, and they usually lessen or even vanish as your body adjusts to the medicine. (They tend to increase each time your dosage is increased, and then settle back down.) Everybody gets some flushing (redness), which is a direct result of vasodilatation, and many get a blotchy rash that seems to come and go. Other common complaints are foot pain, jaw pain, diarrhea, and muscle pain in the calves and feet (*myalgia*). Nausea, vomiting, and headaches also occur. Tylenol can be used to treat the headaches. The foot pain is a dull constant ache that happens when you've been on your feet for a while. Mostly it's on the bottom of the feet.

Doctors don't know why there is "first bite" jaw pain; it has been compared to biting into a lemon. Fortunately, the pain is harmless. To lessen jaw pain (which diminishes the longer you chew), begin a meal by slowly chewing a cracker, piece of bread or a sip of something hot. Jaw pain seems to be related to the salivary glands. Try rubbing your cheeks as you take that first bite. Maureen has found that dairy products stimulate her salivary glands less than citrus or wheat, so she starts a meal with a nibble of a non-stimulating food.

Some patients experience increased anxiety, restlessness or "antsiness" with prostanoids. This may improve over time and only occur after a dose increase. Talk with your doctor and nurse about how to manage this side effect if it is bothering you.

Because epoprostenol also dilates the blood vessels in your intestines, diarrhea sometimes occurs. It can be treated with Imodium AD. Epoprostenol makes you more photosensitive, so avoid bright sunlight. Lightheadedness, restlessness, joint discomfort, abdominal pain, and systemic hypotension (that is low blood pressure) are other possible side effects. Depression has also been reported; if you experience this, you might want to ask your doctor to rule out thyroid problems (which turned out to be the source of some epoprostenol-users' depression).

Some epoprostenol users get a rash on their legs. This is because when blood pools, capillaries break and pigment gets into the skin. Epoprostenol might also exacerbate any underlying skin problems. Your body can reabsorb the pigment, but it can take years. If you have shapely gams but hate that rash, wear tinted hose to hide it.

Rare side effects. Things that occasionally show up down the road include thyroid and goiter problems (usually big nontoxic goiters or nodules). It's possible that epoprostenol may "unmask" a preexisting endocrine or thyroid problem, or that it somehow interferes with communications among cells. Your doctor should monitor you for such developments. A handful of epoprostenol users have developed lung fibrosis or changes in their stomach lining that make them throw up a lot. A thickening of the lining of the stomach (*hypertrophic gastropathy*) makes it hard to eat and keep your food down. Hypertrophic gastropathy can become quite serious. Unfortunately, doctors don't know how to treat it. We're not even sure that it's related to epoprostenol usage.

Osteoporosis has been reported in epoprostenol users; it isn't known if there is a causal link. Finally, a few epoprostenol users have low platelet counts.

Dosage. There are two factors that control dosage: concentration and pump rate. When the concentration is increased, the pump rate is lowered. Doctors still don't know the ideal dosage for epoprostenol. Most adult patients seem to be in the 20 to 40 ng/kg-per-minute range at the end of one year of therapy. (The dose is based on the patient's weight, expressed in kilograms [kg]. For those not used to the metric system, a kilogram is 1,000 grams or 2.2 pounds. A nanogram [ng] is one billionth of a gram.) Children (and especially infants and toddlers) are often on higher doses such as above 80 ng/kg-per-minute and not infrequently as high as 150 ng/kg-per-minute.

Over time, the dosage is sometimes increased. It used to be generally believed that some resistance develops to the drug's effect *(tolerance)*. Now some experts are saying that this is probably not true (others disagree). Some treatment centers used to step up the dosage regularly, whereas others waited for **PH** symptoms to reappear. Even if tolerance really occurs, not everybody develops it to the same degree. Some people seem able to stay at the same dose indefinitely. As mentioned above, children can tolerate much higher doses than adults, and their dosages are sometimes increased more aggressively. Children's dosages must also be increased to accommodate normal weight gains.

Epoprostenol toxicity/overdose syndrome. At first it was thought that the more epoprostenol, the better. Then a beet-red patient who lived in the boonies and had to be followed by phone, stumbled into the Rush Heart Institute, dying, and they did a cardiac cath on her and found that she was in high output heart failure. Epoprostenol makes both sides of the heart pump better - her heart was pumping so much blood that it was failing. The doctors lowered her dose and she improved.

Dr. Stuart Rich and Dr. Vallerie

McLaughlin studied a dozen patients who had developed high cardiac output. They tried reducing the patients' epoprostenol and discovered that the patients' symptoms got no worse. When the medicine was tapered down they did not see any worsening, that is they did not see a rebound effect. The Rush team reduced dosages in tiny steps and reevaluated each patient weekly, using a scorecard of side effects. Deborah, in Texas, felt so much better when her dose was reduced that she was taken off the transplant list.

Dr. Ron Oudiz and his colleagues at Harbor-UCLA also found that after a certain amount of epoprostenol (40 to 60 ng/kg-per-minute), increases in dosage don't help in terms of cardiopulmonary function. Blood is instead shunted through a hole in the heart or through small blood vessels that don't go through the lungs. So only the cardiac output rises.

How can you tell if you're overdosed? It's tricky, because most signs of overdosage are the same as PH symptoms. If you are getting dreadfully fatigued over time *but are not getting shorter of breath*, if you are losing weight, if you have bad diarrhea, trouble digesting food, very red skin, bad belly bloating, or if your cardiac output is too high, then you may be overdosed. Intense jaw and foot pain may be a sign. Aches in shins, muscles and calves, and burning on the soles of the feet might also be dose-related. Some patients have died because their diarrhea was so bad they became malnourished. Note, however, that you can have all the symptoms of overdosage without actually being overdosed; nothing about this disease is simple. So do not try to reduce the dose on your own. Speak with your PH doctor. A cardiac cath will probably be needed (echoes don't measure cardiac output accurately enough; tiny errors get magnified because calculations are geometric).

Who can't deal with epoprostenol? Infused epoprostenol is perhaps the most complicated medicine that patients have ever been trusted to self-administer. But nearly everybody is able to master the mixing, the pump, and potential complications. A tiny handful of patients just can't learn the routine. A few more are sloppy, or have sleepy immune systems, so they get too many infections. Because doctors don't have unlimited time to spend with their patients, a sloppy or noncompliant patient can add greatly to their workload. Doctors who are thinking about offering epoprostenol to a patient will consider things like whether you keep scheduled appointments, whether you can take an active role in your own care, whether you (and your support person) are truly willing to take the time needed every day to mix the medicine and change cassettes; although it seems overwhelming at first, within several weeks, this becomes a 20 minute part of your daily routine.

And the fact that a patient may have abused drugs in the past is not in itself a reason for a doctor to deny a patient Flolan; a chance to save their life may be the motivation he/she needs to quit abusing drugs.

Getting started on infused epoprostenol.
Most PH doctors believe that epoprostenol therapy should only be started in a hospital that specializes in treating PH. Plan on staying a few days, while you learn how to mix the medicine and troubleshoot catheter care. Judging by calls that come in to the PHA Helpline, patients of Doc Outtadate (who learns about epoprostenol by thumbing through his Merck Manual while you wait in his exam room) are much more likely to die or to get sloppy, poor-quality treatment than are those who go to PH doctors with lots of experience treating PH patients on Flolan. We are easy to kill. PHA can supply names of PH centers.

There is so much to tell about handling emergencies, dosage, mixing the medicine, drug interactions, avoiding infections from the catheter, choice of catheter type, etc., that it all cannot possibly be covered here. Many treatment centers have their own epoprostenol

handbook or set of instructions, as does Accredo, the only Specialty Pharmacy that currently provides epoprostenol.

Mixing and storing epoprostenol.
Epoprostenol is supplied in the form of a freeze-dried powder. Once a day (usually), the patient mixes the powder with a glycine buffer solution. Before mixing, the powder and buffer can be stored at room temperature. Once mixed, it has a brief half-life and must be kept cold (but not frozen) even when in use. Epoprostenol must also be protected from light.

Your PH center or health service company will give you mixing instructions-they vary from center to center, so your routine may differ from your PH pal's. Do your mixing at a time and place (that is very clean) where you are free of distractions. The medicine is either placed in one ice-packed cassette (a 24-hour cassette) or is divided into three doses to fill three 8-hour "medication reservoir cassettes." In the latter case, the two cassettes not yet being used are refrigerated. The smaller cassettes are easier to conceal on your body and do not require ice packs while you are using them. Of course, if you use a smaller pack you have to change it three times a day. To make changing cassettes easier, tape a coin to the back of each of your pumps.

At first it will take a long time to do the mixing, but Tessa of Seattle says that after lots of practice she has gotten it down to 10 minutes flat! Ten minutes might be an unreasonable goal for patients who wish to reduce the number of infections they get. What's important isn't your speed but your accuracy.

Interactions of other drugs with epoprostenol.
Your PH doctor should know about all the drugs and supplements you take. When epoprostenol is used with other antiplatelet or anticoagulant drugs, careful INR monitoring is important. Check with your doctor before using aspirin, ibuprofen (Motrin, Advil), phenylephrine (found in many cold medicines), or phenylpropanolamine (a

vasoconstrictor formerly used in decongestants like Alka-Seltzer Plus Night-Time Cold Medicine, Contac 12 Hour Capsules, Dimetapp Cold and Flu Caplets, and Tylenol Cold Effervescent Tablets). Acutrim, Dexatrim, and Stay Trim also used phenylpropanolamine. In November 2000, over-the-counter drugs containing phenylpropanolamine were pulled off store shelves because of epidemiological studies showing it increases the risk of hemorrhagic stroke (phenylpropanolamine, ephedrine, and amphetamine all have very similar chemical structures). It's possible you may still have some of the old formulations in your medicine cabinet, so read the labels.

Epoprostenol (Flolan) providers. In the U.S., epoprostenol is currently available only through Accredo Therapeutics. The Accredo nurses will instruct you on how to mix and use your medication. It is important that a support person (such as a family member or caregiver) also be trained in these processes (and that the caregiver or family member do the mixing once a week because if he/she has to only do the mixing in an emergency, it is likely that he/she will have forgotten how to do it if not doing it on a regular basis).

Accredo Therapeutics provides a "Flolan Education Guide" with instructions on the administration and mixing of epoprostenol. In addition, this guide provides disease state information, proper hand washing techniques, and helpful hints to patients on what to do when traveling. Some PH centers also have their own instructions for epoprostenol patients.

Cost. It is very expensive-starting at about $60,000 per year and going up to over $120,000. As your dosage increases, so does the cost. You can usually get it covered by your private or government insurance (including Medicare) if you are Class III or IV and have "PPH" or PAH associated with the scleroderma spectrum of diseases. (Doctors report that insurance often pays for epoprostenol for many

other types of PAH as well.) Accredo will assist you in getting prior insurance authorization and in monitoring your lifetime maximums. In rare cases, insurance coverage cannot be obtained, and the patient is left with the unpleasant options of paying out-of-pocket for the epoprostenol or seeking help through the maker's patient assistance program.

Patients' reports. Tim was diagnosed with PAH in 1986 when he had a routine x-ray when he applied for a job. He was stable on calcium channel blockers (CCBs) for some years, then started going downhill. He went on epoprostenol in 1993 and at PHA's 2002 conference he reported his PAP to be stable at about 55.

Claudia, a nurse, was told she had less than 6 months to live when she went on epoprostenol. Her pulmonary pressures were around 85. They fell to the fifties, and she was able to work 50 hours a week as vice president of a company doing case management. Sometimes she felt absolutely great, and sometimes she didn't. At the time of the 2002 conference she had begun tapering off epoprostenol and starting on bosentan. She volunteered to help on the original 3rd edition of the *Survival Guide*, but didn't survive to see it published. It really hurts to have to report things like this, to have to change wording to the past tense. But that is the reality of PH. Thank you, Claudia, for looking beyond your own troubles and reaching out to others.

To read the inspiring story of Hannah Carr, a young epoprostenol user, turn to the chapter on Children and PH.

Iloprost (Ventavis)

When prostacyclin is inhaled (in the same manner asthmatics inhale their medicine) its effects are believed to be largely confined to the lungs, which is a real plus because it greatly reduces most side effects. Iloprost, a prostanoid in aerosol form, was approved late in 2003 by the European Commission for sale in all EU countries for the treatment of Class III "PPH" patients. In Europe, iloprost's trade name is Ventavis, and Schering AG is marketing it. In the US, Ventavis was approved for Class III or IV patients in 2004 and is marketed by Actelion.

Clinical trials. The Aerosolized Iloprost Randomized (AIR) Study Group conducted a 3 month, randomized double-blind, placebo controlled multicenter trial of inhaled iloprost 6-9 times per day looking at a combined endpoint (meaning patients had to meet all 3) of 10% improvement in the 6-minute walk test, improved functional class and no clinical deterioration or death. 17% of patients receiving the iloprost met all 3 criteria compared to only 5% of patients on placebo. Overall, the iloprost patients increased their 6-minute walk distance by 36 meters; looking at only IPAH patients the improvement was 59 meters.

A one year uncontrolled open label study of 24 IPAH patients on iloprost improved their 6-minute walk distance by 75 meters and improved their hemodynamics. A long term (535 +/- 61 days) follow-up study of 76 functional class II or III IPAH patients using iloprost was done. The percentage of patients who continued on iloprost without events were 53% at 1 year and 29% at 2 years. The patients with "events" included 14% who died, 9% had a transplant, 33% changed to an IV prostanoid, 23% received additional oral therapies and 17% stopped using iloprost for various other reasons.

Iloprost has also been studied as an addition to bosentan (STEP trial) and was found to be safe. (See the section on Combination Therapy.)

Iloprost is also being tried on persons with Raynaud's disease. (Intravenous iloprost is already approved in Europe for the treatment of severe Raynaud's disease.) Iloprost is also being tried in Japan and Australia.

Side effects. The typical systemic prostanoid side effects (nausea, diarrhea, leg pain) are generally less. Iloprost side effects in some patients (coughing, flushing, headache, and jaw pain) appear to be well tolerated. (If doctors don't see *some* flushing they suspect the dose is too low or your nebulizer is broken.) Those in the iloprost group in the AIR clinical trial reported more serious fainting problems, but fainting was not related to a worsening of their PH.

About nebulizers and inhaling. Iloprost comes premixed in single dose glass vials and is inhaled using a special nebulizer, the I-Neb device. It takes about 10 minutes to inhale the standard 5 microgram aerosol dose. (See section, Lines and Pumps for a discussion of the I-Neb.) Users inhale perhaps 6 to 9 times during the day, and do not usually inhale at night (but some do). The main problem with inhaled iloprost is that its benefits disappear within 30 to 90 minutes, so you have to inhale many times a day, which is a darn nuisance. (Adding sildenafil or other Viagra-type drugs enhances and prolongs inhaled iloprost's effect.)

Effectiveness compared to epoprostenol. The German researchers in the smaller study (Marius M. Hoeper and others) measured mean PAP both before and after inhalations and found quite a difference. In other words, patients did better when exercising right after an inhalation than they did when exercising 2 or 3 hours after an inhalation. After a year of treatment, the patients' mean PAPs *before* inhalation had declined by 23 percent. Immediately *after* an inhalation they saw a mean 42 percent reduction. This post-inhalation reduction is close to the 53 percent reduction in PVR seen by U.S. doctors in patients treated for a year or two with epoprostenol-but epoprostenol's benefit doesn't rise and fall.

Effectiveness compared to sildenafil and nitric oxide. In a very small 2004 prospective study of 10 "PPH" patients, researchers at Ludwig-Maximilians-University Munich, Germany, tried oral sildenafil, inhaled nitric oxide (NO), and iloprost aerosol on each of the patients. They defined a "significant response" as a drop in PVR of at least 20 percent. Seven of the patients responded to iloprost, and 4 responded to inhaled NO with oral sildenafil. The best improvements in hemodynamics and oxygenation were seen with the iloprost.

Iloprost can also be used intravenously and orally. Like epoprostenol, iloprost can be pumped into the heart through a central line catheter. Why would you want to do that, when the biggest advantage of the drug is that no central line is needed? The option is attractive because the drug is more stable than epoprostenol and remains in the body longer. (It shouldn't come as a surprise, however, that most German patients preferred the inhaled version to the IV.) When used intravenously, the side effects are similar to epoprostenol's. In the U.K., iloprost is given both in aerosol form and intravenously, and an oral form of the drug is undergoing clinical trials on patients who have PH triggered by scleroderma.

Which PH patients might benefit from iloprost. As mentioned, "PPH" patients seemed to benefit more from inhaled iloprost than did other types of PAH patients. However, note the U.K. study, above. And Italian researchers have also been looking at iloprost's effects on scleroderma patients (not PH patients). In a 12-month, prospective, randomized, parallel-group, blind-observer trial by Dr. Raffaella Scorza and others at the University of Milan, which involved 46 patients with systemic sclerosis and Raynaud's phenomenon, the cyclic administration of *intravenous* iloprost seemed to control and improve the course of the disease. Note that the study was not focused on PH patients, but if PH caused by scleroderma can be *prevented*, that would be okay, too. These patients were on a sort of weird schedule (approved in Europe for Raynaud's treatment) where they got the drug 8 hours a day for 5 days, and then 8 hours on one day every 6 weeks. Other European researchers

have done little studies suggesting aerosolized iloprost might help selected CREST/PH patients. Iloprost may be a preferred treatment for those with Eisenmenger's/PH, because it affects mostly the lungs, not the whole body. Inhaled iloprost has also been tried in Germany on a dozen patients with portopulmonary hypertension. It decreased their PAPs and PVRs without bad systemic pressure effects.

Cost. In Germany iloprost would cost far less than epoprostenol (although it is still very expensive). Patients starting on iloprost typically use about one ampule a day, which costs about $70 U.S. In Germany, a nebulizer costs about $500. In the US, 1 vial of iloprost (one treatment) is about $33. The nebulizer and supply costs are additional. Ventavis coverage may come from a different part of your insurance than epoprostenol or treprostinil which usually fall under "major medical". Some insurance companies require that the medication is paid through the PBM (Pharmacy Benefit Manager) like oral therapies with the nebulizer covered under a different part, or in some cases, not covered at all. The Specialty Pharmacy helps negotiate this with your insurance company.

Treprostinil (Remodulin)

Treprostinil sodium (Remodulin) was known as UT-15 and Uniprost during its early stages of development by United Therapeutics. (A woman whose daughter has PH founded United Therapeutics.) It is a form of prostacyclin that is stable at room temperature and has a half-life of about 4 hours. It is now taken by both subcutaneous (SC) and intravenous (IV) routes. Remodulin, which comes in multidose vials, is stable at room temperature, but open vials should be refrigerated. Once a vial is open it is good for 30 days. It can withstand undesirable conditions for short amounts of time (less than a day), but check to make sure it's not discolored or looks unusual. If so, don't use it.

Like epoprostenol, treprostinil helps most PH patients. The Remodulin form of treprostinil won its FDA approval in spring 2002 as a "continuous subcutaneous infusion for the treatment of pulmonary arterial hypertension in patients with NYHA Class II-IV symptoms." In 2004 the FDA approved Remodulin for intravenous use in Class II, III, and IV patients who cannot tolerate the subcutaneous infusion and in 2006 it was approved for patients who require transition from Flolan. The Canadian Therapeutic Products Directorate approved Remodulin in the fall of 2002, the drug is approved in Israel, and United Therapeutics has submitted marketing applications in Europe and Australia.

Subcutaneous clinical trials. The study that led to this drug's approval involved 470 PAH patients (either what used to be called "PPH" - including diet pill users - or PAH associated with connective tissue disease or congenital shunts) from the U.S., Europe, Australia, and Israel. The trial was randomized and theoretically placebo controlled (but every patient participant the author spoke with knew if they were getting the real drug because of the site pain!). At the end of 12 weeks, patients who got treprostinil walked farther in a 6-minute walk test than those on placebo: a mean difference of around 16 meters (with a median of 10 meters).

When interpreting these results, several differences from the earlier epoprostenol trial should be considered. The treprostinil trial included many Class II patients who didn't improve as much as the others, because they weren't as sick to begin with. Class IV patients improved their distance by a respectable 54 meters. Most significantly, the average dose of treprostinil was only about 9 ng/kg-per-minute, what most doctors would consider to be a very low dose. In patients who were able to achieve an effective dose by the end of the 12-week trial, results were much better. In addition to walking faster, the patients' breathlessness and other PH

symptoms improved, along with their hemodynamics. The trial did not find any difference in effectiveness between "PPH" and connective tissue disease/ PH patients. The congenital heart disease patients included in the trial did not improve at all during the 12 weeks. (For details, see the paper by Dr. Gerald Simonneau [Antoine Beclere Hôpital, Paris-Sud Université, Clamart, France] and others in the March 15, 2000 issue of the *American Journal of Respiratory Critical Care Medicine*.)

Selected patients on Remodulin who were followed for a year or more have seen continued improvement in their walking distance.

IV clinical trials. Dr. Gomberg-Maitland led an open label 12-week study that transitioned IV Flolan patients to IV Remodulin over 24-48 hours. Of the 31 patients in the study, 27 completed the transition and 4 patients discontinued the study. The patients who were transitioned had no change in their 6-minute walk test distance compared to their walk on Flolan. Dr. Tapson led a 12-week multicenter prospective open label trial of patients started on IV Remodulin (de novo patients, that is, patients new to PAH therapy). Sixteen patients were studied and the average dose at the end of the 12-week study was 41 ng/kg-per-minute. Note that the dose in the SC trial was only 9 ng/kg-per-minute. The average increase in patients' 6-minute walk test distance was 82 meters at the end of the 12-week trial. Patients also showed significant improvement in hemodynamics and 43% of patients improved their functional class.

Post-marketing study. When the FDA approved Remodulin, they asked that a Phase IV post-marketing study be conducted to look for additional benefits of the drug. Dr. Rubenfire led the 8-week study, which took 14 patients who were stable on Flolan for at least 3 months and then randomized them to transition to a placebo drug or SC Remodulin. 93% of the patients in the SC Remodulin group were successfully transitioned. All of the patients (except one) who transitioned to the placebo deteriorated and needed to be restarted on Flolan.

Potency. Some doctors feel Remodulin doses need to be about 2 times the Flolan dose although some patients may be OK with 1.5 times, others may need 3 times or more. As with Flolan, individual doses vary greatly. United Therapeutics has established the bioequivalence of the two routes (IV and SC) of administering the drug. This means that after starting, both routes reach a stable blood level in about 2 hours and the half-life for both is about 4 hours. (Half-life means when the drug is stopped, half the drug is gone from the body in this period of time.)

Intravenous Remodulin. IV Remodulin is given in much the same way as Flolan and has both disadvantages and advantages over SC Remodulin or Flolan. A disadvantage of IV vs. SC Remodulin is the danger of line infections. Any patient receiving intravenous therapy runs the risk of line infections. A recent review by the CDC suggested that infections with gram negative bacteria may be more common in patients using IV Remodulin compared to patients on Flolan. The reason for this isn't known and needs further investigation. It is recommended that patients on IV Remodulin follow the same strict sterile techniques that Flolan patients use for line care management (See the Lines and Pumps section of this chapter) and medication preparation.

The main advantage of IV over SC Remodulin is lack of site pain. Advantages of IV Remodulin over Flolan include its stability at room temperature, meaning no ice packs, it only needs to be mixed and changed every 48 hours and it has a longer half-life which may result in less "rebound PH" and PH symptoms if the drug is accidentally stopped (by a catheter or pump problem). IV Remodulin, like Flolan, uses a permanent tunneled IV catheter. See the section on Lines and Pumps for a discussion of the pumps used for IV Remodulin. Remodulin is usually diluted with saline and placed in the pump cassette or syringe every 48 hours.

The delivery system. Subcutaneous Remodulin gets around the main problem of IV prostanoids (the risk of infection) by avoiding a central line catheter into the central vasculature above the heart. Instead, SC Remodulin is pumped into the fat (usually in the tummy) under the skin (*subcutaneous* fat).

The biggest fear of new users is that they have to poke themselves in the stomach every few days when changing the site with a little needle that's connected by a long, thin plastic catheter to the pump. You can use a bent or straight needle, and insert the needle manually or via an injector. The needle comes out and the little soft plastic catheter remains. Most patients say that it doesn't really hurt much to put in the needle, that it feels more like a little thud. But others compare it to a bee sting. The pain may vary from day-to-day and spot-to-spot.

Although scleroderma patients have used Remodulin with success, those with a lot of skin involvement may have trouble inserting the needle. Portopulmonary hypertension patients may be able to use SC Remodulin, however, asicites is often a problem in liver disease, and the abdomen can be tight as a drum and hard to stick a needle into. Tense asicties may also affect the drug's absorption into your system. Not all portopulmonary hypertension patients have ascites however, and alternative sites can be used. A bit of tape keeps the catheter in place.

A drop at a time, the medicine is delivered under your skin. Many PH centers allow patients to keep the catheter in for extended periods if there is no pain (see the section below on controlling site pain). At least once every 3 days you need to change the medicine cartridge in the pump. You do have to load the cartridge with medicine yourself (using a syringe).

SC Remodulin has fewer risks than epoprostenol from clots, plugging, and a sudden discontinuation of the drug. Site infections are much less dangerous, but site pain (see below) occurs to some degree in everyone.

What happens if the SC catheter falls out or there is a problem with the IV catheter? Because there is a reservoir of the medicine in your subcutaneous tissues, and because Remodulin has a much longer half-life than epoprostenol, there is less risk of PH symptoms quickly worsening if the medication is abruptly stopped. To repeat a warning given in the epoprostenol section: once any prostanoid therapy has begun, it should never be abruptly stopped, nor should the dose be drastically reduced in one big step (unless your doctor says it is necessary). Although Remodulin has a longer half-life than Flolan it is not generally recommended that IV Remodulin users disconnect from their pumps for casual reasons, i.e. swimming. Exposure of the catheter site to water is strongly discouraged due to the risk of line infection which can be life threatening. Your PH doctor may allow you to disconnect from the pump for certain medical procedures or tests, but keeping everything sterile is extremely important to avoid line infections. Please get specific instructions from your PH Center before attempting this!

Dosage. The goal of dosing Remodulin is to improve the symptoms of the disease while minimizing excessive side effects. The dose is individualized for each patient. There are two variables to consider: the concentration and the pump rate. Remodulin comes in four concentrations (1 mg/ml, 2.5 mg/ml, 5 mg/ml and 10 mg/ml). As your doctor raises your dose, he/she will increase the concentration so the syringe will last 3 days. When you change to a higher concentration, you lower the pump rate and then work the rate up as needed to control PAH symptoms. Dr. Adaani Frost (Baylor College of Medicine, Houston) has found that

patients seem to have less site pain at a lower volume (pump rate) even if the concentration is higher.

Researchers in the U.K. reported successfully transitioning a patient with severe "PPH" from intravenous iloprost to subcutaneous treprostinil. The estimated dose equivalence was 1:2.5 (ng/kg-per-min). (Intravenous iloprost is not available in the U.S.)

Side effects. The systemic side effects are about the same as with Flolan, but may be less severe. After using the drug subcutaneously for 6 to 18 months, 30 to 50 percent of Dr. Frost's patients had some jaw pain with the first bite. After 5 months some had mild diarrhea. One patient, Johnny, reports much less jaw pain on IV Remodulin compared to Flolan. A minority experience flushing, headache, nausea, rash, dizziness, edema, itching, or hypotension. There are patient reports of troublesome foot pain similar to Flolan and rare cases of generalized body pain.

The bad news: SC site pain. Eighty-five percent of users report pain where the drug enters their body. It's their biggest complaint about SC Remodulin. Since IV Remodulin goes directly into the blood stream, like Flolan, there is no pain from the drug at its injection site. Doctors don't know why SC site pain happens, but they have a variety of options to help alleviate it. In the big international study, 8 percent of patients dropped out of the trial early because they couldn't tolerate the pain at any reasonable dose. Many doctors don't think site pain is dose related. Others disagree. What is known is that the sensation of pain varies dramatically from patient to patient, and even from site to site on the same patient. The nurse coordinators at your PH Center and the Specialty Pharmacy nurses play a very important role here. With their close support you may be able to solve the pain problem, even if, at first, you think you can't.

The pain is not continuous. After a few

months many patients seem to tolerate the pain better, maybe because they are feeling so much better. Some patients do not have any pain at 6 months, even though they are using four times their original dose. The pain is usually worse the second and third day after a site change. In a European study they found that leaving the site in longer when it "feels good" is beneficial. Incidentally, the amount of redness doesn't correlate with the amount of pain.

Controlling site pain. There are almost as many different possible pain remedies as there are SC Remodulin patients. No one treatment seems to work for everybody, so you need to try many different things. Your PH nurse is your first resource for dealing with site pain. He/she will give you a number of potential pain remedies to try when you start this therapy. Also, you can talk to another SC Remodulin patient either through United Therapeutics Peer-to-Peer program (www.peernetwork.com) or at your local support group for suggestions.

There are three categories of strategies for controlling site pain: site selection, topical measures and oral medications. The most effective thing to do for relief is to try to find a site where there isn't much pain, and then stick with that area for a while. During the clinical trials, patients were told to change their site every 3 days, but most PH nurses and doctors now allow patients to stick with good sites for up to 2-4 weeks. The site does not have to be on your tummy. The needle can go in anywhere you have fat, be it an arm, a leg, or your fanny (a breast isn't recommended). Some women find that their outer thighs or hips are less painful. And we've heard of a guy who finds his lower back surprisingly pain-free. Because the site swells, you may want to have some clothes on hand that are a size larger than you usually wear. Also make sure you don't place the site right under your waistband. There are different types of catheters and different lengths. Ask your PH

center or Specialty Pharmacy nurse about trying another type of catheter. Make sure the needle does not go into the muscle. If that happens the pain is usually immediate and unrelenting. If you are thin, you may have to pinch up some skin to place the needle in a pocket on top of the muscle. Avoid stretch marks as those areas are more painful. Most people find the area right around their belly button to be more sensitive and the sides of their abdomen less sensitive.

Topical remedies are things applied directly to the skin. They range from home remedies to over-the-counter preparations to prescription drugs. One of the simplest and most effective remedies is applying ice packs or hot packs to the site. Susan loves the freezer packs that come with epoprostenol; she says they fit right under her undies. Another effective ice pack is to freeze a folded wet washcloth in a sandwich bag. Let it soften a little out of the freezer and lay it over the painful site. Over-the-counter remedies that help some patients include Preparation H, arnica oil, aloe vera gel, Icy-Hot and other similar products. There are some topical remedies that require a prescription from your doctor. Nasocort spray applied to the site prior to needle insertion helps some patients, perhaps by decreasing the inflammation caused by the drug. Spray once or twice after you've cleaned the injection spot and let dry, then insert the needle. One patient sprayed it in her nose as directed on the package and it didn't help her site pain at all! Lidocaine in the form of patches or in creams may help. It is also used in combination with other ingredients in Zonalon or EMLA cream. One patient finds that a tad of prescription Zonalon cream really helps her with the pain that lingers for 12 hours or so at an old site after the catheter is withdrawn.

An open-label 12-week study funded by United Therapeutics found that pluronic lecithin organogel (PLO) gels (a gooey substance that when mixed with another medicine, helps the medicine go right through your skin) seemed safe and provided pain relief and healing especially at old infusion sites. Most patients were helped by a gel that carried 10 percent Ketoprofen, 5 percent Lidocaine, and 6 percent gabapentin (Neurontin). A couple of patients needed 5 percent Ketamine added to the mix. Ketamine skin allergies are not uncommon, so if your redness or rash seems to increase this may be the cause. Ask for the PLO gel without Ketamine.

Oral pain remedies often help. You don't want to use aspirin or other NSAIDs because they increase the risk of bleeding and also have some anti-prostacyclin effects and can increase fluid retention. Over-the-counter loratidine can help with inflammation or itching at the site. Finally, there are prescription medications to try. Antidepressants like amitriptyline (Elavil) may increase the pain threshold in some patients, meaning it increases their pain tolerance. Others use the anti-seizure medicine gabapentin (Neurontin) or the newer Lyrica, since the pain may be neuropathic in origin. Several centers report that the non-narcotic Ultram (tramadol) is quite effective in some patients and is not habit forming.

A few patients need stronger opioid (narcotic) painkillers. Doctors vary in their willingness to prescribe narcotics for use over a long period of time; some worry about patients becoming physically or psychologically dependent on the drug. Side effects of opioids may include constipation, sleepiness, or nausea One appropriate time to use them might be when you need to increase your dose of Remodulin. Patients report that it helps to take a little narcotic beforehand and to plan to do the increase on a calm day.

Fight fire with fire? If you are the wild and crazy type, you might try eating a lot of hot peppers for a while. Why? Because they contain capsicum, and capsicum depletes a substance that might be causing the pain. (Better run this plan past your doctor first.) If you try the Capsicum Cure, post a note on PHA's message board! What is "a lot" of peppers? Nobody knows. Don't eat so many you get sick. Remember that peppers burn as much going out as coming in and may cause diarrhea, which is already a problem for some Remodulin patients. Maybe this depletion theory is why some people who have been on Remodulin for a long time (without resorting to peppers) no longer have as much pain. It isn't known if this is really true, but a PH doc has wondered aloud if it might be so.

Other things to try include guided imagery, relaxation therapy, acupuncture or acupressure. With their doctor's permission, some SC patients take a soak in the tub for 20 minutes between site changes, with no catheter in place. Have your new infusion ready to go so you can insert it as soon as you come out of the tub.

With regard to a milder sort of site problem: if you get a rash under the little plastic wings that fit against your flesh, try leaving the paper on. Another suggestion is to use a duoderm dressing as a layer between the catheter wings and your skin.

Cost. An analysis in 2003 by Dr. Highland and published in CHEST reported estimated costs for the three available drugs at that time, Tracleer, SC Remodulin (9.3 ng/kg-per-min) and IV Flolan (9.2 ng/kg-per-min). They calculated the total cost for 1 year of each, including things like the monthly blood tests for Tracleer and pump and supplies for Remodulin and Flolan. The 3 day hospitalization cost for intensive training and 6 home health visits were assessed for both Remodulin and Flolan equally. At that time, the annual costs were $36,208 for Tracleer, $89,038 for SC Remodulin and $73,790 for IV Flolan. Currently, most SC Remodulin patients are started at home, not in the hospital. Although this analysis did include the initial Hickman catheter for IV Flolan it did not account for line infections or catheter problems. It also did not include medication costs to treat SC Remodulin site pain.

In 2004, IV Remodulin was approved. While a total cost associated with IV Remodulin has not been published, the monthly cost for the medication can range from approximately $10,000 to $20,000 per month, depending on the dosage amount.

Switching to Remodulin from Flolan and vice-versa. Many patients have switched between Flolan, SC and IV Remodulin. Patients who have had multiple line infections with either IV therapy have changed to SC Remodulin. Patients who cannot tolerate the site pain from SC Remodulin have changed to IV Flolan or Remodulin. Patients on IV Flolan have changed to IV Remodulin for simpler mixing procedures, avoiding the ice packs and to use miniature pumps. Studies have shown that patients requiring transition from Flolan have been successful. There are several ways to transition patients from Flolan including a "gradual transition" or a "rapid switch". Your physician has access to the transition protocols.

Used as a combination drug. When adding bosentan or sildenafil to a Remodulin user's regimen, it may be necessary to lower the dose of Remodulin to avoid increased side effects. Sometimes oral therapies are added to try to decrease the Remodulin dose if there are severe side effects or SC site pain. (See the section on Combination Therapy.)

Accredo Therapeutics, Caremark, and CuraScript provide PH patients with Remodulin. You don't have to be hospitalized to get started on SC Remodulin, although you will need some outpatient training and

monitoring. Starting IV Remodulin is similar to starting Flolan. Initial dosing and up titration can vary from center to center. It is up to your PH center to give you detailed instructions on how to take this medicine. Accredo Therapeutics' number for Remodulin problems is: 1-866-344-4874 (1-866-FIGHT PH). Caremark's number is 1-866-879-2348. CuraScript's number is 1-866-4-PH-TEAM (1-866-474-8326). These numbers should be on a sticker on your pump in case of an emergency. Ask your PH nurse which number to call if you're not sure.

A final word of advice on Remodulin: avoid the midnight plunge. Remodulin pumps-so small that they fit neatly in the pocket of a nightshirt-have a habit of landing in the loo. They usually survive. Ask your PH nurse what to do should your pump take the plunge (it happens during the groggy hours in the middle of the night, so please ask in advance of need). It might be best to clip the pump to your pj's.

Inhaled or oral treprostinil. Clinical trials for an inhaled form of treprostinil are well underway; in fact, enrollment in these studies has closed. A placebo controlled multi-center trial of an oral form of treprostinil (you take pills twice a day) is now underway.

Comparing PH Drugs: Epoprostenol (Flolan), Treprostinil (Remodulin), Bosentan (Tracleer), Sildenafil (Revatio), Ambrisentan (Letairis), & Iloprost (Ventavis)

Although patients often want to know which PH drug is better, it is a little like comparing apples to oranges. It is very difficult to compare a continuous prostanoid to oral therapy. No scientific comparative clinical trials have been done directly comparing any PAH therapies.

In the previous edition of the *Survival*

Guide, we tried to provide detailed comparative information about the different PH treatments, and included some of the results of the clinical trials that studied these drugs individually. It is clear that this is a dangerous and often misleading way to compare these drugs. The Scientific Leadership Council (SLC) of PHA has weighed in on this issue and agrees that it is best for patients to discuss the relative merits of these therapies for their specific case with their health care provider. Certainly, what is best for one patient may not be appropriate for another. Some patients may "push the envelope" by reviewing and discussing the available evidence for each PH treatment with their treating physician, but again this is an individual preference and should not be generalized to all PH patients.

PH is a chronic, long-term disease requiring long term therapy. Things other than how far you can walk in 6 minutes also matter, such as side effects, lifestyle, your individual response to a medication, how you feel on a drug, and cost. Combinations of these and other drugs may work even better. You and your PH team will have to look at the advantages and disadvantages for *you* for each possible approach.

Lines and Pumps

Intravenous Flolan and Remodulin (collectively known as prostanoids) both require a permanent tunneled intravenous catheter. It is made of pliable silicone, and is inserted while in an operating room, with local anesthetic. The catheter is inserted into a large vein, either in your neck or under your collar bone. The end of the catheter that connects to tubing from the pump is then tunneled for several inches under the skin and exits the body at your chest to the right or left of the breastbone (sternum), above your breasts. The tunneling helps to hold the catheter in place and reduce the risk of infection. The hub or end connector is then put on the end of the catheter. Once it has been in

place for awhile, most patients say they don't feel it. You can shower if you properly protect it, but not swim. You can bathe if you keep the catheter exit site above water. It is important to protect the connection between the catheter and the tubing from water as this can be an entrance point for bacteria.

There are several types of catheters in general use: Hickmans, Groshongs, and Broviacs. Groshongs have a valve on the end of the catheter that closes if the infusion stops, so blood doesn't back up. Catheters come with single or double lumens (channels inside a tube). If you have to flush your catheter often, double lumens are more trouble and cause more infections. Also, if you have a little hole in your own cardiac plumbing there is a risk that dangerous air bubbles could pass into blood vessels leading to your brain during flushing. Therefore, most doctors prefer single lumen catheters for PH patients.

In rare cases, such as when a patient needs repeated blood draws and doesn't have good veins, a double lumen may be the catheter of choice, because blood can be drawn through the other lumen. Two lumens could be useful if one clots off, which can occur, but clotting of the tube is unusual with IV prostanoids, and most PH doctors prefer the single lumen because of the reduced risk of infection.

Catheters have two fuzzy "cuffs" to help keep them in place. Normally, the cuffs are inside your body. If one cuff slips out, secure your line with a safety loop and watch it more carefully. Do not try to push the line back in; this could cause infection. If both cuffs come out, the entire line might come out soon, so you should call your doctor.

There are also PICC lines (Peripherally Inserted Central Catheter lines) that go into an arm. The dressings on them only need to be changed once a week and they may have a lower infection rate. But unlike Hickmans, Groshongs, and Broviacs, PICC lines need to be replaced often, and they are therefore not recommended for long term use. If the permanent catheter needs to be removed because of an infection, a temporary dual-lumen PICC is often placed for the IV prostanoid and antibiotics. Once the infection is cleared a new permanent catheter is placed and the PICC is removed.

A note for women: before your catheter is inserted, think about the types of clothes and bras you like to wear, and ask the doctor to take that into consideration when the two of you agree on where the catheter should exit your body. It may be wise to have your bra on when the insertion and exit sites are selected.

Recognizing infection and acting quickly. Central line delivery systems offer germs an easy way to get into your body; they average infections every 2 to 4 years. Every patient is different, though, and some get no infections and others get a lot. If not quickly treated, infections can be life-threatening. If you see any sign of infection (see below), get to a doctor. If a primary care doctor is treating you, ask your PH specialist to give him/her an infection-treatment protocol. Infections can be local, involving the exit site or tunnel or in the blood stream, involving the catheter tip. Local infections are less serious and can sometimes be treated with oral antibiotics, but both should be taken seriously. Infections that start out as minor can become very serious if not aggressively treated early.

Signs of a localized infection are: redness, pain, discharge (pus), or swelling around the spot where the central line exits your body.

Signs of a tunnel infection: Tunnel infections are more serious and may require

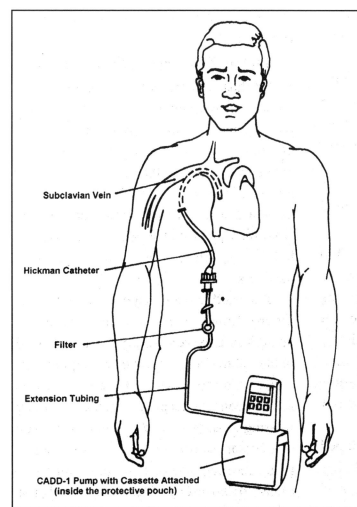

Subclavian Vein

Hickman Catheter

Filter

Extension Tubing

CADD-1 Pump with Cassette Attached
(inside the protective pouch)

Placement of the Catheter for Flolan Infusion

Patients say they no longer feel the catheter once the entrance site has healed. The broken line indicates where the tubing is hidden inside the body.

Illustration by Andrea Rich.

removal of the catheter. You may have a fever and drainage at the exit site. The tunnel area (from the catheter exit site up to your shoulder or neck) is usually red, swollen and painful.

Signs of a generalized infection (sepsis) are: fever, shaking chills, sweats and feeling very weak and ill. Sometimes blood infections are subtle, and can be easily misdiagnosed. Some patients just feel "icky": tired, nauseated, with achy flu-like symptoms, or can have changes in mental functioning such as confusion. Once infections get into the catheter itself, your catheter usually must be replaced (the nasty bugs can form a slimy wall called a "biofilm" around themselves that keeps an antibiotic at bay while the germs work their way along the catheter's wall-ick!).

The first thing the doctor should do if you have an infection is to culture it. This is very important. Drainage from the exit site can be sent on a swab to the lab for culture. Drawing blood cultures from the catheter must be done carefully and quickly so that the infusion is stopped for the shortest possible time. The catheter must be refilled (primed) with IV prostanoid when restarting the pump. Otherwise, it would take many minutes for the drug to reach your blood stream and you may have serious PH symptoms from the lack of IV prostanoid. Once cultures are done, your doctor will then make a guess as to which organism is causing the infection and start you on an antibiotic. When the culture results come back, your doctor can always change the antibiotic if necessary.

Wash away your troubles before they get a toehold. Before working with an IV prostanoid or the catheter, or changing your dressing, use liquid antimicrobial soap to meticulously wash the table or tray you are using as well as your hands. Wipe your work surface with alcohol and let it air dry. Use paper rather than cloth towels. Follow sterile and clean techniques (ask your PH nurse for more detailed instructions). Take off your ring and watch and dig into those creases on your knuckles and under your nails. It takes at least a full minute to do a good job. Don't touch the sink handle after you wash; shut off the sink with a fresh paper towel. Once you're aware of clean and sterile techniques, it becomes a habit. (A side benefit: you'll get fewer colds.)

Many PH physicians recommend that women on IV prostanoids keep their fingernails short and avoid artificial nails. This is because fungus can live under those nail tips and it's harder to clean long fingernails. Chipped nail polish can also harbor fungus and bacteria. Most hospitals prohibit staff with direct patient contact from having artificial nails or even long fingernails because of infection risk to patients.

Avoid touching the catheter site with your fingers. It's a good idea to put on sterile gloves after you wash your hands and to use a sterile swab stick to apply topical antibiotics or antiseptics. Your Specialty Pharmacy can supply central line dressing kits with all the needed supplies in one package. Some centers advise against antibiotic-containing ointments like Neosporin, because bugs become resistant to the medicine in them.

IV Remodulin users may be more prone to infections with bacteria that live in water. At the University of Colorado Children's Hospital, patients use a special technique to prevent bacteria from entering. A closed end cap (BD Q-Syte) is screwed on to the catheter hub and is changed weekly and as needed. Because there is a little gap where the tubing screws together, water can collect there during your shower. When you disconnect the tubing, bacteria in the water can then enter the catheter channel. To

PHA maintains a great deal of information on our website, www.PHAssociation.org. If you are interested in learning more about the availability of treatments around the world, the most updated information can be found in our Therapies Around the World List at www.PHAssociation.org/wwtherapies/.

prevent this, they have patients use Glad Press and Seal while showering or bathing. Tear off a piece of the wrap, fold over both ends to create tabs, sandwich the connection and press the film to make a water tight seal. Wait at least 3 hours after the shower to peel off the film (using those handy tabs you made when you applied the wrap). This makes it important to time tubing changes after your shower. The Children's Hospital also puts a tiny amount of bleach (1/2 tsp to ½ tub-full) in the kids' bath water to kill those water loving bugs. These changes have lowered infection rates for their patients on both IV Flolan and Remodulin.

Dr. Dianne Zwicke at St. Luke's Medical Center, Milwaukee, has her patients disinfect their shower head with a weak bleach solution. Detachable shower heads are soaked in a bucket of bleach solution for 20 minutes every month. If the shower head cannot be removed, the bleach solution is put in a plastic bag and wrapped around the shower head and tied securely. Let the shower run for a few minutes before getting in to avoid getting bleach on you.

Dressing options. The site should be covered with a new sterile bandage. Different patients may require different dressings. There are many to choose from, should you develop an allergy to a particular dressing. Doctors often suggest a transparent dressing like Tegaderm that needs less frequent changing because you can see signs of infection right through it (but if you have been sweating, you will still need to change it daily). Patients who are allergic to Tegaderm may have better luck with Mipore dressings. Another allergy-prone patient adores Tegaderm. It's an individual thing. Allergy-prone patients might also try Primapore pads. Telfa pads and burn dressings don't stick well. A biopatch made by Johnson & Johnson that contains chlorhexidine may help cut the risk of infection. Those with sensitive skin might try a dry, sterile drain dressing with a hole for the tube held in place with paper tape, or knee and

elbow bandages with non-stick pads. Hypafix tape is good for sensitive skin (and is particularly good for making the safety loop).

Many PH centers have changed from povidone-iodine (Betadine) to chlorhexadine (Chloraprep) in response to CDC recommendations. Betadine may still be used by patients who are allergic to Chloraprep. If you are using Betadine, substitute 3 cleanings with 3 Betadine swabs for the Chloraprep step in the procedure below. Each central line dressing kit contains:

> 1 Tegaderm dressing, 4 X 4.75
> 2 4x4 nonwoven gauze dressings
> 1 package of 3 alcohol swabsticks
> 1 pair gloves made of nitrile, not latex, and power free
> 1 earloop mask
> 1 label to mark time and date dressing changed, if Tegaderm used
> 1 1x4 roll of Transpore tape
> 1 Chloraprep applicator containing 3 ml Chloraprep
> 1 folded sterile wrap, 17" x 19"

The 12-step Chloraprep program:
1. Clean your work surface and wash hands.
2. Remove old dressing, taking care not to pull on central line. Peel from edges with one hand while slightly pushing on actual insertion site.
3. Open central line dressing kit using sterile technique. Open Tegaderm dressing (if applicable).
4. Put on mask.
5. Put on sterile gloves.
6. Position supplies so you can easily remove what is needed from your sterile field.
7. Open sterile packets of alcohol swabsticks.
8. Begin cleansing your skin at the central line insertion site using an alcohol

swabstick. Clean in a circular motion, tarting from the center and working out. Repeat twice. Allow to dry. **Do not** blow on site or wave a piece of paper to dry the area faster.

9. Pinch the wings on the Chloraprep applicator. **Do not** touch the sponge. Wet the sponge by repeatedly pressing and releasing the sponge against the insertion site until it is visible on the skin. Cleanse in a circular motion starting from the center and working out.

10. Allow the Chloraprep to dry thoroughly. Again, do not blow on it or wave a piece of paper.

11. Inspect your skin around the insertion site for redness, unusual swelling, any drainage, or pain.

12. Apply the dressing over the insertion site. Place the center of the dressing on first, smoothing the dressing from the center out to the ends.

Safety loop. As a final step to changing your dressing, make a "safety loop" of tubing and tape it to your chest in several places. This way, if there is a tug on the line it will pull the loop, not pull out the catheter. Talk to your PH nurse or doctor for more information on how to create a "safety loop."

Pumps. CADD-1 infusion pumps have been replaced by the *CADD-Legacy 1 pumps*, which have better technology and safety features. This pump is used for both Flolan and IV Remodulin. Your old tubing and cassettes will work with the new pump. If your PH doc approves, change batteries every Monday and tubing Monday, Wednesday and Friday. Some patients find the alarms on the Legacy pump too sensitive, alarming with leaning over or fastening a seatbelt.

The CRONO-5 pump (marketed in the US by Intrapump) is a miniature pump that can be used for IV Remodulin. The medication is mixed in either a 10 or 20 ml syringe. The battery lasts for one month. The tubing is the same as that used with the CADD pump. This pump is good for patients with very active lifestyles, or patients who have difficulty carrying the heavier CADD pump. It is a little more complex to program and medication cannot be taken out of the syringe to prime the Hickman after drawing blood cultures or after a new catheter is placed. (It's very easy to take a little medication out of the CADD cassette for this purpose.) Because the medication is more concentrated than in the CADD pump, care must be taken never to get an accidental bolus of medication. The pump rate is also much slower than with the CADD, so priming a new or "empty" Hickman catheter is even more important than with the CADD because it will take longer for the medication to reach the bloodstream. On the plus side, the pump is small enough to fit into a pocket or cell phone case and light enough so that patients don't notice its weight while walking.

MiniMed 407 C: The Medtronic MiniMed pump used mainly for subcutaneous Remodulin is much smaller than the CADD pump, no bigger than a pocket-sized pager (it was developed for delivering insulin to diabetics). Because the pump is so small, it's easy to conceal. Also, it doesn't make the whirring noise the CADD pumps periodically make. Three watch-type batteries last for one month. Although the pump shouldn't get wet, Medtronic MiniMed makes a waterproof pack, called a Sport Guard that can be used for swimming. Use Vaseline around the edges of the Sport Guard to get a tight seal. It is okay to get the site wet; just keep the pump dry.

CADD-MS 3 pump: This pump is similar to the MiniMed 407 C in that it uses a 3 ml syringe reservoir of medication. It is used for subcutaneous Remodulin and will eventually replace the older 407 C pump that is no longer supported by Medtronic. The same subcutaneous catheters and tubing work with this newer pump.

Carefully selected patients, including some very carefully selected children on IV Remodulin, are now using the MiniMed 407 C or the CADD MS 3 pumps. The 3 ml syringe reservoir holds *undiluted* medication and less than a teaspoon a day is infused through the MiniMed pump. Therefore, the small pump is not for all patients and clotting of the line is a potential serious problem because the line cannot be flushed with this very concentrated Remodulin solution when using the MiniMed pump. Until specialists have more experience using this infusion technique, it must be stressed that the MiniMed pump should be used only in selected patients and only at centers with experience in using it with IV Remodulin.

I-Neb: The device used for inhaled iloprost is called the I-Neb adaptive aerosol device made by Respironics. It runs on rechargeable batteries that are good for about 40 treatments. The nebulizer senses when you take a breath and only delivers medication when you inhale. It currently takes about 10-12 minutes to inhale the standard 5 mcg dose. The medication is nebulized through a mesh that makes very tiny particles that get carried deep into your lungs with each breath. Cleaning the mesh lids must be done with Dawn dishwashing soap and *distilled* water so that the calcium in hard tap water doesn't clog up the tiny holes in the mesh. A new protocol is being introduced that allows for cleaning all the mesh lids at once at the end of the day, saving about 1 hour per day on time

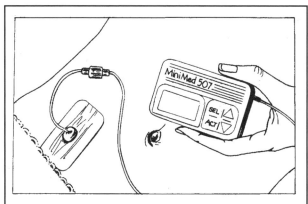

This drawing shows one possible entry site for the Remodulin catheter. The pump itself is small enough to be tucked into a pocket, fanny pack, or sport bra.

Illustration by Andrea Rich.

spent cleaning. Once a week, all parts (other than the motor) are boiled in distilled water. A study is currently underway using a higher power setting that shortens treatment times to about 3-4 minutes. So far, it seems that patients can tolerate the faster delivery of medication. Data from this study will go to the FDA to get approval to change to the higher power setting, hopefully in 2008.

If an emergency occurs. Because of its short half-life, sudden stopping of Flolan is a 911 emergency. Even though the half-life of IV Remodulin is longer, physicians usually recommend treating sudden stopping of IV Remodulin as an emergency, too. Depending on how close you live to an ER or if no one can drive you, IV Remodulin users may need to call 911 to get to the hospital ER. We would not recommend that you drive yourself to the ER.

There is a "How to Handle IV Emergencies" chart at the back of this book!

Keep the number of your Specialty Pharmacy on your pump. Occasionally you may be put on hold. While you are waiting, you can look at Nurse Cathy Anderson-Severson's "How to Handle IV Emergencies," chart, which tells you what to do when particular catheter complications occur. If you have to go directly to the hospital, call your Specialty Pharmacy as soon as you can, using a cell phone or the hospital's phone.

Before you actually need them, let your local 911 responders (probably the fire department) know about your medical condition and medications. Some patients go right to the firehouse themselves to show the firefighters how to help them. Have your PH doctor or health service company brief the nearest emergency room (or provide you with written instructions to show them).

You should know how to do a temporary repair of a damaged catheter (one with a cut, tear, or hole in it) yourself, and stock the repair kit and other necessary supplies. Note that a damaged catheter is an infection risk, so after you've made the repair, call your PH doctor so a permanent fix or new catheter can be arranged.

Wear a MedicAlert bracelet and put a warning on your pump so emergency medical personnel won't stop it. In all probability, they will never before have seen a patient like you, and will make all kinds of dangerous assumptions. Keep a current dosing sheet, list of *all* your meds, and contact information for your PH physician in a sealed plastic bag with your pump. It's hard to think clearly in an emergency; the list will help.

Be prepared for natural disasters: ask your power and phone company for priority help in event of an outage, and keep an emergency kit and medical supplies on hand. Keep an extra pump on hand, as well as fresh batteries, tubing, flushing supplies, dressing supplies, and perhaps an emergency supply of oxygen in case your delivery system breaks down. If you are going quite a ways from your home, your doctor may suggest you take along a little duffel bag with back-up supplies and a pump. Pat Paton, a founder of PHA, keeps a 3-day supply of Flolan, dressings, etc. in an orange plastic cleaning caddy in her hall closet. When she and her husband Jerry have to evacuate quickly (because of Florida hurricanes, medical emergencies, etc.) she grabs the caddy or asks someone else to. It has been a lifesaver.

Hints from fellow patients for IV prostanoid users:

If you go outside in **freezing weather**, protect your pump and tubing from extreme cold. After Flolan is mixed with the buffer solution it can freeze, which isn't good for it or for you.

Avoid sitting out in the sun and shun tanning booths! Not only does prostacyclin make you more sensitive to sunlight, but warming you up also warms the Flolan and makes it less effective.

Make sure there's a "concentration sticker" on your pump telling how many nanograms are to be delivered at what rate. If it's out of date, scratch out the old figures and write in the new. This could save your life in an emergency.

When mixing Flolan lay the vials on their sides after extracting the fluid, so you can easily see if all of the drug has been withdrawn, and which vials are empty.

When traveling, keep your meds and medical paraphernalia within reach-if you check your Flolan as baggage, it might get too hot or cold in cargo, or end up freezing in Fargo while you're frying in Fresno. If you plan to use airplane ice to cool your Flolan cassette, put the cassette in double Ziploc bags, so it doesn't get wet.

Dry Ice while traveling? To keep your ice packs from melting when traveling, ask your doctor if it's okay to put them on Dry Ice in an ice chest (don't put your meds directly on Dry Ice because they will freeze-Dry Ice is more than minus 109.3 degrees Fahrenheit!). Some airlines use Dry Ice to keep ice cream frozen, and may give some to Flolan users.

Free bubble wrap pads. If the ice pack feels too cold against your body, try the bubble wrap stuff that has foil on both sides. It's used to insulate heating and air conditioning ducts. Larry Moody, whose background is in engineering, is the one who discovered how useful this material can be to Flolan users. (His wife, Karen, uses Flolan and had complained of cold legs.) Karen and Larry will send epoprostenol users a pair of pads (or replacement pads) for free. Just send them a request by e-mail or snail mail, along with a single postage stamp, if you can. Contact them at: LarryMoody@direcway.com, or write Larry & Karen Moody, 8268 Stillwater Blvd. N., Lake Elmo, MN 55042. He and Karen have given out hundreds of pairs of pads! Larry says, "In its own little way [giving out pads] gives us a sense of community, while being otherwise surrounded/isolated among people who don't understand this disease."

If you have an MRI scan, keep your pump outside the magnetic field by using several sets of tubing, so its program won't be erased. Some hospitals have an MRI compatible pump that you can be temporarily switched to while you undergo a scan. Be sure to discuss with your PH center if you are having an MRI to have proper arrangements made. Some physicians may allow Remodulin users to disconnect from the pump for the scan. Do not do this without specific instructions from your doctor.

How to reduce pulling. Women might try wrapping the tubing around the middle of their bra. One user clips an ID badge holder (one with an alligator clip) to her collar and runs her line through it. "There have been so many times when the tube has hooked on a door knob, or the arm of a chair, or the dog's floppy ear," she says.

What to do at night. Some hang their pump on the headboard; some tuck it in a partially open night-stand drawer. Make a safety loop with your tubing so if you get up to use the john and forget the pump you will tug at the loop, not the catheter. Some use a tape tab with a safety pin to fasten their line to their pajamas. If your ice pack melts during the night, try using a soft-sided cooler with extra ice packs.

Using IV prostanoids means **keeping track of a lot of times and dates**. Get a calendar or date book, or use the date book on your computer, to note days to change your dose or SC (subcutaneous) site, do a flush, check your

INR, and to record problems or side effects (so you can later tell your doctor). Also jot down the number of days of battery use, tubing use, and site bandage changes.

Once a week fill seven sealable plastic bags, one for each day, with the supplies you will need to mix up your Flolan. When you're ready to mix, just grab a bag.

Combination Therapy

For patients who remain symptomatic on their initial PH therapy, opportunities are now available to add a second drug or third drug to try to improve one's exercise tolerance and symptoms. This is particularly the case if you've had some response to your initial therapy but the response is not satisfactory. However, it isn't as simple as just adding another drug to an existing regimen. Without controlled studies, we don't know what will happen when we add that second or third drug. For example, what, if any, will the additional benefits be, and to which types of patients? What will the side effects be and are they manageable? Is there any impact to other bodily systems? What are the drug interactions? What are the long-term effects? Also, without clinical evidence to support a combination therapy, problems getting insurance approval for one or more of the drugs in the combination therapy can arise.

In most other medical conditions where multiple mechanisms have been identified, such as left-sided heart failure, combinations of drugs have proven to be more effective in treating disease. Unfortunately, there have not been sufficient studies to prove this in the treatment of pulmonary hypertension. In the past, once drug companies got FDA approval for their drug, there was little interest in combination trials. Because combination therapy is now becoming so widespread, it is very important to gather data to provide evidence to support combination therapy. Maybe because of the high PH drug costs and insurance approval issues, we're now seeing more interest in these combination drug clinical trials. Some of these trials are extensions of an earlier trial, sometimes referred to as Phase IV clinical trials. Some of these combination trials begin directly after FDA approval. Some trials are undertaken by research hospitals. Fortunately, results from some of these trials are trickling in.

In addition to these clinical trials, we are hoping to get some valuable information from the REVEAL Registry analysis. Data are being collected and analyzed through the REVEAL Registry which includes information on more than 3000 patients who have WHO Group 1 PAH. Among the plethora of data are the medication histories of all these patients. Hopefully, the registry will provide information about how PAH patients are being treated. The first descriptive papers from this registry are expected in 2008. Through these clinical trials and the REVEAL Registry analysis, we're getting information on the important aspects of the various combination therapies that help us and our doctors to make better, safer and more informed decisions about our care.

Prostanoids in combination therapy. There are several clinical trials investigating a combination of one of the prostanoids (epoprostenol, IV treprostinil, SC treprostinil, inhaled treprostinil, oral treprostinil, inhaled iloprost) with either an ERA (bosentan, ambrisentan, sitaxsentan) or a PDE-5 inhibitor (sildenafil, tadalafil).

Through several trials, we found that generally, when oral PAH medications (either ERAs or PDE-5 inhibitors) are added to prostanoids, there may be an increase in prostanoid side effects, especially if the prostanoid dose is high. This may require a decrease in dose of the prostanoid medication if the side effects cannot be managed.

In the BREATHE-2 study, Bosentan was added to patients stable on Flolan. This was a small study that showed no significant difference

in 6-minute walk distance between the patients on Flolan plus placebo versus the patients on Flolan plus bosentan. The study did, however, provide evidence that this combination was well tolerated.

One retrospective study focused on children with IPAH and PAH associated with congenital heart disease or connective tissue disease who started bosentan with or without IV epoprostenol or subcutaneous treprostinil. It was found that functional class improved in 46% of the patients and stayed the same in 44% of the patients. Hemodynamics were also improved. At 1 year 98% of the patients were alive and at 2 years 91% of the patients remained alive.

In 2006, the results of the small German COMBI trial were presented. The COMBI trial studied the addition of bosentan to inhaled iloprost. 40 patients were randomly assigned to either of two groups: one that was to take bosentan alone or one that was to take both bosentan and iloprost. The trial was open-label and not placebo-controlled. The trial showed no benefit and was stopped early. Three patients in the group that took both bosentan and iloprost suffered severe clinical worsening. It is not clear whether the addition of iloprost caused the worsening, or that these patients had a more severe case of PH or that there was some other related or unrelated reason for the worsening. The study's researchers stated that a larger study may be necessary to conclusively prove whether or not the combination therapy is beneficial.

Shortly after the release of the COMBI trial results, came the results of a small U.S. trial which also studied the safety and efficacy of adding inhaled iloprost to an existing regimen of bosentan. The study followed 67 patients over 12 weeks in a double-blind trial where patients were randomly assigned to either of two groups: bosentan with inhaled iloprost or bosentan with inhaled placebo. In this clinical trial, the researchers found that the iloprost/bosentan combination therapy was well tolerated, that patients' 6-minute walk distance improved, and that both the mean PAPs and PVRs of participants were reduced when iloprost was added.

In the PACES study, Flolan patients who added sildenafil showed decreased clinical worsening with the combination and walked 40 meters farther in 6 minutes than they had at the start of the trial. This study is now in the open label extension phase. Almost all of these patients are on 80 mg of sildenafil three-times-a-day. It is not yet known when the extension trial will close or when data from that trial will be available.

In a small German study, the combination of sildenafil with aerosolized iloprost lowered mean PAPs and PVRs significantly more than did each as a single agent.

In 2006, Actelion sponsored a large trial (VISION) to look at the combination of inhaled iloprost with sildenafil. The study intends to determine if adding inhaled iloprost to an existing sildenafil regimen can reduce the number of iloprost inhalations patients take per day.

Both the inhaled treprostinil (TRIUMPH) and oral UT-15 (FREEDOM) trials are enrolling patients who are on one or both of sildenafil and an ERA (either bosentan or ambrisentan).

Dr. Gomberg-Maitland studied the addition of sildenafil to patients on treprostinil and found the combination improved exercise capacity and was well tolerated in a small group of patients.

Bosentan in combination therapy. A small laboratory study of bosentan and sildenafil taken together has shown an increased blood level of bosentan and a decrease by 50% in sildenafil levels. Although this interaction does not appear to be clinically significant, it may have implications for low doses of sildenafil (20 mg may not be enough in combination with bosentan) and risk of LFT (liver function test) abnormalities. If you are taking both drugs and were thinking you could skip the occasional blood test for your LFTs, think again.

A larger study, conducted by Pfizer COMPASS-2, is investigating the efficacy of the combination of sildenafil with bosentan. The trial is still enrolling patients but is expecting enrollment to be completed in the near future.

Ambrisentan in combination therapy. Currently a multicenter open label clinical trial is underway that is studying the addition of ambrisentan to patients taking sildenafil, epoprostenol, treprostinil and/or iloprost. Patients may be on various combinations of background therapies (for example, sildenafil plus epoprostenol) or ambrisentan may be their first PAH therapy.

Tadalafil in combination therapy. The tadalafil trial is enrolling patients on bosentan and patients new to PAH therapy. This trial will provide data on the combination of tadalafil and bosentan. This trial is currently in the extension phase, where patients are either on 20 or 40 mg daily; after 1 year all patients will go to 40 mg daily of tadalafil. No patients on prostanoids, however, are in this trial.

Looking Ahead: A Cure? Ideas on the Horizon

So much wonderful research is underway that it is now rational to believe that in the not-too-distant future PH can be licked, not just subdued. Cooperation among PH centers (facilitated by PHA's Scientific Leadership Council) has greatly sped the learning process.

A multi-pronged attack against PH is underway that includes basic research, genetic research, unraveling the molecular mysteries of the disease process, and the development of new medicines and ways to deliver them.

Many of us search for new developments on one of the PubMed sites. But once something's published and you locate it, it's often old news.

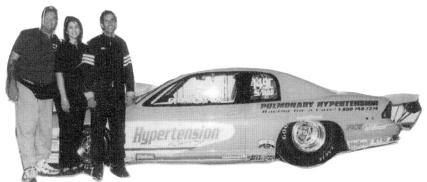

If you want to keep up to date on who is doing what in cutting edge research, join **PHA**, read *Pathlight*, join the PHANews listserv, and attend PHA Conferences. You can also listen to and/or view presentations from past Conferences, which are available for purchase. Call 1-800-748-7247 or the PHA office (1-301-565-3004) for more information.

Someday will we just grow ourselves new lungs in a fat test tube? It's unlikely. Lung "architecture" is very complicated, with an alveolar surface area large as a tennis court, and it's harder to grow endothelial cells than it is to grow some other organs. But who knows? The following are some intriguing new approaches. As exciting as these ideas are, remember that there are still some very basic questions about **PH** to be answered. For example, is our problem the overgrowth of vessel cells or the failure of cells to die like normal cells?

The new ideas that follow are listed, alphabetically and not necessarily in order of merit.

You are not powerless! There is much PH patients and their friends and families can do to try to find a cure. John Sperando and his sister JoAnne Sperando-Schmidt both have FPAH. John asked his friend George Stack (on the right), a prize-winning drag racer (SuperGas class of the Nat. Hot Rod Assn.), to put a PHA sticker on his car. George did far more than that: he dubbed his team "Hypertension Racing," donated his runner-up winnings in 2000 to PHA, and got PH t-shirts and stickers made up that he handed out while asking for donations to PHA. No wonder he was voted NHRA's Man of the Year!

ACE Inhibitors

ACE (angiotensin-converting enzyme) inhibitors are vasodilator drugs (like Accupril). They help prevent the conversion inside our bodies of angiotensin I to angiotensin II (a powerful vasoconstrictor). Researchers at the University of Colorado compared 60 patients with severe idiopathic pulmonary arterial hypertension (IPAH - previously known as PPH) with two normal control populations. They found that a certain genotype, ACE DD, was found in 45 percent of the IPAH patients versus 24-28 percent of the controls. Within the entire IPAH group, mean PAP and duration of PH symptoms were comparable. But here's what's interesting: those with the ACE DD genotype had a better cardiac output and functioned better. Although it is associated with an increased chance of having IPAH, the ACE DD genotype appears to help preserve right ventricular function.

ACE inhibitors are presently used to treat systemic hypertension and heart failure. Would they help some of us too? Doctors don't know; there haven't been any clinical trials with ACE inhibitors in PH patients. Because they block bad hormones that cause blood disease, some experts think that they may offer some benefit to PAH patients. However, adding them to your current regimen may dangerously lower your blood pressure.

Angiotensin II Receptor Blocker

A new type of blood pressure medication that blocks a hormone that causes arteries to constrict has been used in a few PAH patients. Unlike ACE inhibitors, these drugs are selective for angiotensin II receptors. One such drug is valsartan (Diovan). The rationale is the same as for ACE inhibitors, above.

BH4

Tetrahydrobiopterin (BH4) is produced by the body and is one essential ingredient needed for nitric oxide production. Researchers at Vanderbilt are adding sapropterin dihydrochloride (6R-BH4) - an experimental medication very similar to BH4 which our body makes, to patients already on endothelin receptor antagonists. Currently a Phase 1 safety study is looking at various dose regimens, measuring differences in biochemical markers, 6-minute walk tests and quality of life.

Bradykinin Receptor II Agonist

Although still at the rat-testing stage, this compound looks promising. In rats with induced PH it reduced their PAPs and the size of their right ventricles. A new bradykinin receptor B2 agonist, B9972, was used by the researchers (at the University of Colorado and Johns Hopkins).

Dichloroacetate (DCA)

In PAH patients, the pulmonary smooth muscle cells have decreased amounts of certain potassium channels, most predominantly the Kv1.5 channel. As a result, the cell is depolarized, which allows calcium to enter into the cell. (This influx of calcium is much of the rationale behind using calcium channel blockers for patients with PAH). This also seems to contribute to impaired apoptosis (cell death); resulting in over proliferation of pulmonary arterial smooth muscle cells (PASMCs). Dr. Stephen Archer has pioneered much of the work in this area.

DCA causes rapid activation of Kv channels by a tyrosine kinase-dependent mechanism. Dichloroacetate is a very attractive drug to be tested in the treatment of PAH since it has little effect on potassium channels of normal PASMCs. Moreover, it has been tried safely in humans with coronary disease and heart failure.

Dr. Sean McMurtry and colleagues at the University of Alberta, Edmonton, Canada treated rats with DCA. These rats were first treated with monochrotaline (MCT) to induce pulmonary hypertension. These rats were then given DCA 21 days after the MCT was given.

As a result, the rats had 63% decreased pulmonary vascular resistance, 28% decreased medial thickening, and 34% decreased right ventricular hypertrophy (enlargement). Importantly, DCA did not affect normal rats. They also showed a 10-fold increase in apoptosis within the pulmonary artery.

Endothelin Converting Enzyme (ECE-1)

The endothelin antagonists discussed earlier work by keeping endothelin from attaching to spots in the pulmonary vessels where it does its work. Another approach that may help PH patients in the future is a drug that reduces or stops the production of endothelin-1.

Fasudil (Rho-kinase Inhibitor)

Too little oxygen causes blood vessels to constrict (which can lead to PH). A lack of oxygen might cause too little of a substance to be formed that makes the vasodilator nitric oxide. Rho-kinase regulates this decrease. (Note the use of the word "might.")

Fasudil is a Rho-kinase inhibitor, a drug being tried on stable angina patients to reduce their chest pain. Rho-kinase makes smooth muscles more sensitive to calcium, so they constrict more. Fasudil decreases vasoconstriction, increases endothelial nitric oxide synthase (eNOS), decreases inflammation and reverses PH in rats that have been induced with the disease by a substance called monochrotaline. Dr. Yoshihiro Fukumoto of the Kyushu University Graduate School of Medical Sciences in Fukuoka, Japan, and his colleagues studied the effects of the drug in intravenous form on 10 patients with severe IPAH or PH associated with other diseases. They also tried under-the-tongue nifedipine, inhaled oxygen, and nitric oxide. Only the fasudil reduced pulmonary artery vascular resistance. The patients' mean PAPs remained unchanged.

Gene Therapy

There are still many hurdles to leap before there is a gene therapy for PH, but some promising experiments are being done on animals. Trials in humans with PH may be years away.

There are different kinds of gene therapy. One kind is to put good genes into the body to stand in for the faulty ones. This is difficult. In familial PAH, the PAH gene is dominant. You already have one good gene, from your non-carrier parent, and adding another good gene won't overpower the bad one.

There is also the problem of figuring out just where in the body to put the new genes. For example, the gene for cystic fibrosis has to be delivered to the lungs; genes for hemophilia (a problem based in the liver) can be injected into the blood stream. What sort of gene the PAH gene isn't known, nor do scientists know whether it will be necessary to treat every cell. About the best this type of gene therapy can do is to replace 10 to 15 percent of cells.

Then there is what Dr. Kirk Lane, a molecular biologist at Vanderbilt, calls the "new" gene therapy. You add new, good genes to new places to make more of substances that PH patients lack. For example, maybe once a day, or once a month, you might be given new genes to make prostacyclin synthase or nitric oxide.

A company based in Canada, called Endogen, is working on a new kind of gene therapy in which they remove cells from a person, modify the cells genetically, and then return the modified cells to the person's body. By using the person's own cells they avoid the immune system problems you can run into when you use a virus to transport the good genetic stuff. This new technology is called autologous cell-based gene therapy. It has worked in animals with PH.

Gene therapy can be used "farther upstream" to make the stuff that makes the stuff that we have too little of, such as prostacyclin. In an experiment, sheep were given PH, and the PH was then cured using this method. Sheep differ in many ways from humans, of course, and they didn't have PH long enough to develop the vascular changes we have. Still, this is interesting news. The effect lasted as long as 5 days in the sheep.

Experiments (at Tulane University School of Medicine in New Orleans) in transferring endothelial nitric oxide synthase to mice have already been shown to reduce PVR (in mice). In 1996 another research group used an adenovirus to insert human endothelial nitric oxide synthase into rats and also found they did a nice job as a selective pulmonary vasodilator. In other research at Tulane, an adenovirus was used to transfer calcitonin gene-related peptide (CGRP) into hypoxic mice. CGRP helps keep PVR low and modulates pulmonary vascular response to chronic hypoxia. The encouraging results of the experiment suggest another possible way to treat PH. A research group in Japan has transferred human prostacyclin synthase to rats with PH, improving the animals' survival time over that of rats in a control group.

PDGF Receptor-Selective Tyrosine Kinase Inhibitor

PDGF is platelet-derived growth factor, which may play a key role in the development of PH. The PDGF receptor blocker STI571 (imatinib mesylate) has been shown to reverse pulmonary vascular remodeling in 2 different animal models of PH. Because PDGF is known to be a powerful stimulator of cell division, and the progression of PH associated with increased production and migration of pulmonary vascular smooth muscle cells, inhibiting the effects of PDGF may prove effective in reversing pulmonary vascular disease. There are case reports from Germany, France, and the U.S., of imatinib being effective in severe PAH that doesn't respond to other therapies (see "tyrosine

Renin Inhibitors

Renin is an enzyme made by our kidneys. It breaks up angiotensinogen to make angiotensin I, which is then made into the vasoconstrictor angiotensin II. Actelion and Merck are jointly looking at new types of renin inhibitors with the end goal of finding ways to treat hypertension, renal failure, and heart failure. Maybe this will be of relevance to PH patients (see "ACE inhibitors" also).

Selective serotonin reuptake inhibitors (SSRIs), (Prozac)

Medicines such as fluoxetine (Prozac) are taken to treat depression. This medication works by blocking the uptake of a compound called serotonin. Serotonin has been found to cause cell growth of the pulmonary artery as well as smooth muscle proliferation. Using fluoxetine, prevented and reversed PH in rats caused by a substance called monocrotaline. Recently, however, there has been a report of a six times higher incidence of persistent PH of newborns in pregnant women who used fluoxetine after 20 weeks into their pregnancy. It's not known whether fluoxetine directly caused this, but certainly pregnant women should be warned of this significant finding. Researchers in France are currently conducting a trial of the use of escitalopram (Lexapro), another type of SSRI, in PH.

Serine Elastase Inhibitor

Serine elastase is a chemical in our bodies that has been linked to the progression of PH. Dr. Marlene Rabinovitch's research group at the University of Toronto (she is now at Stanford University, California) injected rats with monocrotaline to give them PH, and then undid the resulting muscularization of their pulmonary arteries by giving them an oral serine elastase inhibitor. After 2 weeks, the PAPs and artery structure returned to normal in 86 percent of treated rats, and all the untreated rats were dead. Dr. Rabinovitch says, "The most exciting finding is that we can take a condition that is fatal and reverse it back to where the animals had normal function. There is the possibility of doing this in humans." Dr. Rabinovitch updated the author on this research in the spring of 2004: the synthetic elastase inhibitors they used in the early experiments were found to have toxic effects on the liver. She is still hopeful that naturally occurring elastase inhibitors, perhaps given intravenously, may also be effective.

Simvastatin (Zocor)

Many people take simvastatin to lower their cholesterol. The drug is known to reduce the abnormal growth of endothelial and smooth muscle cells. So a group of Stanford researchers tried it on rats with PH. They found there was less abnormal growth in the vessels of PH rats treated with the drug than in a control group, and also that more nitric oxide was produced in the endothelia of treated rats. (The rats had been given PH by having a lung removed and being injected with monocrotaline.) Johns Hopkins researchers have also been working with rats and simvastatin with encouraging results. Dr. Kawut and colleagues at Columbia are conducting a controlled study comparing the use of aspirin and simvastatin in PAH patients.

Stem Cells & Progenitor Cells

Stem cells can come from embryos or adults (from blood, bone marrow, or the lymph system). They have at least three important qualities: 1) they can renew themselves for a long time by dividing; 2) they aren't yet specialized to do things like contract a muscle or coagulate blood; and 3) under certain conditions they can be turned into cells with special functions. Lately there has been a great burst of interest in stem cells as cures or treatments for various diseases.

An article by Benjamin Suratt and others in the August 1, 2003, *American Journal of Respiratory and Critical Care Medicine* is an example of research suggesting that stem cells harvested from an adult donor's blood and transplanted into the bloodstream of another person can grow into the type of cell needed to repair damage to pulmonary vessels. This might lead to a therapy to grow healthy lung tissue in PH patients.

Dr. Duncan Stewart's team at the University of Toronto, Canada (he is also head of cardiology at St. Michael's Hospital), has done exciting research on rats that have PAH. Endothelial progenitor cells circulate in the rats' bloodstreams, as they do in ours. These are cells that haven't quite decided what to be when they grow up. They are made in the bone marrow and go into the bloodstream where they travel to areas of blood vessel injury and help repair the damage.

Dr. Stewart removed some of these cells, cultured them for 5 days to increase their number, and then reinjected them into the rats' bloodstreams where they went through the "sieve" of the lungs, landed just where they were needed, and formed tiny new blood vessels. The rats' PAPs fell and their heart walls became less thick. This team has also inserted nitric oxide synthase (eNOS) genes into the progenitor cells before reinjecting them into the rats (with positive results). A neat thing about the use of progenitor cells is that they avoid the politics of stem cells. This approach also fits nicely with the design of our lungs, with the way large vessels empty into smaller ones, so the cells are carried right to where they are needed.

Dr. Stewart's team has launched the PHACeT (Pulmonary Hypertension Assessment of Cell Therapy) trial. This is primarily a safety trial to see if patients can tolerate the infusion of progenitor cells that have nitric oxide synthase inserted in them. They aim to enroll 18 patients who have not responded to standard PAH therapy. These patients will receive genetically modified endothelial precursor cells over several days in a gradual dose escalation fashion. The researchers will monitor them to make sure that this type of infusion is safe, that they will not experience any immune system reactions, or any bad effects from blood clots. They will have a Swan Ganz catheter placed in their neck and their pressures will be monitored continuously as these cells are infused. Although the enrollment numbers are still small, Dr. Stewart has observed that in the first 2 patients, there was a slight decrease in the pulmonary pressures, increase in cardiac output, and decrease in the pulmonary vascular resistance. It is the hope that these progenitor cells will repair damaged pulmonary blood vessels and regenerate new vessels. Inserting eNOS into the cells will also hopefully help patients to produce more nitric oxide in the pulmonary circulation. Although the study is in its kickoff stages, it is very exciting to see what will eventually develop.

Tyrosine Kinase Inhibitors (Gleevec)

Imatinib (or Gleevec) is normally used to treat chronic myelogenous leukemia (CML), gastrointestinal stromal tumors (GISTs) and other cancerous conditions. A lot of interest in this medication developed when a case report showed reversal of severe pulmonary hypertension in a German patient who didn't respond to the standard PAH treatments. This medication helps with apoptosis (cell death), and inhibits tyrosine kinase receptors. It's thought that when these receptors are activated, it results in vasoconstriction and proliferation; which is harmful to us patients with PAH. It seems that in PAH and in many cancers, cells do not "die off" as they're supposed to do, which leads to an overgrowth of cells. Therefore, substances that help apoptosis may be beneficial in PAH patients. Clinical trials of the use of imatinib are happening now in the US and in Europe.

Patients in the trials are being monitored carefully for signs of heart muscle damage and resulting left heart failure. Check www.clinicaltrials.gov to see which sites are accepting patients into this trial.

Thromboxane Synthase Inhibitors

At one time there was interest in thromboxane synthase inhibitors or receptor blockers, but interest in them is waning because they cause severe leg pain. A study of one such drug, terbogrel, was stopped because of disappointing results. A patient who was in the trial for about 4 months reports that her PAP fell, but the pain was unbearable. A similar oral drug, cicletanine, is being tried in Europe and is reported to have increased the production of prostacyclin in a small double-blind study. PAPs and total pulmonary resistance decreased significantly in patients getting the real drug. Another rather benign and common drug that can actually decrease the amount of thromboxane is aspirin. Thromboxane is a lipid that plays a role in platelet inhibition. Thromboxane levels are also increased in PAH patients. There is a lot of good evidence that show the benefits of using aspirin in coronary artery disease. Dr. Girgis at Johns Hopkins and Dr. Kawut at Columbia are conducting a trial to study its effects on PAH patients (See simvastatin section). If proven effective, perhaps aspirin might end up being the cheapest medication used to treat PAH (wouldn't that be lovely!).

Vasoactive Intestinal Peptide (VIP)

VIP is a neurotransmitter with a role in electrolyte and water secretion. In animal models, treatment with VIP decreases pulmonary arterial pressure and pulmonary vascular resistance. It also decreases smooth muscle and platelet activation. In mice where VIP was "knocked out," they eventually developed PAH with an increase in right ventricular systolic pressure as well as the small vascular changes that are seen in patients with PAH. More work needs to be done in this area to see if VIP will eventually be a beneficial treatment for PAH.

Should You Join a Clinical Trial?

Without the clinical trials over the past decade or so, we would still be dying in droves. Clinical trials are carefully designed experiments to test the benefits and safety of new treatments and are the only way we will eventually find a cure for PH. The trials advance the interests of PH patients *as a class*, but do not necessarily serve the near-term interests of a particular patient. So those PH patients who participate in trials are truly heroes.

A trial isn't begun until after laboratory studies have already suggested that a drug may be promising. During a trial, medicine (which might not otherwise be available) is provided free, as are the necessary medical procedures and doctor visits. You will get a lot of close monitoring, so if you deteriorate you can be pulled out of the trial and given another treatment. This is extremely important to remember as your PH physician does not want to put you in harm's way, so they will be sure to take you out of the trial if there is a concern. After the placebo-controlled phase of the study, if the results are promising you are often allowed to continue to receive the study drug, at no cost, until the drug is approved or the company gives up on it. Some of your regular follow-up visits and blood tests may also be free while you are in a study.

If you join a trial, you are exposing yourself to some unanticipated risks, such as a toxic reaction or troubling side effect. Clinical trials are experiments, not FDA-approved treatments. In randomized, controlled, double-blind trials some patients get a placebo or no treatment at all while others receive the trial medication. You, and everyone involved in your care is 'blinded', or doesn't know if you are on the study medication or not. So you may be denied, for a time, a drug that would help you. Going without treatment carries risks.

The FDA says you cannot switch from one *investigational* drug to another unless you are off the first drug for at least 30 days. (Flolan, Remodulin, Ventavis, Tracleer, Letairis and Revatio are no longer considered investigational drugs.)

Not every trial is suitable for every patient. Ask a lot of questions before you join up and for a frank appraisal of the risks. You have every right to say "no thanks", even if your doctor suggests you join a trial. Read the consent form carefully, and then ask more questions if the form isn't clear or comprehensive. A consent form is not a contract; you can drop out of a study (or be dropped) at any time.

When you are in a trial, your relationship with your doctor takes on aspects of "researcher-subject" as well as "doctor-patient." You should politely ask the doctors involved in the trial to tell you who is paying for it. Insurance companies won't pay for drugs and procedures used as part of a trial, and universities won't usually find the money, either. This means the cash typically comes from a drug company or the national government. Money is usually paid on a "per patient enrolled" basis. An ethical approach is for a research group to put any excess, after covering costs, into a PH research fund. You should also *very nicely* ask if anyone on your PH team has a significant financial interest in the outcome of a trial (e.g., owns shares of the sponsoring company). Many doctors own stock funds, and if your doc owns shares of, say, Vanguard's health fund, that's not the sort of thing that is likely to cause bias. Most doctors probably have only a vague idea of which companies their mutual funds invest in. It is common, by the way, for drug companies to pay doctors consultant fees to help design studies, etc.

There are four phases of clinical trials.

Phase I uses healthy volunteers and looks for the best ways to administer a drug, unacceptable side effects, and the maximum tolerated dose. In Phase II the drug is given to more people, this time people with the disease being studied, while its safety is still examined and preliminary evidence of its effectiveness is sought. If things look good, a Phase III will be done that involves far more patients, with a focus on finding out about the drug's effectiveness and side effects. FDA approval is sought after a successful Phase III. After FDA approval, when the drug is on the market, a Phase IV study monitors its safety and effectiveness for the general population. Phase IV trials might also be done in patients whose type of disease doesn't match the type of disease for which the treatment was approved.

Resources to help you find a trial and decide whether to sign up. When you are afraid you are dying it may be difficult to think clearly about joining a clinical trial. Force yourself to ask the hard questions, and talk options over with persons you trust. For more information, see "How to Find and Survive a Clinical Trial," *Pathlight*, Winter 1998, p. 5 (reprinted from *Consumer Reports*, December 1998). See, also, "A Study Guide to Scientific Studies," Jane E. Brody, *The New York Times*, p. B11 (science section), August 11, 1998. A supposedly comprehensive registry of clinical trials is available through the federal National Library of Medicine at www.clinicaltrials.gov (search for "pulmonary hypertension"). You might also try the National Institutes of Health at www.cc.nih.gov (or call 800-411-1222). Also check out the advice on the FDA site: www.fda.gov/oashi/aids/fdaguide.html.

When PH doctors suggest you consider joining a trial, they try to make sure that it's a win/win trial: it should be a fair deal for you, with you getting out of it things that benefit you. This might include the right to use the drug prior to FDA approval, even if you got the placebo during the trial.

Surgical Treatments

Surgery can help PH patients in several ways. It can help correct congenital heart problems, and help patients with heart failure due to IPAH/FPAH and connective tissue diseases. Old scarred blood clots can be removed in patients with PH due to such clots. And, perhaps most importantly, PH patients who are doing poorly in spite of other treatment may benefit from lung or heart/lung transplantation.

Fixing Your Heart's Plumbing

Many congenital heart problems can be surgically corrected before PH develops or while it is still reversible. The trend is to treat congenital heart problems earlier (sometimes even before a baby is born). But some adult hearts are also fixable. Don't be surprised if you, an adult, are referred to a pediatric cardiologist! They are the ones with the most experience.

If surgery is too risky, drug treatments are still possible and may help you feel much better (see Chapter 5). For example, intravenous epoprostenol may help PH patients with some types of congenital heart disease and may also convert a nonoperable patient into a candidate for repair surgery or transplant.

Non-Surgical Closure for ASD: Plugging a Hole in the Heart

Although doctors insist this isn't a "surgical" procedure, patients think of it as surgery, so it is included in this chapter. Holes in the heart (congenital defects) such as atrial septal defects (ASDs) can lead to PH. Although these are best fixed when you are young, sometimes a hole isn't found until later in your life. You might then face a tough decision: should you have the hole closed, or is the damage already done? PH doctors and pulmonologists can help you decide by trying medicines to see what happens to the flow of blood in the lungs during a right-heart catheterization. If the flow of blood is still mostly from the left side of the heart to the right (from the left atrium to the right atrium, in the case of an ASD), or if medications such as inhaled nitric oxide can lower pulmonary pressure and increase flow from the left side to the right side, it might be possible to close the hole.

Hole closures are done today with gizmos like the Amplatzer™ closure device. It looks like two little umbrellas. (There are similar "generic" gizmos called "clamshell devices.") They are inserted, closed, during a catheterization. Once in place—with an "umbrella" on each side of the hole—they are popped open and squeezed together, covering the hole. Cool, huh? This is now common practice. It works well in carefully chosen patients and is a lot easier than open-chest surgery. Success depends on having a hole that is not too big for the umbrellas to cover, and on whether covering the hole lowers pulmonary pressures significantly.

Atrial Septostomy

For a very few PPH patients who have right ventricular failure in spite of maximal treatment with medicines, or who are fainting a lot, a doctor might consider an atrial septostomy. This procedure might be done to keep the patient alive until a transplant is available. A catheter with a balloon on its tip is poked through the dividing wall (the *septum*) between the two upper chambers of your heart, making a hole. The hole allows blood to pass from the right side of the heart without having to go through the lungs. This is called right-to-left shunting, and it relieves pressure on the right side of the heart, which might otherwise fail due to the high resistance to the flow of blood through the lung's blood vessels. There have been publications about the use of this procedure in treating PH patients. While this procedure is done at several centers, it's still risky and can have a high mortality rate. Afterwards, levels of oxygen in your blood will fall (because blood is bypassing your lungs), so you will most likely need supplemental oxygen. A septostomy only relieves symptoms; it does nothing to cure PH. Look for a doctor with lots of experience doing it on IPAH / FPAH patients.

Balloon Angioplasty

It's too early to say much about the use of this procedure (where a balloon catheter is inflated inside an artery to increase its diameter) on PH patients. Dr. J.A. Feinstein and colleagues at Children's Hospital, Harvard (Boston, Massachusetts) reported in 2001 on 18 patients with chronic thromboembolic PH whose clots were not reachable by surgeons, or who couldn't have surgery because of other medical problems. The patients underwent an average of 2.6 procedures and 6 dilations. After an average of 3 years of follow-up, their 6-minute walking distances improved from 209 to 497 yards, and their mean PAPs fell significantly. This was a nonrandomized, uncontrolled study. German researchers have also reported a couple of chronic thromboembolic PH cases that they successfully treated with balloon angioplasty. But no randomized studies comparing this technique with medical therapy for such patients have been done.

Pulmonary Thromboendarterectomy: Roto-Rootering the Lungs

When PH is caused by a blood clot (or clots) in a pulmonary artery, a surgical procedure called a *pulmonary thromboendarterectomy* (throw that phrase out at parties!) may restore almost-normal blood flow to the lungs. This is one of the very few types of PH for which there presently is often a cure.

Most clots form in the legs, break off, and travel to a lung (such clots are called *thromboembolisms*). If these clots do not dissolve on their own (most do), and if they lodge in the large arteries of a lung, they age and become almost like scar tissue (*chronic thromboembolic disease*).

A founder of PHA, the unsinkable Dorothy Olson, had a thromboendarterectomy at the age of 69. She says the gunk removed from her looked like "a bunch of bubble gum," not blood, and she has a photo to prove it!

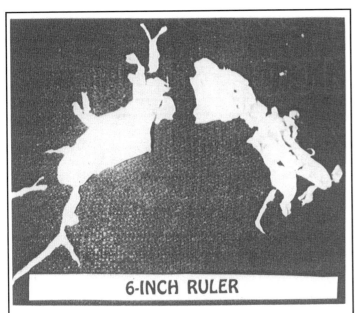

6-INCH RULER

Dorothy's clot after it was successfully removed.
Photo used with permission of Dorothy Olson.

A CT scan, MRI, or an angiogram can reveal the existence of a clot and give doctors information about where it is, so they can determine whether it can be removed. Reading angiograms can be tricky, because radiologists are used to looking for acute pulmonary embolisms, not chronic ones. Dr. Richard Channick says that in about a third of the cases they see they still aren't sure if an operation is feasible, so they use a fiber optic tool called an angioscope to give them a better look at the inner wall of a clotted artery. For a truly inside view, you can watch the television screen along with your doctor. Still, there is uncertainty in a remaining 10 percent as to whether clots are operable. It is the practice of this team to explain the assumed higher risk to these patients and offer them the chance to try surgery.

Sometimes doctors suggest prostacyclin, sildenafil, or inhaled iloprost therapy prior to a thromboendarterectomy to improve right-heart performance and reduce pressures. There have been no controlled studies of the benefits of doing so, but it seems sensible. German researchers tried inhaled iloprost on 10 thromboendarterectomy patients both before and after their surgery. It didn't do any good before, but after surgery it improved early postoperative hemodynamics.

Pick a team with experience. There is a steep learning curve on this operation, so you want guys with experience. A pulmonary hypertension multidisciplinary team is best, and they should do at *least* one such operation a month. More is better, because beginners have a mortality rate of maybe 20 to 40 percent. The University of California, San Diego (UCSD) Medical Center, where doctors pioneered this procedure, has done the most thromboendarterectomies—about 1,400 since 1990. The mortality rate for their more recent cases is around 4.4 percent. The Mayo Clinic had a 19 percent mortality rate in their first 21 patients, but only 4.5 percent mortality for the last 43 they did (as of February 2003). In the U.S. you also can check out the Cleveland Clinic and a few other places. There are half a dozen or so centers in Europe that do thromboendarterectomies. You can find one in Paris, northern Italy, Austria, and England; there are three centers in Germany. The center at University Hospital, Mainz, Germany, which has done about 300 procedures over a 12-year period, may hold the European record.

It is possible for a center to manipulate its mortality rate by accepting only those patients most likely to survive—this practice may discriminate against people with clots farther downstream from the big pulmonary arteries, folks who may well be helped by the operation. (Diagnosing what is smaller artery [*distal*] disease is tricky; sometimes such clots are very operable.) Once again, it's up to you to ask lots of questions and pick your center carefully.

The major cause of mortality is that not enough of the clot can be removed, so pulmonary pressures remain high and the right side of the heart gives out from the stress of the operation. If only part of a clot can be reached, it may still lower pressures enough for a patient to get on a transplant list or be treated with epoprostenol. There is not a lot of experience as to how patients with these persistent clots do when treated with standard PH medicines, but there are reports that in patients with limited benefit from surgery, or with worsening PH years after surgery, some of the PH medicines may help. Inhaled iloprost and intravenous epoprostenol have been used for patients like this with different degrees of success. So far, no one has looked at how large numbers of these patients do with medicines like bosentan.

Who qualifies. Whether a clot can be reached surgically is the most important factor in deciding whether to operate. Other considerations are how healthy a patient's heart is, what other diseases the patient has, and the patient's age. UCSD has successfully operated on an 86-year-old. Obese patients are more likely to die from the operation.

The big chill. During the thromboendarterectomy the body is cooled way down and blood flow might even be stopped for up to 20 minutes. Dorothy, with her sparkle and wit, is living proof that this process need not turn you into a zombie. A midline incision is made through the breastbone, and you go on a heart/lung machine. It takes only about an hour to remove the clots, but the cooling down and warming up process makes this a 6-to-8-hour surgery.

Filter tips. Before removing a clot like Dorothy's, the surgeon puts a filter (usually a "bird's nest" type filter) in the main vein draining blood from the lower part of the body (the *vena cava inferior*). You can't be on anticoagulation drugs during the surgery because you might bleed too much, so the filter catches clots that might otherwise join those already blocking the lung vessels. It also helps protect you from clots after the

operation. Patients are kept on an anticoagulant for life. UCSD targets an INR of 2.5 to 3.5, a bit higher than is usual for patients with PH caused by other things. This level of blood thinning has been proven superior to lower doses.

To learn more about pulmonary embolisms and their symptoms see the traveling section in Chapter 12.

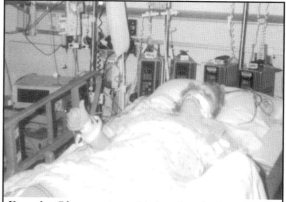

Dorothy Olson post-op. It's her thumb that matters, not the tubes!
Photo used with permission of Dorothy Olson.

Postoperative life. The operation is not particularly painful, but patients feel wiped out for a few days afterwards. A hospital stay of 7 to 10 days is typical. Most patients are Class III or IV prior to surgery. Of those who survive the operation, two-thirds have improved to Class I or II. In most cases the improvement remains indefinitely. (For more info, see Chapter 7.)

Obesity Surgery

For morbidly obese persons unable to lose weight by other methods, obesity surgery (a.k.a. gastric bypass or bariatric surgery) to alter the digestive process by reducing the size of the stomach and/or bypassing part of the small intestine has increased in popularity. Obesity is associated with the worsening of PH and its symptoms.

So why not have obesity surgery? Well, it's not the cure-all some think, and it's dangerous. Even in people without breathing problems, the overall mortality rate of 1 to 2 percent for gastric bypass surgery is nothing to sneeze at. And in those with respiratory insufficiency (e.g. sleep apnea and obesity hypoventilation syndrome) it may be around 2.4 percent. It would probably be much higher in PH patients, should such a study be done. The procedure has been done successfully on a tiny number of desperate PH patients, but for heaven's sake, consult with your PH specialist if you are thinking about trying this. The NIH says 10 to 20 percent of patients operated on have complications that later require more surgery, and that nearly 30 percent have post-operative nutritional deficiencies. You have to learn to eat right and take vitamins, and will still need to avoid overeating. Your new "pouch" will stretch over time, and many patients regain about 5 pounds a year.

Transplantation

Some of the following information and recommendations on transplantation are from a supplement (July 2004) to Chest: *"Diagnosis and Management of Pulmonary Arterial Hypertension: ACCP Evidence-Based Clinical Practice Guideline." Thank you,* Chest!

A transplant is an option when medical treatments for PH are no longer helping you. About 150 lung transplants are done each year on PH patients at one of the 70 or so trans-plant centers in the U.S. (The introduction of prostanoid therapies is probably mostly responsible for the drop in the percentage of PH patients among all lung or heart-lung transplant patients from 13 percent in 1991 to 4 percent in 2001.)

When you get a transplant you are trading one disease for another, because you will have to take immunosuppressive drugs for the rest of your life so your immune system doesn't reject your new lungs. On the other hand, transplant recipients often enjoy a vastly improved quality of life for 5 to 7 years, or even longer. IPAH/FPAH has not been known to recur in a transplanted lung, but other problems related to rejection of the organ and infection can limit the quality and duration of life.

As one transplant surgeon put it: "We're still at the square-wheel stage of understanding the immune system and organ preservation." Lung transplants are not as easy or successful as heart transplants. The lung is the only organ open to room air, so everything we breathe in affects it. The surgery is also difficult. Big breakthroughs in transplant science are not expected in the near future. Artificial lungs are still science fiction, and lung transplants from animals remain unrealistic.

There are four types of transplants for the treatment of PH: heart-and-lung; bilateral-lung (two single lungs); single-lung; and living-donor lobes. They all involve considerable risk (see Chapter 7). Different transplant centers prefer different approaches. Once you pick a transplant center, they will not ask you if you would like one lung or two, and what about a heart? Instead they will use their own criteria to match your disease process with appropriate organs. The truth is, there haven't been any randomized studies proving that PAH patients do any better or worse with any of these approaches. For example, centers disagree on whether heart-and-lung offers any survival advantage over the lung(s) only approach.

Heart-Lung Transplants

A heart-lung transplant is seldom done for PH any more, because an enlarged but otherwise healthy heart can recover when the lung problem is solved. Hearts as big as footballs can recover! The first lung transplant ever (1981) was a heart-lung transplant done on a woman with "PPH." Heart-lung transplants have the advantages of not requiring as much fancy sewing by surgeons. They can also cure many kinds of congenital heart disease along with the PH. If you have complex congenital heart disease, this may be the best option for you.

The way organs are allocated in the U.S. means you have to wait much longer for a heart-lung transplant. Even in patients with congenital heart disease, it is faster and sometimes more effective to fix minor problems in your own heart at the time of surgery and transplant only lungs.

Bilateral-Lung Transplants

Most transplant centers now prefer to do bilateral-lung transplants for those with PAH, because things generally go more smoothly after the operation. With a bilateral-lung transplant, there is a greater reserve when something goes wrong. Furthermore, with a single-lung transplant there is a chance of a ventilation/perfusion mismatch (where the majority of the flow will go to the new, more easily expanded lung) causing post-operative complications. The down side is that you have to wait longer to get two lungs (you might die while waiting), and it is a longer, more difficult operation. A study at Johns Hopkins of 57 PH patients (both primary and secondary PH) found that bilateral-lung transplant is the treatment of choice for IPAH patients. If you have PH associated with another disease the situation is less clear: if you have a mean PAP greater than 40 mm Hg, you *might* do better with a bilateral-lung transplant, and if your PAP is less than that you *might* do better with a single-lung transplant. Whenever possible, experts believe that children should get a bilateral-lung transplant, because it appears to give them a greater chance of long-term survival (by avoiding the development of chronic rejection).

Single-Lung Transplants

A single-lung transplant is easier to do, and people can do just as well, short-term, on a single lung. You won't have to be on a bypass machine as long. You are more likely, however, to have a ventilation/perfusion mismatch when most of the blood flow goes to your new, unobstructed lung. But the survival statistics for single-lung and bilateral-lung transplantees are not dramatically different, and there are times when the single-lung option clearly makes sense. For example, an older person who would not be eligible for a bilateral-lung transplant may be happy to get a single lung. Or, a situation might arise where lungs become available that are a match for two desperate PH patients on the same transplant list, and the patients and doctors agree to give one lung to each.

Lobar and Living-Donor Transplants

For people the right size who might not survive until whole lungs become available, there is a fourth option: lobes of lungs, rather than whole lungs. It is possible to transplant lobes of lung from living or dead donors. Most transplant organs come from cadavers, but donated cadaveric lungs can be used only 10 to 15 percent of the time. Cadaveric lungs deteriorate faster than any other organ prior to removal from the donor and are vulnerable to infection and other problems. Furthermore, there simply aren't enough to go around. The Organ Procurement and Transplantation Network reports that from 1998 to 2003 there were 11,019 lung transplants in the U.S. Only 219 of these were living-donor transplants. The number of living-donor procedures declined from a high of 29 in 1998, to 13 in 2002, and 10 in 2003.

With a living-donor transplant there is a shorter waiting period, the operation can be planned in advance, and the organ is outside a body for a shorter time (only about half an hour vs. up to 4 hours for a cadaveric transplant). The operations are expensive, although doctors have had success in getting many insurance companies and Medicare to pay for them.

Living-donor transplants are possible because each of us has five lobes (three on the right, two on the left), which are more than we really need to get along well. The diseased lungs are removed from the patient and replaced with donated lobes. It always takes two living donors. Usually the lower lobes are donated. The first living donor lung transplant was done in 1990 by Dr. Vaughn Starnes, then at Stanford University. He has since moved to Children's Hospital, Los Angeles (which is affiliated with the University of Southern California), and that center has done the most of these transplants. In 1993, the first bilateral living-donor lung transplant was done in an adult patient with cystic fibrosis. Most are still done for cystic fibrosis, not PH. (New operations, unlike new drugs, do not have to be approved by any government agency. It's up to hospitals to make their own rules and to do follow-ups and reports on donors and recipients.)

Patients between 20 and 50 kilograms (44 to 110 pounds) seem to be the best size match for lobe transplants, whether living-donor or cadaveric. As children grow, lung tissue can expand. But a child may outgrow his transplanted organs and need another transplant later.

How recipients do after getting their lobes. Most recipients are able to go back to school or work. As with any transplant, the person receiving the organ(s) must take immuno-suppressive drugs for the rest of his/her life

and deal with all the risks of rejection and infection. USC data suggests that mortality is a little higher in their living lobar transplants than in cadaveric ones.

Ethical issues. There are obvious ethical issues with living-donor lobar transplants. It takes three people (two of them healthy) on three operating tables in three operating rooms undergoing dramatic, risky surgery. In spite of all the precautions a hospital takes, a donor might feel coerced into giving up part of his or her lung (a parent has been known to lean hard on a child to donate a lobe to the child's brother/sister). Tension between doctors and social workers has been reported, with social workers hyper-alert for any sign of ambivalence on the part of donors, and surgeons raring to operate. It's best that the two donors and the recipient each have their own doctor, to help avoid conflicts of interest.

Who makes a good living donor? The best donors are related to the recipient, in excellent health, nonsmokers, and able to pass a psychosocial assessment. Although USC will transplant a lobe from each parent in select situations, it's a complex issue. Someone who may need every ounce of his/her lung capacity on the job, such as a police officer, fire fighter, or pilot, will not be accepted as a donor. Donors must be old enough to legally give consent.

How safe is it to be a donor? Although no lobe donors have been reported to die, this is always a possibility. Just going under anesthesia carries risks. A donor might also become handicapped, or have lung problems later in life. Complications have been reported, such as hemorrhage requiring blood transfusions, nerve injury, abnormal heart rhythms that needed surgical correction, pneumonia, temporary heart rhythm problems, and infections of the area around the heart (*pericarditis*).

On Lung Transplantation in General

The biggest problem: deciding when to transplant. Ironically, while the use of prostanoids and other new **PH** drugs have made it possible for many PH patients to avoid or delay transplantation, the success of these drugs may also have resulted in more extremely sick, higher-risk transplant patients. The better condition you are in before transplantation, the more likely a satisfactory outcome.

When other therapies do not help, if you are Class III or IV and there is a clear downward trend in your health, or if your PH is so advanced that it is unlikely that other therapies can help you in time, a transplant may be your best option.

Your pulmonary artery pressures alone do not determine whether you should have a transplant. There are patients with systolic pressures over 100, and who have big right ventricles, who are nevertheless doing well clinically. Conversely, because pressures can fall as a heart begins to fail, a transplant might be the best option for someone with pressures considerably under 100. Your PH doctor can advise you if and when to begin this process.

When to get listed. It's somewhat easier to decide on when to "get listed," because you can ask to be put on hold if you get near the top of the list and are still doing well. At some centers you may slip back a little on their list if you go "inactive." (If you are still on a list when an organ is offered and you pass it up, you may forfeit some months.)

UNOS says about 3,890 Americans were waiting for a lung transplant in 2003, but only 800 to 1,000 lungs are available each year. Historically, 30 to 40 percent of PPH patients waiting for a lung transplant died while still waiting (new drugs have improved these statistics). Many doctors like all their Class III or IV patients to be evaluated for transplant and to get on a list so they can start accumulating time, just in case. This disease can quickly turn nasty on us; a PHA member suddenly started getting worse and tried to get on a list, but was unable to hang on long enough for his insurance company to get around to approving his transplant workup. Bonnie Dukart, PHA's past president, wrote an article for *Pathlight* while she was awaiting transplant, urging her fellow patients to get listed earlier and to learn more about the listing process. (Bonnie died of heart failure soon after her transplant. Her article may be read in the spring 2001 *Pathlight*.)

How waiting lists work. Once approved, you get on the national transplant waiting list. The United Network for Organ Sharing (UNOS) matches donor organs with recipients based on blood type, length of time on the list, and (somewhat) chest size. Your chest size is a function of your age, sex, height, and race. Unlike transplants for most other diseases, the sickest lung disease patients are not moved to the head of the line. In other words, even if your doctor gives you only a week to live, that fact won't put you on the top of the list. This is illogical: although someone with emphysema can be stable for a relatively long time, PH patients can go downhill fast. A special exception has been made for pulmonary fibrosis patients, who get a 3-month handicap, and PH docs would like to see us get this head start, too. PHA's Scientific Leadership Council has been trying hard to get UNOS to revise their wait-time policy. (But see p. 135!)

There are about 70 different lung transplant centers in the U.S., and waiting times and rules differ. For patients with "PPH" the waiting time, as of January 2003, was a little over 3 years at some big centers with long lists. At smaller centers (doing 20 to 30 transplants a year) the waiting list may be only a year. This is still a very long time when you can feel yourself dying. Patients occasionally put their names on more than one list (some centers think this practice is very unfair and do not allow it). UNOS has divided the country into regions for transplant purposes, and you cannot put your name on more than one list in the same region. You must also live close enough to a center that you could get there within the allotted time after you are notified that an organ is (or organs are) available and be willing to get your long-term care from the institution that transplants you. At least one high-volume transplant center (Washington University) requires the patient to move to the St. Louis area prior to transplant, to participate in an intensive rehab program. If you move to another region, you can apply the waiting time you have already accumulated to your new center, but you will be dropped from your old center's list. This is what Bonnie Dukart had to do because the center near her home had too long a list. Some insurance companies will allow you to be evaluated at more than one center, some won't.

The waiting time and process of getting listed is usually even worse outside the United States, and fewer organs are available. If you live outside the U.S., you can get more information at www.ishlt.org, which is the website of the International Society for Heart and Lung Transplantation. Five percent of the patients listed with ISHLT have IPAH; 10-20 percent probably have PH secondary to another disease. Most of those receiving a heart-lung transplant have PH secondary to another disease.

Look for a center with good all-around expertise. Search for a center that has a really good transplant team, not just a star surgeon. To pull through, you're going to need good pulmonologists, anesthesiologists, critical care nurses, etc. Ask about the quality of organs the center accepts, whether the organs come from nearby or far away, and learn about the

institution's post-operative care. Talk to folks they have transplanted and network with other transplant patients. A list of all lung and heart-lung transplant centers in the U.S. is available from Second Wind (see Resources). A list of Medicare-approved lung and heart-lung transplant centers is available on the website of the Health Care Financing Administration (www.hcfa.gov/ medicare/lunglist.htm). Most big centers have their own websites with information on their doctors and programs. (NEWSFLASH! See p. 135.)

Here are some things a transplant center may not tell you: if a center doesn't have a high enough success rate, it loses its ability to transplant Medicare and some private insurance patients. So some centers simply refuse to accept very sick patients, even those who might well survive the process. On the other hand, a center has to do a minimum number of transplant operations every year to stay approved. This might tempt them to transplant somebody who might live longer if given drug therapy instead. The lens of self-interest might make a transplant seem more appropriate than it actually is.

A center has to balance these sometimes-conflicting pressures. A new transplant center that does not yet have Medicare approval (and therefore has a smaller patient pool to select from) may be willing to transplant a riskier patient. Sometimes a new center may be staffed by experienced transplant doctors and / or team members who had to leave their certification behind when they left their old center (it's centers, not individual doctors, who are certified by Medicare).

Who are the best candidates for lung transplants? This is not quite the same as who qualifies, although the categories overlap. Most of those removed from transplant lists are done so for "psycho-social" reasons. They may smoke, or be addicted to drugs, or frequently miss their doctor appointments, or be passive, indecisive types. Because there are nearly always some bumps in the road when you have a transplant, transplant teams look for the right mental attitude: people who have a reason for wanting to live (such as raising their kids), people with determination and a positive attitude who won't be put off by the need to take lots of meds. They also consider whether you will have family or friends to help you out after your transplant, and will be able to get to your transplant center for follow-ups.

Who qualifies for a transplant? Not everyone can get on a transplant list. (Lobar transplants have some different requirements—see the section above.) Different centers have different criteria. A general requirement is that the potential recipient has an "end-stage" lung disease likely to result in death within a year or two. It used to be that persons over a certain age were seldom considered, but the age limits have softened (some cynics say the age limits were raised as the pioneering transplant surgeons themselves grew older). The age cut-off for PH patients is often lower—to be considered for a bilateral-lung transplant you must generally be under 60 to 65 years old; for a heart-lung you must generally be under 55 years old. Exceptions are made. A 67-year-old PH patient reportedly got a lung transplant and is doing just fine. If you have a "cut off" birthday while you are listed, the powers that be might allow you to remain on the list. There does not seem to be a lower age limit, although it is not known how immuno-suppressive drugs will affect a child's growth.

If you have active hepatitis B or C, or HIV infection, a center might refuse to list you for transplant, because the immunosuppressive drugs you must take will make your infection worse. But sometimes a lung that wouldn't otherwise be used because the donor, too, has hepatitis C can fit the bill. If you are currently a smoker or substance abuser, some centers won't consider you. Other red flags that make you a less than optimum candidate are being very weak or ill with poor nutrition, blocked arteries, severe liver or kidney dysfunction, poorly controlled diabetes, and bad osteoporosis with bone pain. Cancer, (other than localized skin cancer) rules out a transplant. But if your cancer was years ago, and there is no sign that it has returned, then you can still be considered. Some cancers are more likely to come back when you take immunosuppressive medicines.

Obesity is another risk factor; there is a tendency to gain weight on the steroids you must take post-transplant. Excessive weight also means a greater chance of lung and wound infections and less ability to walk, so clots are more likely to form. It's hard to lose weight before you have a transplant, when you barely have the energy to wiggle your toes, but it sure can help!

Transplant and scleroderma or lupus. Patients with scleroderma/PH do not do as well after transplantation as those with "PPH." Many transplant centers are reluctant to operate on scleroderma/PH or lupus/PH patients because the disease affects many organs, not just the lungs. The heart and kidneys, for example, may be injured and not working well. Many scleroderma patients have very bad disease of their esophagus (the swallowing tube). This usually means that food, acid, and bile from the stomach end up in the lungs. This is bad enough when you have normal immunities and coughing ability. But when your immunities are suppressed because you are recovering from a major operation and are taking immunosuppressive drugs, and when you no longer have your natural coughing reflex (because the nerves are cut between your newly transplanted lungs and your brain), a sick esophagus is a HUGE problem. So most transplant centers look at all these things carefully and make transplant decisions on a case-by-case basis.

Transplant and PH/liver disease patients.
Liver disease usually precedes the development of PH in patients with liver disease/PH, and many liver disease/PH patients are denied *liver* transplants because their PH is so bad it puts them in a high-risk category. Historically, over half of liver transplant patients with PH did not know they had the PH until they were in the operating room getting prepped for liver transplant! This will be less true now, with better diagnosis, although it's still easy to miss. And if it is missed (and not treated), the transplant patient will die about a third of the time, which is way above the normal 7-10 percent mortality rate for liver transplants. Patients with higher pressures (mean PAPs above 50) have a 100 percent likelihood of death with a liver transplant. Those aren't good odds.... Even picking only patients with lower pressures (under 45) still results in the death of a third of them.

Most centers won't do a liver transplant on a PH patient because they don't know if the PH is reversible. So can you get a heart-lung-liver transplant? Don't count on it. There are patients who have had heart-lung-liver transplants with good outcomes, but it might be better to go on intravenous epoprostenol and try to get your lungs and liver in better shape to optimize your condition before surgery. There are a few known cases, however, where epoprostenol caused patients' spleens to grow huge and their platelet count to drop further. So doctors go easy on the epoprostenol in liver patients.

Who does well? Those with lower mean PAPs (especially those with PAPs under 35), lower mean vascular resistance, and a lower trans-pulmonary gradient. To better your odds, you may need to start using epoprostenol months or years before your transplant; it won't help to start it with the first incision! You will need to continue on the epoprostenol after the operation, and there is no ready answer for how long you need to stay on it. Many patients have been weaned from epoprostenol, however, after a successful transplant.

Other problems with lung transplants in liver disease/PH patients are that the meds you have to take after a transplant can be very toxic to the liver.

By the way, those patients whose PH is discovered in the OR when their liver transplant is about to happen, end up having the transplantation cancelled. They then get their PH treated. So far, only a few have improved enough that they became good candidates for liver transplantation. But new PH medicines (see Chapter 5) give more reason for hope.

Transplant and congenital heart defects.
People with PH and congenital heart defects do not do as well after lung transplants as those with "PPH," because there is more than one surgical problem. Dr. Victor Tapson, at Duke University, said in 2002 that his group has a better 3-year survival rate for bilateral lung transplants in "PPH" patients than they do for transplants in congenital heart disease patients (90 percent—but many of these heart disease patients have gotten a single lung). Most centers have about an 80 percent survival rate.

The transplantation process. It begins with an evaluation. This will probably take a few days and can be done in a hospital or on an outpatient basis, and often includes a heart catheterization, an echocardiogram, lots of blood tests (to determine your blood type and the functioning of your liver, kidneys, and immune system), pulmonary function tests, a ventilation-perfusion lung scan, a chest CT scan, and a MUGA heart scan (to see how well both the left and right sides of your heart are working). The transplant team will also do tests to find if you have a tubercular, bacterial, viral, or parasitic infection that might flare up when your immune system is suppressed by anti-rejection medications. They may screen you for cancer. If you have to wait a long time to get an organ (or organs), most of the tests will have to be repeated, probably at least once a year, to keep the information current.

Take along a good book, your knitting, or your iPod, because you'll be sitting in a lot of hospital corridors. On the up side, you get to be the center of attention, and the whole process is darn interesting. The transplant team usually includes a social worker (who can help with questions about paying for all this) and a psychologist.

The phone call. When you get the phone call saying organs are available, things happen fast. Legally, you still have the right to say, "No thanks." But lungs deteriorate rapidly, so a delay might deprive someone else of the chance of living. Shirley was sitting watching TV and quilting when her beeper went off—for the first time in 26 months! It was just in time, too. Her doctor had told her she couldn't make it another week. Shirley had practiced what to do and had her insurance cards, backup epoprostenol, oxygen, and clean underwear ready to go.

Luksha needed a double-lung transplant in 1991. When she got the call that lungs were available she had to be flown from Jacksonville, Florida, to Pittsburgh. A plane with her nurse and doctor aboard was held up in Jacksonville by airport officials who wanted to search it for drugs. Thinking clearly in spite of the drama, Luksha called a television channel and told them how her life was at stake. A reporter called airport management. Minutes later Luksha was on her way. (Nine years after her first transplant, rejection set in and she had a second, single-lung transplant. She now does volunteer work to better the lives of transplant survivors.)

The actual transplant. You'll probably be in the operating room for 5 to 9 hours. Patients often report that they remember no pain from the actual operation. When you awaken in the Intensive Care Unit (ICU), you will have what patients call a "zipper" on your chest. This new scar will run down the center, or laterally across your chest just under the breasts, or be off to one side. Where it is depends on the type of transplant you had. You can always lie and tell the guys or gals in the locker room that you got the scar in a knife fight in Khartoum. The truth, however, might be more impressive.

Recovery period. About 10 percent of lung transplant patients die during, or shortly after, the transplant. If you are in the lucky 90 percent who make it, you will probably wake up with a breathing tube down your trachea, and it will stay there for as little as 3 to 4 hours or as long as several weeks. Make your family swear they will take no photos until the tube comes out! Also warn your loved ones that when they first see you after the operation you'll probably look really bad, like you're dying, even if the operation was a total success and you're actually doing great.

Most patients are able to walk by the third or fourth day after they enter the ICU. Some patients are discharged in a week; some require a month or more to recover. According to the Duke Transplant Center, 2 to 4 weeks after transplant the average patient can walk a mile, and in about 6 weeks it is as safe as it ever is to have sex. Most patients, the Center says, can go back to work about 3 months after the operation.

As is true of patients successfully treated with calcium channel blockers or other PH drugs, lung transplantees usually find that the size and function of the right ventricle of their heart becomes much more normal.

Post-transplant problems. A whopping 80 to 85 percent of those who survive a transplant have a good functional status afterwards and can do normal activities without difficulty. Fifteen percent can't be totally independent, and a few need lots of help.

Most patients, however, do not work following their transplant (although among those who survive 5 years, 40 percent work full or part time, compared to around 30 percent after one year).

Transplant failure may be due to the failure of the primary graft to heal, acute rejection, or chronic rejection. Rejection is the tendency of your body's immune system to try to kill your new organ because it is different from "you." Lungs are more immunologically sensitive than most organs, so rejection is more of a problem. Acute rejection, perhaps triggered by a virus, can happen at any time, but is most common during the first month after transplant. When treated early, it is curable. Because rejection is often asymptomatic at first, lung biopsies are done regularly (after the first year, once a year may be enough). Too much anti-rejection medication can hurt the kidneys, but too little can allow chronic rejection to happen. It sometimes feels funny to be feeling good—better than you remember ever feeling—and then have your doctor tell you that your breathing tests and your lung biopsy show rejection. When you have been sick for a long time with a disease you are familiar with (PH), you have to relearn what normal is, so you can tell when your new lungs are sick. This can be sort of scary for patients.

The major long-term cause of death is chronic rejection (a.k.a. *bronchiolitis obliterans*). Bronchiolitis obliterans involves the formation of nodular masses (made up of fibrotic tissue and granulation) inside the small air passages in the lungs. A very small pilot study found that treating bronchiolitis obliterans with the antibiotic azithromycin (Zithromax) was well tolerated by patients and improved their lung function significantly. There are several lines of research underway to try to solve the bronchiolitis obliterans problem. For example, the anti-rejection drug rapamycin (originally developed in 1975 to treat yeast infections) might help. Rapamycin works through a different mechanism than calcineurin inhibitors like cyclosporine. Dr. P. Ussetti and others at Clinica Puerta de Hierro in Madrid, Spain, tried it on seven lung transplantation patients showing chronic rejection or toxicity associated with calcineurin inhibitors (common immunosuppressive drugs) with encouraging results. (See Chapter 7 for transplant survival statistics and a bit more information on bronchiolitis obliterans.)

How well will my new lung(s) function?
Healthy folks very seldom use their full lung capacity; even a single lung can usually supply you just fine. A lung transplant can transform somebody from near dead to near normal. A panelist at the 2000 conference told how she went from a wheelchair and eating icy pops in bed (the only things she had the energy to eat) to being able to care for her two kids when her husband, a long-distance trucker, was on the road.

Side effects. You will notice a difference in your resting heart rate. Before transplant it may be around 60 beats per minute. Afterwards it may be 100. It may also take your heart longer to speed up when you start exerting yourself. This is because the vagus nerve, which governs the heart rate, is not reattached after transplant. Fortunately, the body has another (chemical) way to signal the heart to speed up. It just doesn't work quite as fast.

Your voice might also sound different, because your vocal cords may be mechanically affected, or a nerve to them might be injured. Another possibility is that you might have a sense of breathlessness as the cilia (threadlike projections) inside your new lungs wiggle about trying to clear secretions. There is no way to reattach certain nerves to your new lung or lungs, so you will not feel like you need to cough, even when secretions fill your lungs. Therefore you have to consciously cough a lot and take deep breaths. There is a bit of evidence, however, that lungs and hearts sometimes reconnect nerves on their own.

The most serious side effects come from the medicines you have to take afterwards, for life, to prevent rejection. There are lots of pills to swallow. Some take 12 pills a day, some 40. It's an individual thing. A combination of drugs like cyclosporine and corticosteroids are used to weaken your immune system. This means that you are less able to fight off infections and diseases caused by bacteria, viruses, and fungi. The drugs might run about $3,000 a month or more (transplant centers usually have a staff person to help you figure out how to pay for the operation and drugs). Cyclosporine can cause flushing, hair growth (on the face, arms, and body), swollen gums, a fine hand tremor, headaches, high blood pressure, and numbness in hands and feet. Side effects of azathioprine (Imuran) can include mild, temporary hair loss; nausea, vomiting, and diarrhea; and the growth of tumors. Corticosteroids (such as prednisone) can boost your appetite, round out your face and abdomen, increase stomach acid and acne, weaken leg muscles, and cause sweating, joint pain, bone thinning (osteoporosis), and eye problems.

When listed like this, the side effects of immunosuppressive drugs seem more over-whelming than they usually are in real life; not every patient experiences every side effect. Other drugs and things as simple as increased exercise can counter some of the side effects. Doctors are learning to use multiple drugs to get a maximum anti-rejection effect with minimum toxicity. New approaches to controlling the immune system are also being explored. Pfizer is working on a drug code-named CP-690,550 that targets an enzyme (JAK3) found only in immune cells. It seemed to work as well in monkeys as conventional immune-suppressing drugs (that attack cells throughout the body) with fewer side effects. It's now being tested on people with psoriasis, before being tried on transplant patients.

Patient reports. Shirley Jewitt shared her experience with a single-lung transplant at the PHA 2002 conference. It was a bit over a year since she'd had the operation, at age 57. Before her transplant she fainted periodically and was close to death. She weighed 204 pounds when she was evaluated and had to shed 70 pounds to get listed. It took more than 2 years for a lung to become available; she credits epoprostenol with keeping her alive during this time. Following the transplant, Shirley was hospitalized for a month. Now all her PH symptoms are gone, she renewed her California realtor's license (passing the test with a higher score than before she became ill). She plays 18 holes of golf twice a week and crews on a 42-foot sailboat. To get the whole story, you can find her book about her transplant, *I Call My New Lung Tina,* in PHA's website store.

Sharren Yamron wrote about her *second* lung transplant for *Pathlight.* It was a 3-year wait and there were many false calls because she and her husband lived far from Johns Hopkins. They would get part way there—or even have Sharren prepared for surgery—before learning that the organs weren't in good enough condition. But she finally got a new lung. "The breathing tube and ventilator were hell," she says. "I smiled from ear to ear when I got that thing out." A year after her surgery she leads a normal life, with moderation. She is an active PHA volunteer, running the support group in Pittsburgh and answering calls to PHA's hotline. She hopes to make people aware of their right to a second transplant.

A final word. If you are considering a transplant, be sure to check for any updates on the Consensus Statement on lung transplantation by PHA's Scientific Leadership Council, which is posted on the PHA website. Now that the results of the Human Genome Project are out, the floodgate is opened for new therapies. To quote one lung transplant surgeon: "Not one of us wants to be doing transplants 40 years from now."

LATE-BREAKING NEWS

In 2005, the United Network for Organ Sharing (UNOS), changed the way organs are allocated to transplant patients. In the new method, instead of giving organs based on the length of time on the waiting list, each patient was given a specific lung allocation score.

The score is supposed to take into account how sick the individual is. It is derived from clinical predictors of survival that is reported on a scale of 0 to 100 (0 being the least ill and 100 being the most ill). For more information on how this new system might affect PH patients, see the article on page 285 & 286.

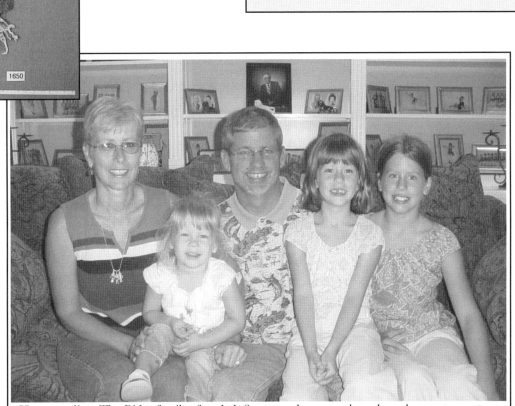

Happy ending. The Rider family after dad- Scott - underwent a thromboendarterectomy at UCSD in 2003. He put off the operation until Sarah (on his lap) was born.
Scott, being a guy, sent a photo of HIS clot (above-left), which is bigger than Dorothy's (p. 123)--in fact, he says it's the second largest ever removed!
Photo used by permission of the Ennis Daily News.

Tell Me, Doc,
How Long Do I Have?

Because how you feel is one of the best indicators of how things are going, you have "inside information" as to how long you will survive—be sure to share it with your PH specialist! This chapter lays out some generalities, but you are an individual, not a statistic. The mortality predictions are based on "averages" or "means" that may or may not apply to you. Each of us is unique, and new treatments seem to come along every year or so.

Only a decade ago, the prognosis was much worse. PH patients were told the disease would most likely progress rapidly and they would soon die, probably from chronic right ventricular failure or sudden death (perhaps from really slow heart action, *bradycardia*, or an outright cessation of heartbeat). The *Merck Manual* published in 1987 dourly predicted that a person with "PPH" would die two to five years after diagnosis. Children usually died within a year of diagnosis, according to Dr. Robyn Barst.

The past few years have seen tremendous advances. Even if you have to be pushed in a wheelbarrow to get to your initial visit with a PH specialist, it's how severe your PH is *after your treatment gets well underway* that matters the most. (The prognosis for children still varies a bit from that for adults. See Chapter 8.)

As you are reading the statistics, keep in mind the difference between mean (average) and median (the middle number of a string of numbers, where half are above, and half below

the median). A cluster of early deaths, or a few very long-term survivors, can jerk an "average" number around.

Also keep in mind the shifting definitions of PPH, SPH, and IPAH (see the Glossed-Over Glossary). In different studies, these terms may include or exclude different groups of patients, and researchers aren't always careful to spell this out. The *Survival Guide* usually uses the term the researchers used, unless it seems pretty clear that the researcher would have used a different term under the newer definitions.

Long-term survivors. Many PH patients are either approaching or well past the "20-years-since-definitive-diagnosis" mark. At the 1998 PHA International Conference, we formed the first long-term survivors' support group. Eight years was the threshold for group membership. About 15 of us showed up, a decent turnout. By the 2000 conference, so many patients could pass the 8-year test that we felt our club was, well, getting less *exclusive*, so we considered redefining "long-term" to mean 10 or more years.

Long-term survivors are a diverse lot: male and female; saints and sinners; young and old; and from a variety of ethnic backgrounds. As of 2000, those of us who showed up for the meeting were still mostly *primary* pulmonary hypertension patients. What kept us alive? Many responded well to CCBs. The blockers tend to work better on IPAH/FPAH folks than on patients with PH associated with another illness. And the blockers were available years before epoprostenol was around. Others had a transplant or underwent a thromboendarterectomy. At least one man was on nitric oxide therapy. More of us were using epoprostenol in 2000 than in 1998.

Spontaneous recovery? Even without treatment, a tiny percentage of adult "PPH" patients plod along year after year, for a decade or more. Spontaneous recovery, however, is exceedingly rare. If a treatment is available that works for you, use it! Remember that, untreated, this serious disease feeds on itself, and the prognosis is dreadful.

CDC Mortality Data on "PPH"

An interesting survey using Centers for Disease Control and Prevention mortality data (the CDC collects the death certificates of all U.S. citizens) blew some long-standing notions about who dies from "PPH" right out of the water. When adjustments were made for the age of the deceased, it was found that a greater percentage of blacks than whites died of "PPH," more women than men (this was already known), and that infants had the highest mortality rates. After childhood, death rates increased along with age. In other words, "PPH" appeared to cause death more often in infants, blacks, and especially in elderly black women, who were apparently dying at an

Annual Age-Adjusted PPH* Mortality Per One Million Population in the U.S. from 1979 through 1996, by Race and Gender

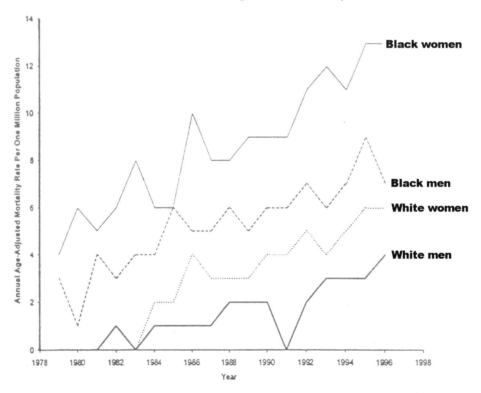

* (ICD-9 rubic 416.0)
From Chest (Mar. 2000) *117(3):796-800. Used with the permission of D.E. Lilienfeld, L. J. Rubin, and* Chest.

astonishing rate of 13 deaths per million U.S. citizens by 1996 (the deaths per million *PH patients* would, of course, be far higher).

The authors of this survey speculated that the overall increase in mortality found for all groups between 1979 and 1996 might be attributed, in part, to the introduction of anorexigenic diet pills, to the increased number of persons who are HIV positive, to improved diagnosis, and to heightened awareness. The researchers cautioned that it isn't known whether the changes in the death rates had anything to do with the incidence of the disease in the U.S. population. A lot more research needs to be done to find the true incidence of this disease.

General Things Doctors Consider in Making a Prognosis

It's frustrating that many studies apply only to those with the poorly defined term "PPH." But some of the "PPH" studies probably included patients who got PH as a result of diet pill use, HIV infection, taking illegal drugs, and maybe even some missed congenital heart disease and/or thromboembolic disease. Even if you have another form of PH, things that are bad signs in "PPH" patients are probably not good signs for you, either. As you will notice, many of the prognostic indicators overlap, and the studies are maddeningly inconsistent in the types of patients they include and the way they measure results.

The type of PH you have and the treatment you are receiving. What is known about how longevity relates to the types of PH is spelled out below, under specific headings. Types of PH come first, followed by a look at the success of various treatments on various types of PH.

The severity of your symptoms and your functional classification. The severity of your symptoms can tell you a lot. The worse your symptoms, the worse your prognosis. This applies to all forms of PH. As explained earlier, the symptoms a PH patient has place him or her in one of four classes. In IPAH / FPAH patients, the higher (worse) your classification before you start treatment, the more likely you are to die sooner. And the lower (better) your class, the more likely you are to live. Before epoprostenol was available, functional class I or II patients lived a median of 6 years, while functional class III patients lived 2.5 years, and class IV lived only 6 months.

Sleep-disordered breathing. It isn't known which comes first, the periodic cessation of breathing (*sleep apnea*) or the worsening of PH, but preliminary data has found an association.

Pericardial effusion. The presence of fluid in the cavity around the heart suggests a poor prognosis.

Things apparently *not* associated with longevity. Study results are conflicting and blurry, but it seems that, at least in patients with "PPH," age, sex, and the length of time between when you first experienced PH symptoms and when you were diagnosed do not reveal much about how long you will live.

The NIH Registry: the Grim Granddaddy of "PPH" Mortality Studies

To prove how wonderful their new drugs or treatments for PH are, researchers compare their results with what they call "conventional therapy." This means treatment with only oxygen, diuretics, warfarin, calcium channel blockers, and sometimes digoxin. The definitive survey was done by the National Institutes of Health (NIH) Registry, which collected data on 194 "PPH" (their term) patients from 1981 through 1985, and found the median survival time back then was only 2.8 years. (Remember that epoprostenol, the first real treatment other than transplant, wasn't approved by the FDA until 1995.) The NIH Registry showed the following with conventional therapy:

Survival at 1 year:	68 %
Survival at 2 years:	48 %
Survival at 3 years:	34 %

Survival According to Type of PH

Thanks to Chest *for allowing us to use some statistics in this section that appeared in their not-to-be-missed July 2004 supplement, "Diagnosis and Management of Pulmonary Arterial Hypertension: ACCP Evidence-Based Clinical Practice Guideline."*

Congenital Heart Disease/PAH Patients

In general, patients with congenital heart disease/PAH do not deteriorate as fast as "PPH" patients do. This is also true for congenital heart disease/PAH patients treated with epoprostenol. Here are some figures for patients with Eisenmenger's syndrome (none of these patients were transplanted):

1-year survival	97 %
2-year survival	89 %
3-year survival	72 %

Chronic Thromboembolic PH (CTEPH) Patients

Unless your clots are removed surgically, if you are in Class III or IV, your chance of survival is poor.

Fenfluramine/PAH Patients

Rush Heart Institute doctors compared 10 patients who had PH triggered by diet pills with 70 IPAH patients who were similar in age, symptoms, treatment, and hemodynamics, but who had not taken diet pills.

	Used fenfluramine	Did not use fenfluramine
1-year survival	50 %	88 %
3-year survival	17 %	60 %

Dr. Stuart Rich calls the disease triggered by diet pills worse and more resistant to treatment than sporadic IPAH. Some other doctors strongly disagree. It is possible that the sickest patients were sent to Rush because it is a premiere referral center. Note that there were only 10 diet pill users in the study. As discussed earlier, drug treatments can still help, even if results aren't as spectacular. Furthermore, the above figures do not consider the transplant option.

HIV/PAH Patients

The overall survival of HIV/PAH patients is similar to that of IPAH/FPAH patients. HIV/PAH patients who are not sick from their HIV die mostly from their PAH, not necessarily from infections related to their HIV. In a prospective, case-controlled study of 19 HIV/PAH patients published in 1997 by Dr. M. Opravil and others (University Hospitals in Zurich, Switzerland), HIV/PAH patients survived a median of 1.3 years (versus 2.6 years for HIV patients without PAH). This is really depressing, but the outlook is better when patients use antiretroviral therapy and infused epoprostenol.

Another group of researchers (Dr. Hilario Nunes and others, Université Paris-Sud, Clamart, France) looked at 82 cases of HIV / PAH and in 2003 published these overall survival rates:

1-year survival	73 %
2-year survival	60 %
3-year survival	47 %

Those in functional Classes I-II at time of diagnosis did better:

1-year survival	100 %
2-year survival	90 %
3- year survival	84 %

Those in functional Classes III-IV at time of diagnosis fared worst, of course:

1-year survival	60 %
2-year survival	45 %
3-year survival	28 %

Within the group of Class III and IV patients, those with a CD4 lymphocyte count of over 212 cell mm(-3), (i.e., those not sick from their HIV), and those who used epoprostenol infusion and combination anti-retroviral therapy did better than the others.

IPAH Patients

If only "conventional therapy" (pre-epoprostenol drugs, see above) is used, a higher mean right artial pressure and/or mean PAP, and a lower cardiac index all suggest a worse prognosis. In a study of 81 patients with severe IPAH who were followed for 3 years, and who participated in a randomized epoprostenol clinical trial, the presence of a collection of fluid around the heart and an enlarged right atrium were associated with a worse prognosis.

Biomarkers (found from a blood test). (The following studies apply only to IPAH patients.) The evidence supporting the prognostic usefulness of these tests is still fairly weak. Brain naturetic peptide (BNP) levels are thought to rise because of an overloaded right ventricle, and it appears that elevated levels of (BNP) are a bad sign. In one study, patients with BNP levels below a median value of 180 pg/ml were a lot more likely to still be alive 2 years later. Using an analysis with different cutoffs/breakpoints, 70 percent of patients with baseline BNP levels under 150 pg/ml survived at least 2 years, compared to 52 percent of those with higher levels of BNP. It is also a bad sign if your BNP levels don't decline after you start treatment for IPAH.

Other researchers have looked at a protein in the blood called the von Willebrand factor (a.k.a. coagulation factor VII, a congenital bleeding disorder). IPAH patients and patients with PAH/congenital heart disease who have too much von Willebrand factor have been

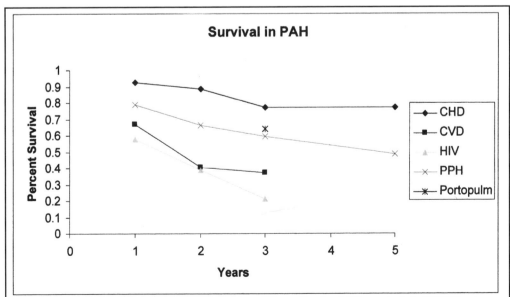

From "Prognosis of Pulmonary Hypertension, "Terry Fortin, M.D. et al., July 2002 Chest supplement on "Diagnosis and Management of Pulmonary Arterial Hypertension: ACCP Evidence-Based Clinical Practice guidelines. Used with permission.

found less likely to still be alive a year after their diagnosis than those without the excess factor.

Cardiopulmonary exercise testing (CPET). Dr. Roland Wensel (Deutsches Herzzentrum Berlin, Germany) and others studied 70 IPAH patients and found that their peak oxygen uptake (how much oxygen their heart is able to deliver to their body) during exercise and also their peak systolic blood pressure strongly predicted who would survive. Those less likely to live had both low peak oxygen uptakes (less than 10.4 ml/.kg(-1)./min(-1), and systolic blood pressure of 120 mm Hg or lower). Such patients had only a 23 percent chance of being alive a year later. Patients with one or neither of these factors had a 79 percent and 97 percent chance, respectively, of being alive.

Dr. Giuseppe Paciocco and colleagues at the University of Michigan in Ann Arbor reported in 2001 that in the 34 moderately symptomatic "PPH" patients they followed for a median of 26 months, oxygen desaturation during exercise and the distance walked in 6 minutes were linked to mortality. Patients who walked 300 meters or less in 6 minutes were 2.4 times more likely to die than those who walked more than 300 meters. A patient's arterial oxygen saturation dropping by 10 percent or more at the end of their 6-minute walk test meant they were 2.9 times more likely to die than those whose saturation did not drop as much. When PVR was adjusted for, each percent decrease in arterial oxygen saturation meant a 27 percent increase in the likelihood a patient would die.

Doppler right ventricular index above the median. This is a calculation made during an echocardiogram of how well the right ventricle of your heart is working. It is also called the "Tei" index. If you have IPAH and your index is elevated, it suggests a poor prognosis.

Pericardial effusion. If you have IPAH, a collection of fluid inside the sac that surrounds your heart suggests a poor prognosis and a significantly increased chance of death.

Pulmonary function tests (PFTs). In IPAH patients, researchers at Harbor-UCLA Medical Center have found that PFT results correlate with the severity of the disease, but it is not yet known if these tests can tell you anything about how long you will live. For scleroderma/PAH patients, a DLCO (a type of PFT) may have prognostic value. See the section below on Connective Tissue Disease / PAH Patients.

Six-minute walk test (6MWT). How well you do on a 6MWT can reveal a lot about how long you will probably live. Three studies have reached this conclusion. In an "unencouraged" test (where patients were not urged to walk faster or farther) reported on in 1996, Dr. Robyn Barst and others followed 81 patients with "PPH" for 12 weeks and found that nonsurvivors walked about 195 meters (plus or minus 63 meters) and survivors walked 305 meters (plus or minus 14 meters). Other researchers followed this same group of patients for several years (after most had begun treatment with epoprostenol), and found that those who had walked less than 153 meters before treatment were less likely to have survived.

Dr. Shoichi Miyamoto and others at the National Cardiovascular Center in Osaka, Japan, looked at 43 "PPH" patients who underwent *encouraged* 6-minute walk tests. They divided the group according to the median 6MWT distance of 332 meters, and found that after 21 months (plus or minus 16 months), those in the group that had walked over 332 meters (363 yards) were more likely to still be alive than those who had walked less far.

The data from other types of exercise tests, such as treadmill tests, haven't been studied well enough to make predictions. Nor is there good data on the prognositc value of 6MWT for PH patients who do not have IPAH. Furthermore, some patients might not try very hard—something their doctor can often detect by how they do on the "Borg Perceived Exertion Scale," which tries to quantify pain and effort on a scale of 1 to 20, the latter being extreme exertion. It considers factors like leg discomfort and labored breathing. So if you walk fewer meters than hoped for, don't panic. Talk it over with your specialist.

PAH Patients

At the 2003 meeting of the American Thoracic Society, Stanford University researchers reported on their efforts to identify patients who would survive for at least 3 years following their diagnosis with PAH. They looked back at the records of 88 patients, and found that these groups were 97 percent certain to survive without transplantation: (1) PAPs or right ventricular systolic pressures under 60 mm Hg; (2) PAPs or right ventricular systolic pressures in the range of 61-80 mm Hg *plus* no need for loop diuretics (a class of diuretics that includes Lasix, Bumex, Demedex, etc.); and (3) PAPs or RVSP greater than 80 mm Hg *plus* no need for loop diuretics *plus* being in Class I or II. Patients who fell into one of these three categories were *fifteen times* more likely to survive than those who fit none of them.

Portopulmonary Hypertension Patients

The mean survival after diagnosis of PH related to portopulmonary hypertension used to be only 15 months (1996), but epoprostenol has probably improved the survival rate.

Connective Tissue Disease/PAH Patients

According to the Scleroderma Federation website, "the course of mild to moderate PH in scleroderma patients is still unknown, and it's possible that it may persist unchanged for long periods of time." However, scleroderma/PAH patients do not appear to live as long as IPAH patients, even if their hemodynamic numbers are similar, and even with epoprostenol therapy. When scleroderma patients die, it is usually from pulmonary disease, particularly pulmonary vascular disease.

Dr. Cathy Morgan and other researchers at the University of Manchester, UK, identified predictors of "end-stage" lung disease in a 2003 report that looked at the medical records of 561 scleroderma patients. "End stage" was defined as: 1) death; 2) PH requiring continuous ambulatory iloprost; or 3) pulmonary fibrosis requiring continuous oxygen. From 1982 to 1997, 24 patients reached "end stage." Cumulatively, 4 percent reached this point at 5 years, 6 percent at 7 years, and 12 percent at 14 years. If a patient had normal lung function at baseline, they were at very low risk. The "end stagers" were much more likely to have been in the lowest third of either diffusing capacity or forced vital capacity at baseline, and to have protein in their urine. The findings of blood tests and the extent of skin disease were not relevant. According to other researchers, if the ability of your lungs to diffuse carbon monoxide (DLCO) is less than 45 percent of what is predicted for you, and you don't have interstitial fibrosis, it may mean your prognosis is even worse.

One PH expert called the survival curve of scleroderma patients prior to the use of epoprostenol as "horrific." Patients with CREST/PAH had a reported 2-year survival of 40 percent, compared to 80 percent for

CREST patients without PH. Those with PAH and diffuse or limited scleroderma had about a 50 percent survival rate at 2 years. Other researchers reported a 2-year survival rate of 40 percent in systemic scleroderma/PH patients. If a systemic sclerosis/PAH patient has DRw52 (an HLA antigen) he or she is less likely to survive.

A quarter to half of PAH patients with systemic lupus erythematosis (SLE) were alive 2 years following their diagnosis of PAH. (But some of the studies on which this statement is based were done prior to the use of epoprostenol.)

Mixed connective tissue disease/PAH patients tend to have either scleroderma or SLE as their most prominent disease, and would follow the mortality patterns of those diseases.

For rheumatoid arthritis/PAH patients or dermatomyositis/polymyositis/PAH patients, the prognosis isn't known.

Survival According to Type of Treatment

Atrial Septostomy Patients

A survey of the literature found four reports of this procedure, involving only 55 PH patients. Forty-two of them survived at least 30 days or until they checked out of the hospital.

Bosentan (Tracleer) Users

At the American Thoracic Society (ATS) annual meeting in 2003, Dr. Vallerie McLaughlin presented data collected from 27 PH centers and involving 169 IPAH

patients or patients with scleroderma/PAH who were followed up to 39 months. Before starting on bosentan most patients were Class III, but a few were Class IV. Here is what she found:

1-year survival	96 %
2-year survival	89 %
3-year survival	86 %

Some of the patients used only bosentan; all used it as a first-line therapy, but after 2 years about 20 percent were on another therapy either in addition to, or instead of, bosentan. There is no follow-up data on what Class the patients were in after 39 months on bosentan. After a while, some patients added epoprostenol. Two patients died while on combination therapy (none died who got a placebo), but the study was too small to draw any conclusions as to the safety of the drug.

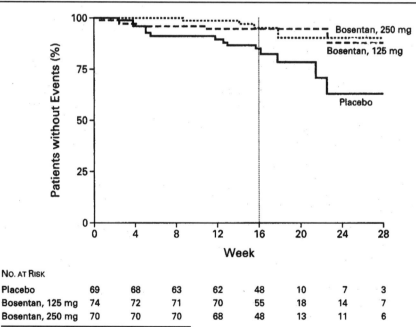

No. at Risk							
Placebo	69	68	63	62	48	10	7	3
Bosentan, 125 mg	74	72	71	70	55	18	14	7
Bosentan, 250 mg	70	70	70	68	48	13	11	6

Kaplan-Meier Estimates of the Proportion of Patients with Clinical Worsening. Clinical worsening was defined by the combined end point of death, lung transplantation, hospitalization, or discontinuation of the study treatment because of worsening PAH, a need for epoprostenol therapy, or atrial septostomy. P<0.05 for the comparison of the bosentan groups with the placebo group at weeks 16 and 28 by the log-rank test. There was no significant difference between the two bosentan groups at weeks 16 and 18 (P=0.87).

Copyright © 2002 The New England Journal of Medicine.

Patients Using Calcium Channel Blockers (CCBs)

Papers published in *Circulation* in 1987 and in the *New England Journal of Medicine* in 1992 gave a small group of "PPH" patients their first cause for hope. In the second study, Dr. Stuart Rich and his colleagues treated 64 Class III and Class IV patients with high doses of CCBs. All of those who responded well were still alive 5 years later. For purposes of this study, "responder" means a patient whose mean PAP fell by 39 percent, and whose pulmonary vascular-resistance-index also quickly fell by 53 percent. Dr. Rich said his responders—who also took warfarin—were still going strong more than a decade later. He also said that some Class II patients might respond even better to the blockers.

Other research found that patients who responded only moderately well did not live significantly longer than those who responded very little. As mentioned earlier, there is lots of disagreement as to what constitutes a good response. At most, one out of five IPAH patients "passes" an acute vasodilator test.

If you do not respond well during an acute vasodilator trial, or if you have secondary PH, it isn't known whether your vasodilator responsiveness is linked to your probable longevity.

Epoprostenol (Flolan) Users

No one disputes that epoprostenol significantly prolongs the life of PAH patients, but different studies show somewhat different results. Most indicate that, 5 years after beginning treatment with epoprostenol, between 55 and about 68 percent of patients are still alive.

Vanderbilt researchers followed 91 PAH patients treated with epoprostenol at their institution between June 1995 and August 2001. They found that epoprostenol significantly improved survival. Predictors of increased mortality included being above the median age of 44 years when the disease began, being in Class IV at baseline or follow-up, and having scleroderma.

"PPH" patients in functional Classes III and IV have a much better prognosis if they use epoprostenol. In scleroderma/PAH patients, epoprostenol doesn't seem nearly as helpful. In patients with other types of PH, there just isn't enough data to say for sure how epoprostenol affects survival.

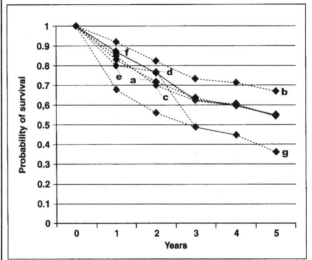

Probability of survival among PAH patients treated with epoprostenol (a-f) vs. untreated patients (g). (a) 195 sequential patients with PAH of various types who started treatment with epoprostenol prior to January 2001 (unpublished data). (b) 97 sequential patients with PPH and full right-heart hemodynamic studies at epoprostenol initiation prior to January 2001 (unpublished data). (c) 178 patients with PPH receiving epoprostenol treatment over period of 8 years. (d) 162 patients with PPH receiving epoprostenol over period of 10 years. (e) 59 patients with PPH treated with epoprostenol. (f) 17 patients with PPH treated with epoprostenol. (g) patients enrolled in the National PPH Registry.
From Advances in Pulmonary Hypertension, Vol.1, No. 3.

Here is a summary from the *Chest*, July 2004 supplement on "Diagnosis and Management of Pulmonary Arterial Hypertension: ACCP Evidence-Based Clinical Practice Guidelines," of what percentage of "PPH" patients survive with, and without epoprostenol (using the grim NIH Registry "conventional therapy" figures for comparison):

	1 yr	2 yrs	3 yrs	5 yrs
"Conventional therapy"	77 %	52 %	41 %	27 %
With epoprostenol	87 %	72 %	63 %	54 %

Similar results were reported for 162 consecutive patients treated with epoprostenol by Dr. Vallerie McLaughlin and others at Rush-Presbyterian-St. Luke's in Chicago:

87.8% 76.3% 62.8%

After the first year of therapy, those patients were more likely to survive who moved to lower functional classes and saw improvements in their exercise tolerance, cardiac index, and mean PAP (this is hardly surprising). But if a patient had IPAH and had been treated with Flolan for at least 3 months and was still in functional Class III or IV, he/she was less likely to survive a long time. Other bad omens in her study included: 1) having a history of right-heart failure and a baseline 6-minute walk of less than 150 meters (remember that cutoff points have varied in different studies); and 2) the absence of a fall of at least 30 percent in total pulmonary resistance compared to baseline. An elevated baseline mean right atrial pressure was another bad sign.

Even if you are in a group less likely to survive, you may be an exception. Judy was on epoprostenol for over 4 years before she began to see a downward trend in her high pressures. "At our home," she said, "we have the philosophy that we will live 'life' and not 'death.'"

A 12-week prospective study of 81 patients done by Dr. Robyn Barst, Dr. Lewis Rubin, and others (*New England Journal of Medicine*, February 1, 1996), found that those treated with epoprostenol survived longer (all of them survived) than those treated with conventional therapy (80 percent survived). (The "conventional therapy" included CCBs, but lumped together patients who responded well to them with patients who did not.) There has not been a head-to-head comparison of CCBs and epoprostenol from day one of treatment, but a study by Dr. McLaughlin and others concluded: "Indeed, were it not for the complexity and expense of the delivery system, epoprostenol might be considered first-line therapy for all patients with primary pulmonary hypertension."

On the surface, the survival figures for epoprostenol do not look as impressive as those in the CCB study. But the epoprostenol studies included only those who didn't respond well to CCBs, so the patients in the studies were usually much sicker. Remember that less than 20 percent of PH patients respond well to CCBs, while nearly all respond to epoprostenol (although the initial response might not be dazzling). Furthermore, patients with right-heart failure cannot take CCBs because of the risk of worsening or death. So very sick people are included in the survival figures for epoprostenol. Finally and unfortunately, some patients using epoprostenol die because they are unable to stop using the street drugs that caused their PAH.

Another retrospective study, this time of 178 patients (led by Dr. McLaughlin and published in 2002) looked in more detail at how functional classification affects the longevity of patients using epoprostenol:

Class when epoprostenol use started	3-year survival	5-year survival
Class III	81 %	79 %
Class IV	47 %	27 %

After a mean of 17 months of epoprostenol therapy:

Class I or II	89 %	73 %
Class III	62 %	35 %

Class IV had a much lower 24-month survival rate of 42 percent.

Predictors of a worse than usual outcome for patients using epoprostenol included being older (above a median age of 44 in one study), being in functional Class IV before or after treatment (as opposed to Class I, II, or III), and having scleroderma.

Iloprost Inhalers

Schering, AG, in Berlin, Germany, (the makers of iloprost) funded S. Nikkho and others to look at how 40 "PPH" and 23 patients with PH associated with another disease were doing after 2 years of inhaling iloprost. The first 3 months of the study were randomized, and two control patients and two patients using iloprost died. Another four died during the long phase of the trial. Three of the eight patients who died had "PPH," the others five had PH associated with another disease. These results were much better than expected.

Treprostinil (Remodulin) Injection Therapy

In 2002, United Therapeutics reported that a preliminary analysis of 843 PAH

patients treated with Remodulin had a 3-year survival rate of 69.83 percent.

Thromboendarterectomy Survivors

This is the procedure described in Chapter 6 where specialists surgically remove clots from the lungs of patients with chronic thromboembolic PH. Doctors at UCSD, San Diego, CA, have done over 1,400 of these procedures since 1990, while steadily improving their techniques. In 2003, they reported a mortality rate of only 4.4 percent for the last 500 patients they operated on. Many survivors were essentially cured of their PH. A 6-year survival rate of 75 percent, with several patients living longer than 15 years, was reported by Dr. Carol J. Archibald and colleagues at UCSD (1999). As discussed in Chapter 6, in some patients not all of the clot can be removed, and these patients must still take a PH medicine. Doctors at Mayo in Rochester, MN, report that their mortality rates have improved, and since 1997 the operative and hospital mortality in 42 patients was only 2 percent. (A hospital's mortality figures can be influenced by the type of patients they accept.) The Mayo doctors also saw improvement in the size and function of their patients' right ventricles. A broader survey of 19 uncontrolled reports from various centers (spanning the years from 1992 to 2002) found a 30-day "post-operative" mortality among 802 patients of 14 percent. The causes of death appeared to be inadequate clot removal (persistent PH), hemorrhage, inability to remove a patient from bypass, and sepsis.

UCSD researchers mailed questionnaires to over 420 patients who had undergone a thromboendarterectomy at least a year previously. Their ages ranged from 19 to 89 years, with a mean age of 56. This is what the 308 who responded said:

+ 56 patients could walk "indefinitely."
+ The median distance others could walk was a mile.
+ Of the working population, 62 percent of those unemployed before the operation were able to return to work.
+ 10 percent used oxygen.
+ 93 percent were in Class I or II.

These are hardly "mortality" figures!

Transplant Recipients

A heart-lung, single-lung, or double-lung transplant may well improve your quality of life and might lengthen your life. Any transplant is a high-risk operation, of course. As of 2003, centers worldwide had done over 13,453 lung transplants for various forms of lung disease; some of these were retransplants. About 1 out of 10 transplanted patients died before leaving the hospital. One-year survival is roughly 75 percent. Two-and-a-half-year survival is roughly 60 to 65 percent. An informative (but depressing) website is maintained by the International Society for Heart and Lung Transplantation (ISHLT) registry. Click through their PowerPoint slide presentation and you will discover that about half of "PPH" patients live 4 years post-transplant. If you consider only those who survive the first 3 months, however, about half live 7 years or longer. (Patients with PH associated with another disease are not broken out as a group.) You will also find that mortality is higher among lung transplant patients with elevated levels of bilirubin or creatinine (common in PH patients), a need for supplemental oxygen pre-transplant (also common in PH patients), or a pre-transplant pulmonary artery systolic pressure above 40 mm Hg. If the donor or recipient is older than is usual, this can also increase the risk.

Doctors have found that PH patients who receive a transplant are more likely to live longer than comparable PH patients who receive "conventional therapy." In other words, they live longer than those poor souls did who were listed in the old NIH study. But today there are many drug treatments for PH, so transplantation is appropriate only when drugs are not effective. As a whole, most experts would probably say that transplant recipients survive about as long as patients using epoprostenol. This does not mean that if you pick one of these choices right after you are diagnosed you are likely to get the same outcome. Five years on epoprostenol followed by a transplant, if necessary, is probably the best choice. (As discussed in the previous chapter, there are a few PH patients who need to go straight to transplantation.)

Which is better: one lung, two lungs, or a heart and two lungs? Docs speaking at PHA's 2002 conference said the longest living "PPH"/lung-transplant patient they knew of lived 13 or 14 years. A heart/lung recipient lived about 19 years. But these are, of course, the exceptions. Cold statistics tell a less rosy, but still encouraging story.

In 2003, the International Society for Heart and Lung Transplantation (ISHLT) looked back at the numbers for lung transplants done for all reasons, not just PH, and found a slight advantage for double-lung transplants at least up to 9 years following the operation, but the difference between the survival of single-lung and double-lung recipients wasn't statistically significant.

Here are the ISHLT survival figures for the recipients of lung transplants:

	1 yr	3 yrs	5 yrs	9-10 yrs
Single-lung	65 %	50 %	43 %	23 % (9 yrs)
Double-lung	70 %	55 %	45 %	20 % (9 yrs)
Heart-lung	65 %	45 %	40 %	25 % (10 yrs)
IPAH				
heart-lung	70 %	50 %	40 %	25 % (10 yrs)

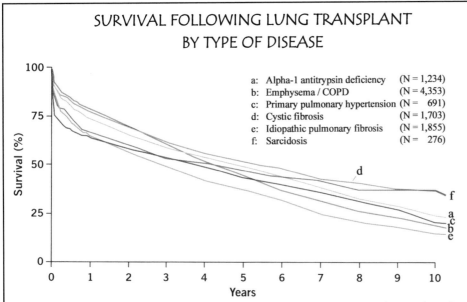

SURVIVAL FOLLOWING LUNG TRANSPLANT BY TYPE OF DISEASE

a: Alpha-1 antitrypsin deficiency (N = 1,234)
b: Emphysema / COPD (N = 4,353)
c: Primary pulmonary hypertension (N = 691)
d: Cystic fibrosis (N = 1,703)
e: Idiopathic pulmonary fibrosis (N = 1,855)
f: Sarcidosis (N = 276)

UNOS/ISHLT registry data showing actuarial survival for all lung transplant patients by diagnosis (January 1990 to June 2001). Note higher early mortality for recipients with primary pulmonary hypertension compared with other diagnoses. From www.ishlt.org.

Heart-lung transplants for congenital heart disease/PH have about the same survival rates as for IPAH. Dr. John Conte and colleagues at Johns Hopkins Medical Institutions in Baltimore, Maryland, reviewed all the lung transplants they had done for "PPH" and PH associated with other diseases and reported in 2001 that bilateral lung transplantation for "PPH" gave a survival advantage at all points up to 4 years. For patients with PH associated with another disease, the choice was not as clear, but the researchers thought that if their mean PAP was greater than 40 mm HG they *might* do better with two lungs; if it is under that, they *might* do better with one.

The first heart-lung transplant was done at Stanford University in 1981. In 1999, Stanford doctors reported an operative mortality rate of 18 percent, and actuarial survival of 72 percent at 1 year, 67 percent at 2 years, and 42 percent at 5 years. Seventy percent were still free of obliterative bronchiolitis at 5 years. Stanford researchers say bronchiolitis obliterans seems to occur less frequently with heart-lung transplants than with lung transplants, and that survival statistics are "comparable." The most frequent causes of death for heart-lung transplants are infection, bronchiolitis obliterans, and accelerated coronary artery disease.

Several groups of researchers have concluded that bilateral lung transplantation can be safely used on congenital heart disease / PH patients who need only simple repairs, and that heart-lung transplants are best when repairs are complex.

When you are looking up survival statistics, note what period is covered. If data includes people transplanted back in the 1980s it may give a misleading impression, because the development of better immunosuppressive drugs has since improved survival rates. Fewer single-lung transplants are being done now, and this also reportedly improves rates of long-term survival.

The conventional wisdom is that we PH patients do not generally do as well as the average lung transplant recipient. It is said that emphysema and cystic fibrosis patients who undergo transplants generally have a better survival rate than do PH patients. This may be incorrect. A study published in 1999 by Dr. Bryan F. Meyers (Washington University School of Medicine, St. Louis) and others found that although PH patients have a higher early mortality rate, their long-term results are similar to, or even a tiny bit better than, those for transplants done for other diseases. The study reviewed 10 years of clinical experience at that hospital and 450 lung transplants on 443 patients. The 1-year survival rate of all transplant recipients was 83.6 percent; the 5-year survival rate was 52.9 percent. Five years out, 25 percent of lung recipients were still free of bronchiolitis obliterans.

It's hard (if not impossible) to compare transplant survival studies because of the great number of variables. Another study found that the kind of PH you have does appear to affect your chance of survival. Dr. Ulrich Franke and other researchers at Friedrich-Schiller University in Jena, Germany, looked back at 10 years' experience with lung and heart-lung transplants. They compared 63 "PPH" transplant recipients with similar people who were transplanted because they had Eisenmenger's or PH secondary to chronic pulmonary embolisms. Their study, published in 2000, found that the patients with PH secondary to chronic pulmonary embolisms were much more likely to be alive 1, 3 and 5 years after transplant. Only 35 percent of "PPH" transplant recipients were alive 5 years out.

Transplantation is riskier in persons with severe right-side heart failure, ascites, an enlarged liver, or really high levels of bilirubin in their blood. It is also riskier if you are more than 20 percent above your ideal weight. However, the Cleveland Clinic group looked at the obesity question, and found that while it is associated with a greater short-term mortality, it does not affect long-term survival.

When you ask a transplant center about their survival rates, specify survival for PH patients, and also ask about the survival rates for patients who have your type of PH. Try to find a center with really good pre- and post-surgery care. Nurse friends can be a great source of information on this—they know which facilities are understaffed and which attract the best nurses and other members of transplant teams.

What goes wrong. Whether you get one lung or two, or a heart and lung, the biggest early killers are infection and acute graft rejection. Infection is always a problem, because working lungs are continually exposed to dirty air. Sometimes the site where the airway is attached just doesn't want to heal well. Accelerated coronary artery disease (a form of rejection) may be a problem when a heart is included.

Long-term, the biggest cause of death is bronchiolitis obliterans. Dr. Vibhu Kshettry and others at the University of Minnesota, Minneapolis took a look back at 107 lung transplants and found that patients who are transplanted because they have "PPH" are more likely to develop bronchiolitis obliterans, and to develop it sooner, than the average lung transplant patient (*Chest*, September 1996).

ADULT LUNG TRANSPLANT RECIPIENTS: CAUSE OF DEATH
(Deaths from January 1992-June 2002)
Source: ISHLT/UNOS

CAUSE OF DEATH	0-30 Days (N=937)	31 Days-1 Year (N=1,345)	Over 1 Yr. to 3 Yrs. (N=1,096)	Over 3 Yrs. to 5 Yrs. (N=572)	Over 5 Yrs. (N=456)
Bronchiolitis	5 (0.5%)	74 (5.5%)	313 (28.6%)	185 (32.3%)	142 (31.1%)
Acute rejection	46 (4.9%)	27 (2.0%)	21 (1.9%)	4 (0.7%)	2 (0.4%)
Lymphoma	1 (0.1%)	44 (3.3 %)	23 (2.1%)	9 (1.6%)	18 (3.9%)
Malignancy, other	—	27 (2.0%)	52 (4.7%)	43 (7.5%)	40 (8.8%)
CMV	1 (0.1%)	56 (4.2%)	17 (1.6%)	4 (0.7%)	2 (0.4%)
Infection, non-CMV	220 (23.5%)	521 (38.7%)	284 (25.9%)	113 (19.8%)	79 (17.3%)
Graft failure	286 (30.5%)	236 (17.5%)	175 (16.0%)	99 (17.3%)	58 (12.7%)
Cardiovascular	108 (11.5%)	58 (4.3%)	36 (3.3%)	24 (4.2%)	21 (4.6%)
Technical	78 (8.3%)	37 (2.8%)	12 (1.1%)	1 (0.2%)	2 (0.4%)
Other	192 (20.5%)	265 (19.7%)	163 (14.9%)	90 (15.7%)	92 (20.2%)

However, others disagree and this question remains unanswered.

If you have only a mild case of bronchiolitis obliterans you can still enjoy a very good quality of life. But if your bronchiolitis obliterans is severe, your quality of life is awful. Things are particularly grim if you got only a single lung. With present therapies, doctors can stop the progression of bronchiolitis obliterans about 50-60 percent of the time. Doctors now have an arsenal of about 10 anti-rejection drugs they can pick from and mix to reduce side effects and increase effectiveness for particular patients. Better therapies may be available in a few years.

The chart on p. 150 includes lung transplants done for any reason. There is much less data on transplants done just for PH, PAH, or IPAH.

Factors *not* significant for 1-year mortality for adult lung transplants (done for any reason, not just PH):

- Recipient factors: hospitalized, $pCO2$, gender, chronic steroid use, transfusions, history of malignancy, recent infection requiring IV drug therapy
- Donor factors: gender, clinical infection, history of hypertension, history of cancer, COD
- Transplant factors: procedure type, ABO compatibility, HLA mismatch, year of transplant

Source: ISHLT/UNOS, 2003.

Transplanting children. It is riskier to transplant children, so epoprostenol therapy is often used to delay transplantation and allow the child to do more growing. Many doctors think children should receive bilateral lung transplants whenever possible, to reduce the risk of bronchiolitis obliterans.

Survival of lobar transplant recipients. As of 2001, the 1-year survival rate for pediatric patients at Children's Hospital (affiliated with the University of Southern California) was about 80 percent. For 2 years, it was about 78 percent. In 2003 about half of lobar transplant recipients were still alive at 7 to 8 years. Children did slightly better than adults. Apparently, the better HLA typing that resulted from using a related donor did not make much difference in how well a recipient did. Dr. Vaughn Starnes, a pioneering transplant surgeon, looked back at 123 lobar transplants from *living* donors between 1993 and 2003 (done mostly because of cystic fibrosis). One-year actuarial survival was 70 percent, 3-year survival was 54 percent, and 5-year survival was 45 percent. Patients who were intubated prior to transplantation did the worst. Age, sex, reason for transplantation, donor relationship, etc. didn't influence survival.

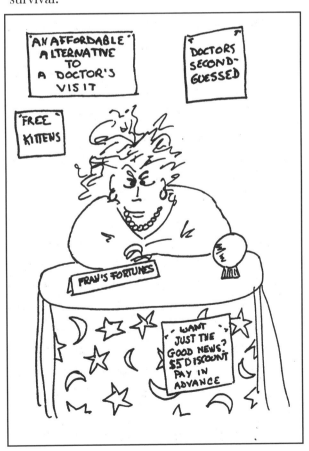

Dr. Michael Bowdisy, also at Children's / USC, looked at patients who had received lung transplants from 1993 to 2002 and lived longer than 90 days. Of these, 59 got a lobe and 43 got two cadaver lungs. (Ninety-five percent of these patients had cystic fibrosis, not PH.) At 3 years there was no difference in survival statistics between the two groups. They did about the same in exercise tests, rates and types of infection, risk of rejection, and lung function.

Since infection is, thus far, what has killed most of their patients, the Children's/USC team hopes to improve long-term statistics in living-lobar transplants by backing off on immunosuppressants and being more aggressive in treating infections with antibiotics. They think this might be why obliterative bronchiolitis is not the leading cause of death for recipients of lobes from living persons.

Warfarin (Coumadin) Users

As shown in the graph below, patients who respond well to CCBs might slightly increase their survival rate if they also take warfarin. For those who do not respond to CCBs, the use of warfarin appears even more important. (As detailed in Chapter 4, existing studies on the impact of warfarin on PH patients are somewhat flawed.)

A 1997 retrospective European study by H. Frank (University of Vienna, Austria) and others of 173 patients also found that anticoagulant therapy improved the odds of survival in "PPH" patients, along with improving their quality of life. Those who used anorexigenic diet drugs were particularly benefited by anticoagulation.

Kaplan-Meier Survival Estimates, According to Presence or Absence of Response to Calcium Channel Blockers and to Concurrent Use of Warfarin. Overall survival was significantly improved by warfarin therapy (P = 0.025).

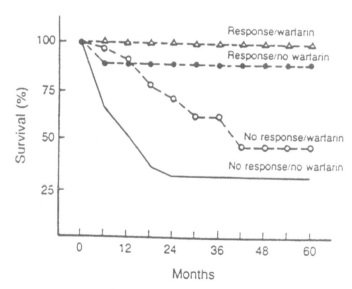

From S. Rich and others, "The Effect of High Doses of Calcium-Channel Blockers on Survival in Primary Pulmonary Hypertension," The New England Journal of Medicine (July 9, 1992) 327(2):76-81. Copyright © 1992 Massachusetts Medical Society. All rights reserved.

If Treatment Fails: Congestive Heart Failure

I'm allergic to writing in the first person (elsewhere in the book I hide under the alias Abigail), but here it seems necessary. While my cursor blinks, I've been remembering what it was like when I was experiencing severe congestive right-heart failure.

I was diagnosed with IPAH in 1983, but had gone without treatment because I was unwilling to undergo a transplant, which was the only treatment then available. (Don't try doing this yourself. I am extremely lucky to still be alive.) Ten years later, in 1993, my heart was in fibrillation and I could barely stay conscious. My doctors told my husband to call our daughter home from college.

I knew I was very sick. I had gained a lot of weight (fluid) over a short period. Even with supplemental oxygen I was weak and dizzy and there was an annoying pounding and gagging sensation in my swollen neck veins. My right ventricle was huge. My legs and ankles were swollen in spite of support hose. My abdomen bulged out and my liver area hurt. My shortness of breath when moving about was awful, and it didn't entirely go away when I was resting. My pulse was over 200.

Except maybe for the high pulse rate, my symptoms were fairly typical. "Congestive" means that when less blood is pumped out of your heart it backs up, and fluid from your blood seeps into your tissues and collects in organs like the lungs and liver. It can be the end game.

But I had been keeping up with the medical literature, and had found an article in the *New England Journal of Medicine* by Dr. Stuart Rich in which he described his success in treating PH patients with CCBS. I asked the University of Washington to try them on me. They worked. (Incidentally, today doctors would not give CCBS to a patient as sick as I then was. There are now safer alternatives, like epoprostenol.) Today it takes a sharp eye to tell I'm disabled.

But I want to go back to that night when it appeared I was about to die. What would it have been like if the doctors had not been able to stabilize me enough to try the blockers? What if the medicine had not worked? While the doctors were clustered around me I was very concerned, but not particularly scared. Deep in my core I knew everything would be all right, whatever happened.

This belief probably stemmed from an odd thing that happened to me way back in 1983, just before I was first diagnosed. (It was, in fact, the incident that led to the catheterization that diagnosed my IPAH.) My husband, my daughter (who was then only 8 years old), and I were on a Thanksgiving car trip and stopped at a mountain pass. When I got out of the car to walk around, I passed out. I stopped breathing, my husband says, and he could find no pulse. To get me out of the wet snow and mud, he carried me to the car and laid me across the front seats. While he tried to revive me, I floated above the scene looking right down through the metal roof of our car at that poor unconscious woman. I felt wonderful. There was a warmth on my back and it seemed as if my very molecules were loosening so that I was expanding into the universe.

Then my little girl screamed "Mommy! Mommy!" and I had to squeeze back into that body to soothe her. It was so cramped and limiting.

I don't know what to make of all this. But we seem to come equipped with what we need to deal with the entire course of our lives, including the end. It is a great comfort to me to know this.

Children and PAH

Children are not just small adults when it comes to PAH. Their prognosis, treatment, and coping strategies all differ. There is no minimum age for PAH; babies can even be born with the disease. It was once thought that the difference in the incidence of PAH in males and females wouldn't kick in until puberty. But with the exception of infancy (where congenital heart problems are the big cause of PAH), little girls are twice as likely to have PAH as little boys.

In spite of PAH and/or an epoprostenol pump, if needed, many children of all ages with the disease lead normal lives. They dance, take gymnastics, play sports, bicycle, roller blade, and slam their bedroom doors.

You must be your child's advocate. Parents said this over and over at a PHA conference workshop. It is not uncommon for a parent to save a child's life by asking questions, insisting, getting the child to a PH center, and by finding a PH specialist both they and the child are comfortable with. One mom said the experience had turned her into a "mother tiger." There is no one, she said, who will stand up for your child's welfare more than you will. "It sometimes takes getting angry," she said. "It sometimes takes being demanding. And that's not my personality at all. It's been a real challenge for me." A mom in the UK was told by her local doctor that her baby boy, Jack, would die of PH, and that she should not bother looking on the Internet for information because she would only find

rubbish and false hope. Fortunately, Jack's mom did a simple search and quickly learned about PHA-UK and the specialists and treatments that were available. Jack had the highest pressures recorded in a child of his age, his parents were told, and he was the youngest ever fitted with a central venous line and given epoprostenol treatment in the UK. When Jack turned three in late 2003, he was still on epoprostenol and was matchday mascot for the Australian Legends vs. the Doncaster Dragons rugby game. He kicked off for the Dragons.

Genes and PH

Familial PAH (FPAH)

If there are two or more persons in your family with PAH, you are said to have "familial" PAH. It used to be included in the category *primary* PH (PPH) along with idiopathic PH (IPAH), a term used when the disease does not run in a family and no cause for it is known. Sometimes people with IPAH have genetic mutations like those in FPAH.

Having FPAH does not mean your children are doomed to have the disease. Here's how it works: if one parent carries a PAH gene, his or her child has a fifty-fifty chance of inheriting the gene. The PAH gene is dominant, so it takes only one to create a predisposition to the disease. *Even if a child inherits a PAH gene, the child still has only a*

10 to 20 percent chance of actually developing the disease. Nevertheless, because of the severity of the disease, if it runs in your family all your children should be watched for symptoms, and perhaps even clinically or genetically screened for the disease.

If your child is the only one in your family known to have had IPAH, at least one expert recommends clinically screening your other children every 2 years, even though the odds are really against them getting it. Other experts feel this is being overly cautious.

Genetic testing is available for those with FPAH and even IPAH, but researchers do not yet know all the mutations that encourage or discourage the disease. For more information, see Chapter 3.

Down Syndrome and PAH

Nearly 8 percent of adults with Down syndrome have PAH. Although Down syndrome is genetically based (an extra chromosome is involved) it is not related to the genes that cause PAH. The much higher incidence of PAH among those with Down syndrome, as compared to the general population, is mostly due to the heart defects that often go hand-in-hand with the syndrome. It can also be linked to respiratory problems, like upper airway obstruction or sleep apnea, that are seen in many Down syndrome patients.

When congenital heart problems are surgically corrected, the outcomes are fairly similar for children with and without Down syndrome, except for large heart defects such as ventricular septal defect or complete atrioventricular septal defect, where Down kids have a worse time of it both before and after surgical repair.

Obstructive sleep apnea (OSA) is fairly common in children with Down syndrome. Children's Hospital in Los Angeles studied 53 children with Down syndrome in 1991 and found that 45 percent had OSA (a considerably greater number had this or another type of breathing problem while sleeping). The presence of OSA was not affected by age, obesity, or whether a child had congenital heart problems. The researchers concluded that OSA often goes unrecognized. A more recent study (1997) by doctors at Children's Medical Center in Atlanta, GA, suggests it would be wise to periodically test Down syndrome patients for OSA. They report success in surgically correcting the structural problems that contribute to OSA.

Can a Woman with PAH Have a Baby?

It seems very unfair that PAH is a disease that often afflicts women of child-bearing age. This means the question of pregnancy is frequently raised. For a woman with PAH, pregnancy is contraindicated because it is associated with life-threatening risks for both mother and baby. When a woman with PAH becomes pregnant, she is putting both her own life and that of her potential baby at risk. For those who survive, their PAH often worsens during pregnancy and remains worse after delivery.

The danger exists even during the first trimester, when your heart begins to beat more frequently, your blood volume and cardiac output increase (including blood flow through your pulmonary arteries), and your systemic blood pressure falls. At about 5 months, these changes peak. When you deliver the baby, your heart must work even harder. The most dangerous time is immediately following delivery, when hormonal changes can contribute to the danger.

A review of reports published between 1978 and 1996 that looked at maternal deaths within 35 days of delivery, found that the death rate for patients with "PPH" was 30 percent, for Eisenmenger's complex patients 36 percent, and that for patients with other forms of PH it was 56 percent.

Because of the potentially catastrophic risks to both mother and child, PH doctors do all they can to help their patients not get pregnant. If a patient does become pregnant, they recommend a therapeutic abortion. When a patient's personal beliefs rule out abortion, then doctors treat her PAH as aggressively as possible, and follow her closely both during and after her pregnancy. The mother may have to be hospitalized a long time.

Epoprostenol, calcium channel blockers, and nitric oxide therapy may help pregnant PAH patients survive, although the risks remain very high regardless of treatment, including risks to the baby, both from the mom's problems and possibly from the medications prescribed to treat her PH (see below).

Pregnancy is also dangerous for a woman who has had a lung transplant. Some lung transplant recipients have had a baby and lived, but, as a general rule, pregnancy is strongly discouraged for transplant recipients.

Keep in mind that if you are being treated for PAH, your medicines might harm your fetus. Warfarin (Coumadin) is very dangerous to a pregnant woman's baby. There are reports of birth malformations, spontaneous abortions, stillbirths, and babies with low birth weight and growth retardation. It is unknown whether prostanoids can cause birth defects and other pregnancy-related problems. Endothelin receptor antagonists, such as bosentan (Tracleer), are also known to cause birth defects. The would-be mother is faced with a terrible choice: continuing on her meds, which could harm her baby, or stopping the meds and putting herself (and thus her fetus, too) at great risk.

Still, some women decide to take the risk. In an article in *Glamour* magazine (April 2004) Shawn Saline tells how, when treatment reduced her pulmonary pressures, she took the risk and birthed a healthy daughter and later a son. She admits that she was incredibly lucky. JoAnne Sperando-Schmidt, a member of PHA's Board of Trustees who has FPAH, looked at the hard, cold facts and decided not to have children. Her aunt, who like JoAnne had FPAH, died because of a pregnancy.

Adoption and surrogacy. If you have the energy to raise a child, adoption is a much better idea. Women with PAH have been accepted as adoptive parents. Jeannette and her husband adopted twin boys after she was successfully treated with a calcium channel blocker. Surrogacy is also a possibility. Lise (a PH patient) and her husband wanted a baby who would be genetically related to one or both of them. They arranged for a surrogate mother to have their child. It was decided that it was too risky (and the odds of success too low) for Lise to donate an egg, so they settled on "traditional surrogacy," the artificial insemination of the surrogate mother. They are delighted with the results (see *Pathlight*, Summer 1995). Andrea (who is on epoprostenol) and her husband Chris also went the surrogacy route. Tests showed Andrea was in no danger of passing her FPAH on to a child, and that she could endure the egg retrieval procedure. Andrea and Chris were birth coaches to their surrogate mother when their daughter, Shea Elizabeth, arrived in May 2002. Their story was told in the *Boston Globe* and reproduced, with permission, in the August 2003 issue of PHA's *Persistent Voices*.

How to avoid getting pregnant. PH, like any serious chronic illness, can affect your monthly cycle. If your PH worsens, it might possibly bring on an early menopause. Many women with Class III or IV PH stop having menses and cannot get pregnant. On the other hand, PH professionals have seen cases where epoprostenol appeared to restore menstrual cycles. The regularity of your periods is not, however, directly related to the severity of your PAH.

Even if you think you aren't fertile, don't take chances. Of course you can "just say no," but that's usually not an acceptable (or necessary) solution. There is, as yet, no consensus among PH specialists as to what is the best form of birth control, although the barrier method (condoms for men and/or a diaphragm with spermicide in women), or a vasectomy in the male partner for a woman in a monogamous relationship are thought to be the two safest methods.

A survey of 23 PH specialists in Europe and North America found them almost evenly divided on whether birth-control pills are acceptable for a woman with PH, even if the woman is taking warfarin to help prevent the clots that these pills may predispose her to. There is concern among some doctors that estrogen might worsen PH. If you do use birth-control pills, use those with the lowest-possible effective dose. There is a potential interaction (nothing is known for sure) between endothelin receptor blockers and birth-control pills. If you decide on the pill, and have to take antibiotics for some reason, they may decrease the effectiveness of the pill until your next period occurs.

Another option is one of the newer intrauterine devices (IUDs), such as Mirenaâ, which have a lower risk of bleeding. A prophylactic use of antibiotics during insertion and removal is recommended.

It is sometimes recommended the PH patient or his / her partner consider the option of surgical sterilization. Tubal ligation is acceptable *if* a patient does not have severe heart failure. This may be too radical a

solution when a woman is young and has not yet had her family; medications and technologies may be found in time to make pregnancy less risky for her.

For more information, see the Consensus Statement on birth control on PHA's website.

Hormone replacement therapy (HRT). The same survey of PH specialists found that 65 percent of them felt that HRT was acceptable in post-menopausal women with PAH. But the benefits of such therapy, except for the control of specific menopausal symptoms like hot flashes, are being increasingly questioned.

PH and the Newborn (PPHN)

Newborns sometimes have PH because their lungs don't get enough oxygen. This is called persistent pulmonary hypertension of the newborn (PPHN). When the umbilical cord is cut and a baby takes its first few breaths a lot happens fast: the arteries to the baby's lungs expand, allowing blood in, and the fluid that has been filling the lungs' air sacs is pushed out. Things can go wrong. A lack of oxygen can cause an infant's pulmonary arteries to constrict (a normal state in a fetus, but not in a newborn). Pressure then backs up and blood flows into a patent ductus arteriosus (see Chapter 3), or through a hole in the wall between the upper chambers of the heart. A stressful delivery can trigger PPHN. Or the baby may suck meconium (its first feces) into its lungs. Some congenital conditions can cause PPHN, and sometimes no cause at all can be found.

PH in newborn infants usually clears up fairly quickly, although it occasionally persists for several weeks. A PH specialist should follow infants until all signs and symptoms of their PH have resolved. When the PH persists, further treatment is needed.

Near-term or full-term babies do a lot better when they inhale the gas nitric oxide (NO). The FDA has approved this gas for full-term infants. It might have saved the life of Jessica, in Montana, who was born with typical symptoms of PPHN: rapid breathing and heart rate, bluish skin, flaring nostrils, and "grunting" while breathing out. After 8 weeks in the hospital, Jessica went home, and is thriving. With NO, babies are less likely to need to be put on a machine that increases the amount of oxygen in their blood, and less likely to develop chronic lung disease. In infants with less than 34 weeks of gestation, the use of NO is still investigational.

When a critically ill infant in Germany did not respond to NO, doctors used iloprost, instilled endotracheally and inhaled, which helped the baby a lot. This is of interest because up to 30 percent of infants don't respond well enough to the NO treatment. Other researchers have expressed a desire to study phosphodiesterase inhibitors (think Viagra) as a possible PPHN treatment. It is already being used in Canada and India for PPHN, and clinical trials are underway in the U.S.

Indomethacin (used to treat premature labor and an excess of amniotic fluid in the bag of waters) and naproxen (used to delay a birth) may be linked to an increased likelihood of PH in newborns. (These drugs are also used as pain relievers—see the next paragraph.) Cocaine abuse by a mother has been reported to cause persistent PPHN.

A 2001 study out of Wayne State University (Detroit, MI) found that far more pregnant women than expected, or than reported in maternal histories, used nonsteroidal anti-inflammatory drugs (NSAIDs like ibuprofen, naproxen, indomethacin, and aspirin). The researchers learned this by analyzing 101 infants' first poop. Women who used NSAIDs while pregnant were more likely to have babies with PPHN and low Apgar scores. Much more needs to be done to warn would-be mothers of this danger. It is possible, of course, that the conditions that prompted the women to take painkillers might also have affected the development of the fetuses. A multi-center study is underway to look for links between PPHN and maternal exposures to smoking and to NSAIDs. At present, smoking appears less dangerous to a fetus than NSAIDS, as far as developing PPHN is concerned. However, smoking is implicated in 20 percent of low-weight births.

Children's Symptoms

Early PH symptoms are much the same as for adults: exercise intolerance and dyspnea (gasping for breath, a worried expression, blue-tinged lips and nails, etc.). But because children run around more, they are more likely than adults to get dizzy or faint with exertion, and to show obvious breathlessness. Sarah's first big clue that something was wrong came in the second grade when she blacked out in gym class, doing push-ups. Children's vascular systems are more reactive than adults'—more likely to both relax and constrict—and constriction can cause a pulmonary crisis. And children's hearts are usually strong, so heart failure is not a typical early symptom.

Other symptoms can include fatigue, paleness, breathlessness, "asthma" symptoms, pounding or too-rapid heartbeat, chest pain, poor appetite, profuse sweating, rapid breathing, seizures, and "failure to thrive."

Like any serious illness, PH can affect a child's growth. No direct link between PH and growth problems is known, but because PAH is often associated with thyroid problems, PH docs recommend a blood test at least once a year to screen for thyroid problems, which can affect a child's growth.

Because they are diagnosed earlier, children are more likely than adults to still be only in Class II when the disease is detected. Still, Dr. Robyn J. Barst, Director of the Pediatric Pulmonary Hypertension Center at New York Presbyterian Hospital (New York City), says children are often misdiagnosed for several years as having asthma, seizure disorders, or psychiatric problems. She believes more children probably have PH than is realized, because deaths are mistakenly attributed to pneumonia, asthma, seizures, or sudden infant death syndrome.

What About Ritalin and PH?

Medicines similar to Ritalin may trigger PH. If your child has Attention Deficit Disorder and PH runs in your family, be wary of Ritalin. If it must be used (during the school year, for example), proceed very cautiously and only with your PH doctor's consent, and consider testing your child for PH before you begin. There have been no scientific studies; this recommendation is based on the knowledge and gut instincts of a pediatric PH expert.

Drugs to Treat PH in Children
(listed alphabetically)

Beraprost

There is little information on how this pill-form prostanoid works in children. Although beraprost is available in Japan, it is not being clinically developed in the U.S.

Bosentan (Tracleer)

An open-label study (no placebos) looked at how safe and effective bosentan appeared to be in 18 children with either "PPH," or PAH/congenital heart disease patients, ranging in age from 3 to 15 years. There appeared to be

few bad side effects (the study lasted only 3 months, however). Mean PAPs fell, even in the patients who were also using other PH drugs.

Calcium channel blockers (CCBs)

Dr. Barst has treated kids with PH for over 25 years, and has found that treatments used on adults also work for children. She and her colleagues know for sure that long-term vasodilator use helps the children live longer. Those who respond well to an acute vasodilator test generally do fine on CCBs. Here's some good news: kids are twice as likely as adults to respond really well during a vasodilator trial: a whopping 40 percent are good responders! There are reports of many children doing well for a long period on CCB therapy, although frequent follow-up is essential, because some children stop doing well on CCBs and need more aggressive therapy, such as a prostanoid. A child's dosage in relation to his or her weight is often greater than an adult's.

Epoprostenol (prostacyclin, Flolan)

Intravenous epoprostenol is at least as effective in children with severe PAH as it is in adults with "PPH." When children are on epoprostenol their pressures often continue to fall over several years. Adults, on the other hand, usually do all the responding they are going to do in the first years. Epoprostenol has saved the lives of many children with PAH. Tegan, a teen in the UK, was so sick her doctors didn't dare attempt a transplant, so they started her on bosentan and, later, epoprostenol. She is now so well that there's no need to think about a transplant. Her doctor, Professor Dan Penny, says that epoprostenol is "a liquid-gold drug from our point of view." At PHA conferences, flocks of little kids with epoprostenol pumps tucked into backpacks dart all over the place.

What about using epoprostenol on kids who are still only Class I or II? Doctors just don't know how well the medicine works on the less sick. Dr. Barst's intuition tells her that because epoprostenol works so very well in so many different ways, it may be good for less sick kids. She hopes that by getting pressures close to normal earlier in life, children can do better long-term. In coming years, the availability of less intrusive forms of prostanoids may encourage doctors to try them on the less sick. Treprostinil (Remodulin), a prostanoid that has a longer half-life and that doesn't have to be refrigerated when it's in a pump, looks like it will be an effective treatment for some kids with PAH. Because it's usually delivered (by needle) into fat under the skin instead of by a catheter into a vein (like epoprostenol), there's much less risk of dangerous infection.

Dosage. This varies a lot in children, and some tolerate higher doses than adults: although 30 ng/kg/minute can be right for one child, another child might need a dose of 150 ng/kg/minute. Dr. Barst has also found that, with cooperative children over 6 years of age, 6-minute walk tests and bicycle tests can reveal small changes in exercise capacity before they are obviously symptomatic. Repeat catheterizations are recommended to adjust meds.

Overdosage. An eight-year-old who soils her pants nine times a day might be overdosed. Cutting back on her medicine may allow her to go to the mall with her friends—an important part of a kid's life! The difference between the right dose and too little can be tiny (and the difference in the patient's symptoms dramatic). Some kids may also need medicine to control diarrhea. Talk it over with your PH specialist. There does not seem to be this problem with calcium channel blockers.

The symptoms of overdosage are pretty much the same as they are in adults (see Chapter 5) and sometimes mimic the symptoms of PH. General fatigue suggests an overdose; shortness of breath is probably PH, not an overdose. (General fatigue can also be caused by a line infection, even if the child has no fever.)

Is Flolan forever? If you have ordinary hypertension and you take medicine that returns your blood pressure to normal, you can't stop taking the medicine if you want to enjoy its benefits. This seems to hold true of PH, as well. Whatever caused the PH is still there. Children with normal pressures have been taken off epoprostenol, been okay for a while, and then their symptoms returned. More than one parent who thought epoprostenol was doing their child no good, because the child's pressures didn't come down, has asked that the epoprostenol be stopped. When this was done, the children's pressures rose, suggesting that the epoprostenol was keeping them from getting worse. The children went back on epoprostenol.

It's possible, however, that in the future some children on epoprostenol will be able to switch to other PH drugs now under clinical development, or even to Remodulin. Some adults have already been weaned from epoprostenol, and are keeping their pressures down with other PH drugs.

Iloprost

There is not yet good data on the response of children to this drug. Doctors in Turkey have tried both inhaled and intravenous iloprost in children with PAH secondary to congenital heart disease. Both forms lowered the children's mean PAP and PVR; not surprisingly, intravenous iloprost also caused a big decrease in the children's systemic blood pressure.

Inhaled Nitric Oxide

Inhaled nitric oxide (NO) has proven to be of great use in treating PPHN (see discussion, above). Its benefit has been shown by multi-center, randomized, clinical trials. In 1999 the FDA approved NO for use in full-term babies. Researchers followed "NO babies" for 5 years, and found no late complications.

Multi-drug Therapy

Like adults, many children are taking more than one PH drug with good results. You may find, however, that many insurance payors will not approve more than one drug at a time.

Phosphodiesterase Inhibitor

Sildenafil (Viagra) has been used to wean infants from nitric oxide, and there are also small, encouraging studies of its use in children with "PPH" and with congenital heart disease/PAH. It is usually taken in an oral form, although in infants it has been used intravenously. Sildenafil is currently being clinically evaluated. A recent trial of sildenafil vs. placebo in adults with PAH in India revealed significant improvement in exercise capacity after just 6 week s of use. This, and many case reports of children getting improvement from sildenafil, is encouraging. Stay tuned.

Treprostinil (Remodulin)

There is little information on the use of subcutaneous treprostinil on children, but experts have used it in children as an alternative to epoprostenol (see section above on epoprostenol).

Warfarin (Coumadin)

Although children were not included in clinical studies of warfarin, children with PH *who have right-heart failure* are generally put on blood thinners. There are exceptions: a bad candidate might be a 15-year-old boy who lives on a farm, rides horses, and works with dangerous machinery. Children without right-heart failure can be cautiously anticoagulated. In most patients, a doctor will probably shoot for an INR around 1.5 to 2.0. But different levels are needed for different children. A lower INR may be advisable for a really active 7-year-old, or if a child's PH is very mild, or if the child has a blood factor that makes her/him bleed more easily. Children who have blood that clots easily may need higher doses and may also need to take a short-acting blood thinner, such as heparin, when warfarin needs to be temporarily stopped (e.g. for an operation or dental work). Parents should know what level of anticoagulation the PH doctor is shooting for, and ask for the results of each pro-time check.

Interaction with antibiotics. It seems that little kids are *always* on antibiotics! Some drugs, like erythromycin, really react with warfarin, making its effect more powerful. One mom found this out the hard way when her little girl fell against a table: the whole side of her face turned purple and stayed that way for 6 weeks. Flagyl, Zithromax, amoxicillin, and other drugs can also affect INRs. But it's a very individual thing. Different children react differently to different drugs.

It's usually better to have an INR that's too low than one that's too high. So if your child has an INR problem when taking antibiotics, your doctor may want to lower the dose of warfarin, or even stop it altogether, while your child is on the other drug.

Other PH drugs might also interact with warfarin, so you always need to discuss your child's warfarin usage when adding or stopping drugs.

Lung Transplants

To quote "Dr. Jackie" (Jacqueline Szmuszkovicz, Children's Hospital, Los Angeles), "Lung transplantation is the *last* option, and it's an *option*, not a requirement." In other words, it's not necessarily appropriate for everyone. Lung transplants are considered only when all other remedies have failed. It is now an accepted, not an investigational procedure, but it comes with no guarantees. If you are considering a lung transplant for your child, pick a site that specializes in them.

Many children who need a lung transplant have congenital heart defects. Older children may have had an injury to a lung, or have "PPH" (10 percent), or cystic fibrosis (the most common reason). The survival statistics for lung transplants in children are about the same as those for adults, although far fewer are done.

A child may be a candidate for transplantation if the child is on epoprostenol yet still fainting, or has lots of fluid in his/her belly that doctors can't get under control. It's wise to get on the transplant list if your child is Class IV. You can always go inactive, and keep accumulated time (for more information on transplant lists see Chapter 6 and the box on page 135). The wait for lungs from a cadaver in Los Angeles can be 2 or 3 years for a child. Historically, nearly half the kids who needed lungs did not survive long enough to get them. Your child may be turned down for a transplant if he is infected with organisms resistant to antibiotics, has certain heart, liver, or kidney problems, has a systemic disease like HIV, is in the middle of a viral infection like the flu when a cadaveric organ becomes available, or if you, the parents, can't provide adequate social support or appear unlikely to comply with medical requirements.

A part of an adult lung from a cadaver is sometimes used, although smaller "cadaveric" lungs from children are a better physical fit. Sometimes cadaver lobes from child donors are given to neonates. Not-too-complicated heart repairs can be done at the same time as a transplant. A heart's enlarged right ventricle usually shrinks back to a normal size after a transplant. It's more difficult, in children, to do a single-lung transplant. The majority of doctors now seem to favor double-lung transplants anyway.

Living-donor lobe transplants. Parents, relatives, or family friends can each donate a lobe to a child with PH (see Chapter 6). Living donors must be 2 to 20 inches taller than the recipient. Blood types must also match, but Rh factors aren't considered. The biggest advantage of using living donors (it always takes two donors) is that you don't have to wait. Your child would have to spend more time on a lung machine (to allow the new lobes to expand more), and more time in the hospital (about 4 weeks) following surgery. Dr. Marlyn Woo, who works with post-transplant patients at Children's in LA, says living-donor lobe recipients have greater mortality during the first month, but thereafter have less acute and chronic rejection. At their center they have an 87 percent survival at one year, compared to a nationwide survival of children who get lung transplants of about 63 to 75 percent at one year. Around half the transplant recipients live at least 5 years. Once children have recovered from the operation, there are no exercise limitations. It isn't known for sure how immunosuppressants affect overall growth. Some patients have grown a foot and a half since their transplant, and their new lobes seem to grow along with them. Research is continuing, but most doctors think that the air sacs do not increase in number, but instead grow bigger, trapping more air.

Prognosis

Unfortunately, if PAH in children is not treated, the disease seems to worsen more quickly than it does in adults. When you consider persons of all ages, the greatest mortality rates for "PPH" are found in infants, but the lowest rates are found in treated children who survive infancy. Today, with treatment, younger children appear to have a better prognosis than adults. It isn't known exactly why this is true, but it could be because children are diagnosed earlier, because their pulmonary arteries are more responsive to the new medicines, or because until about 8 years of age there is still some capability to grow new vessels. The age at which a child is diagnosed with PAH correlates with the success of medical treatment: the earlier the diagnosis, the more likely the child will do well.

Dr. Barst and her colleagues found these survival rates in the era of using CCBs and epoprostenol (but not bosentan, which wasn't available until more recently): 97 percent survival at 1 year, 97 percent survival at 5 years, and 78 percent surival at 10 years. For children being treated with PH medications alone, the treatment success rates were: 93 percent medication treatment success at one year, 86 percent medication treatment success at 5 years, and 60 percent medication treatment success at 10 years. The difference in the two sets of figures is because children who underwent transplantation or who had an atrial septostomy were not considered to have had a "treatment success" with medications alone.

Day-to-Day Living

It's really important to allow your child with PH to live a normal life. If you coddle your PH kid too much, your other children might wish they, too, were sick (one little boy actually voiced this wish aloud to his dad). Try not to ignore your spouse; a strong marriage is good for everyone in the family.

Right after the diagnosis it's not uncommon to feel almost as bad as if your child had died. As one mom put it, she lost her "normal" child. You go through stages of mourning like denial, depression, and anger. And then you start to cope, and the sun comes back out.

Talk with your child about how important it is to tell you if he/she has chest pain, feels dizzy, nauseated, or has constipation or diarrhea. No one likes to talk about constipation or diarrhea, but all these complaints need to be attended to.

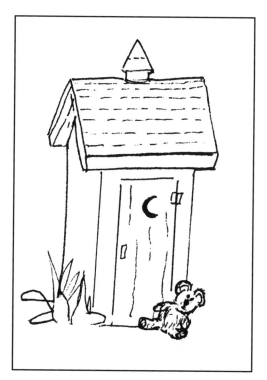

Make sure, too, that your child knows there is no reason to feel "embarrassed" about having PH when they are around their friends, even if they use an epoprostenol pump. You might tell them this secret: if they treat their illness as no big deal, their friends will follow their lead. Other people tend to see you as you see yourself.

Stress and PH

Stress is bad for PH. It can come in many forms: pain (like site pain and foot pain), anxiety, anger, tension, fear, etc. Adrenalin causes pulmonary pressures to rise. When kids have a cardiac catheter in place and they get upset and start crying, doctors can literally watch pulmonary pressures rise.

But you have to raise your kids, including those with PH, the way you think they should be raised. Long-term, this will reduce the stress in their life. Kids will cry. They will get hurt. Scary things do happen, but we can cope with them. Mattie's Flolan line came out on the L.A. freeway, and another time a gerbil in her backpack chewed through the Flolan tubing! But Mattie's still with us, and is doing great. As Leslie, the mom of a teenager with PAH says, keeping a positive attitude is the best medicine.

What to Tell the Kids

When someone in the family has PH, what should you tell your healthy kids? Children know something is wrong. If they can use a computer, they probably already know anything about PH that you are trying to hide from them. Don't lie to them, but consider their age in telling them a version of the truth. They may need counseling or a family member to talk with about their fears. More cuddles seem to help. They may become more concerned than necessary if they themselves get sick. One young boy in a PH family broke his arm. A few days later, his class was painting. He refused to paint because he thought that if his arm got paint on it, it would get infected.

Colds and Flu

An ordinary cold can be serious for a PH patient. Teach your child to wash his hands before touching food, his mouth, or his face (cold germs can even sneak in through the eyes). Tell your pediatrician about any cold, even before it gets "serious"; pediatricians need to use aggressive antibiotic therapy to treat respiratory tract infections in children with PH. Ask your doctors about the new antiviral therapies to nip flu and colds in the bud.

If you or another family member has something contagious, be considerate of your PH patient. When you have a cold, merely speaking splatters germ-laden droplets into the nearby air. Consider wearing a facemask when you are near the child. Teach everyone to cough into their elbow, not their hand. A hand sanitizer that contains ethyl alcohol, not antibiotics, can be used when hand washing is impractical.

All children should get an influenza vaccine every year (unless there's a reason, such as an allergy, not to). In fact, *everyone* in the family should get a flu vaccine. (The vaccines aren't 100 percent effective, so you want to try to avoid bringing the bug home.) In addition, everyone in the family should be vaccinated against pneumonia. The vaccine is effective in up to 70 percent of people, and may last a lifetime. But those at high risk of pneumococcal infections (like PH patients) may want to be revaccinated every 5 years.

PH doctors also recommend aggressive treatment with antipyretics such as Tylenol when a child with PH has a fever (over about 101 degrees F), because fever increases the demands on your child's heart and lungs; it's as if your child is running a marathon 24/7. Don't give your child aspirin or another NSAID without first talking it over with your PH doc.

Another good idea is to strengthen your child's immune system with a healthy diet. Some pediatricians recommend vitamins to help keep your child healthy. Check with your PH specialist to learn if your child needs to be on an iron supplement. Preventing constipation, either with diet alone (or with medical therapy, if needed) is also important, because straining during bowel movements puts more strain on the heart and can cause children to faint. A healthy diet should also include adequate amounts of water, particularly during sports activity and in hot weather.

Taking Pills

It's not news that kids don't like swallowing pills. One creative mom taught her five-year-old to swallow them by first practicing on mini M&M's. She then moved on to regular M&M's in a spoonful of applesauce or ice cream, and from there to real pills. If the pill your doctor prescribes is in a time-release form (such as Procardia XL), do not cut it apart or crush it, as that will destroy the time-release mechanism and possibly cause a drug overdose.

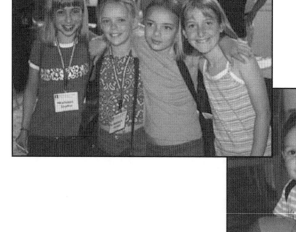

At PHA's 2004 conference in Miami.

Because it's so easy to forget which pills you've taken, use a segmented pillbox (or boxes—one for morning, one for evening) to help you and your child remember what to take and when to take it. As soon as your child is old enough, he/she should learn what each medicine is for, and how to take it.

At School

Discuss your child's condition with his/her classroom teacher, gym teacher or sport coach, principal, and school nurse (if the school has one) so they are familiar with the disease and its treatment. For questions related to PAH or if there is an emergency involving epoprostenol (Flolan), make sure the school knows who to contact: Accredo Therapeutics at 1-866-344-4874 (1-866-FIGHT-PH); or TheraCom at 1-877-356-5364 (1-877-FLOLAN-4). For questions related to treprostinil (Remodulin), have the school call Accredo Therapeutics at 1-866-344-4874 (1-866-FIGHT-PH), Caremark (1-866-879-2348), or Priority Healthcare 1-866-474-8326 (1-866-4-PH-TEAM), as appropriate.

If your child is on anticoagulants, let the school know that the child can take Tylenol but not aspirin or other NSAIDs. Because of your child's special vulnerability, ask the school to notify you when contagious illnesses are going around. And check with your doctor to learn whether the school should keep oxygen on hand. Make sure an emergency number is on the back of your child's pump, along with the dosage and pump rate. Your health service company may be willing to help you educate the school staff. The Spring 2003 issue of *Pathlight* (available on PHA's website) has a sample form letter you can hand to personnel who work with your child.

Ask your child's teacher to treat her like any other student; the other students will usually follow the teacher's example. Some parents visit their young child's classroom every fall to explain an infusion pump and its alarm, and answer classmates' questions. This saves the child from repeatedly answering the same questions. If your child approves, consider showing the pump and even a corner of the catheter dressing. Just because a child has PH doesn't mean he/she can't participate in gym class. You and your PH specialist need to discuss what activities your child can do.

911 Calls

Contact the fire department paramedics or other EMTs who serve the area(s) where your home and the child's school are, and discuss PH emergency procedures with them. If your child is on Flolan, and if the delivery system has failed, be sure the dispatcher sends someone who can place an IV in a child. If your child is old enough to understand, teach him/her when and how to call 911. Stock a repair kit for your type of catheter and size of lumen, because the emergency room you go to might not have it.

Those Terrible Wonderful Teenage Years

Although a younger child might just accept the pump and tube as normal, during the self-conscious teenage years it hurts a lot to be different from peers. It's really, really important for parents to keep the lines of communication open with their PH teenagers.

Teens with PH are at extra risk from S.A.D. (Sex, Alcohol, & Drugs). We're not talking about morals, only about facts.

Sex. If a girl with PH gets pregnant, it might make her PH a lot worse or even kill her. (See the section above on "Can a Woman with PH Have a Baby?") Even if she survives pregnancy, caring for a baby might be too big

a burden on top of her PH. Sterilization is too extreme a measure, because a cure for PH or treatments that make pregnancy less risky may be found while the patient is still of child-bearing age. Birth control pills can cause clotting, so they often aren't recommended. A girl with PH who is sexually active needs to talk to both her gynecologist and her PH expert before choosing an appropriate birth control method (see pages 157-58).

Boys with PH need to consider the dangers of becoming a father too early. It's easy to father a child (witness the 6 billion humans now aboard the planet), but it takes lots of energy to care and provide for your new son or daughter in the way you'd like to. Raising kids is stressful, and stress can worsen PH. If your girlfriend gets pregnant it could be very hard on your health. Fatherhood certainly isn't ruled out by PH, but you need to wait until you can handle the challenges.

Alcohol. Binge drinking can be dangerous for us. A little alcohol now and then probably won't hurt, however, as long as you keep your INR (anticoagulant) levels steady. If you are on vasodilators you'll get light-headed pretty fast, so take it slow and drink plenty of water to prevent getting dehydrated (unless you are taking diuretics). If you binge drink and vomit and get dehydrated you might end up with pneumonia, be very, very sick, and could even die.

Warfarin (Coumadin) is broken down by your liver; binge drinking can waste your liver and make your INR levels too high. Here's a worst-case-but-quite-possible scenario: you're tipsy, coming home from a party in a car driven by a friend who is also loaded. There's an accident. You hit your head on the windshield. You bleed a lot inside your skull because of the blood thinner you take. You die or have a crippling stroke.

Drugs. Methamphetamines can easily kill those of us with PH. One PH expert predicts that the soaring teen use of this family of drugs may cause as big an epidemic of PH as did the diet pills. Its not just street drugs that are a problem. France has gone a step further and taken all amphetamines off the market. They are still legal in the U.S., by prescription, but maybe they shouldn't be.

Sports. Some teens with PH can participate in sports, some can't. It depends mostly on how well you respond to treatment. When Jessica was in tenth grade, just walking to class made her breathless, in spite of using Flolan.

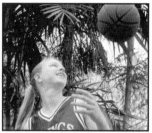

But this courageous girl stuck it out, usually completing a full day of school. And despite her PH, as a child she was able to care for her mother, who had fatal scleroderma. That's an accomplishment worth many sports trophies.

Hannah Carr, who is 17 at the time this is being written, has been on epoprostenol since she was 7 years old. The medicine has returned her pulmonary pressures to normal, and now she uses only a very low dose of epoprostenol plus calcium channel blockers. Hannah is an aggressive basketball player (forward and guard) and co-captain of her team. When she plays, she wears her pump in a small beltpack under her jersey. On the court, she doesn't use the ice packs. She also plays golf and softball. Sure, like many epoprostenol patients she gets an infection now and then and has to be hospitalized to receive antibiotics through an IV. And her catheter has been replaced more than once. One of her parents is always present during her basketball games, just in case the line cracks or comes out. But most of the time, Hannah says, she barely notices the pump.

Hannah isn't the only PH patient active in sports. Fifteen-year-old Sara Galligan, who uses Tracleer, also loves basketball. Because of active young women like Hannah and Sara, WNBA player Debbie Black became a PHA spokesperson, helping to raise awareness. Both Sara and Hannah have been able to shoot some hoops with Debbie!

College. Many PH patients go to college. It's a lot more interesting and fun than junior high or high school, and by the time you're a freshman there will probably be better ways to control PH. On your college application essays you can write about how heroically you've dealt with your PH. The admissions committee at your dream university may think you're handicapped and give you a handicap! You might also try to snag one of those scholarships for the disabled (even if you feel great on your PH medicines).

Helping Hands

Networking. Many parents of children with PH find the parents' message board on PHA's website very helpful (www.phassociation.org). If you call our 800 number (1-800-748-7274) and ask for a member of PHA's Children's Committee to call you back, PHA can put you in touch with other parents and children coping with this disease.

Kids like to do their own networking, too. Some parents coordinate their child's visit to

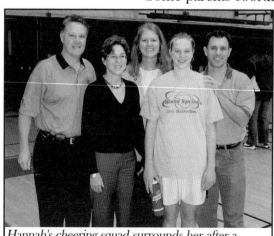

Hannah's cheering squad surrounds her after a basketball game. From left to right: Jack Stibbs; Dr. Robyn J. Barst; Linda, Hannah, and Austin Carr.

the PH doc to coincide with the visits of other children of similar ages with PH. You can use PHA's message boards to do this. The PHA website also has a chat room every Tuesday at 8:30 EST, 5:30 PST, for youth with PH, but please remember that everything you hear in the chat room may not be correct. If you're unsure, ask your PH doc. Children and teens at the biannual PHA conferences often form lasting friendships with others who really understand what they are going through. Many keep in touch later as pen pals or by e-mail.

Make-A-Wish Foundation. Children with PH between the ages of 2-and-a-half and 18 have had their wishes granted at no charge through the Make-a-Wish Foundation. Some take a trip to Disney World in Orlando, FL. Others have chosen to get their bedrooms redone, go on shopping sprees, get a computer, meet celebrities, etc. Joey Nelson, 4 years old, had a neat new playhouse built for him, complete with a wrap-around porch and chair swing. (Joey is training to be a Jedi knight.) Amber Spencer, 18, who has Down syndrome and PH, got to fly from Iowa to Los Angeles to meet the twin sitcom stars Mary Kate and Ashley Olson ("Full House"). Call 1-800-332-9474, or visit www.wish.org, to learn more, and see *Pathlight*, Summer 1997. If you decide on a trip, ask your doctor if your child needs supplemental oxygen aboard the airplane.

Summer Camps. Many states have summer camps for children with chronic illnesses. Check with your nearest children's hospital or pediatric cardiologist. A list of such camps appeared in the Spring 2003 issue of *Pathlight,* which is available on the PHA website. (One change from the list—the Painted Turtle Camp was told by a cardiologist that the altitude of their camp was too high for most children with PH.) Two young girls on epoprostenol attended a camp in Florida for a week at no charge, where the nurses mixed the drug daily and cardiologists were on site around the

clock. See *Pathlight*, fall 1997. Cassie, who also uses epoprostenol, went to Paul Newman's Summer Camp in Connecticut where she rode horses, climbed rocks, and did arts and crafts. She said the experience gave her a chance to "be normal." (See more about Cassie at the end of this chapter.) For a list of which camps serve what special needs, go to www.kidscamps.org. If you don't want to fill out an information form and wait for a response, you can often paste the camp name into a search engine such as Google and learn more about it right away.

Free transportation to medical care. If you are otherwise unable to get to the medical care you need, there are organizations that will fly you and your child for free, nationwide (and occasionally in Canada). Flying can be difficult for many PH patients, but a national Angel Bus Program offers transportation to sick needy children. Kimberly, a toddler with PH, rode such a bus from Akron, OH, to New York City. See "Free Transportation" in Chapter 14.

Helping Out

Never underestimate the power of children and teenagers to move mountains. By sharing their stories with others, giving emotional support to PH friends, designing cards for PHA to sell, writing stories for PHA publications, and even doing things like raising money for PHA while trick-or-treating, PH kids have contributed a lot. Cassie Tessier in New England raised over $600 trick-or-treating, and Camille Freede put together a cookbook to sell to raise funds. Children can also help out at fund-raising garage sales, and maybe add a little to the take by having a lemonade stand to one side. Thank you!

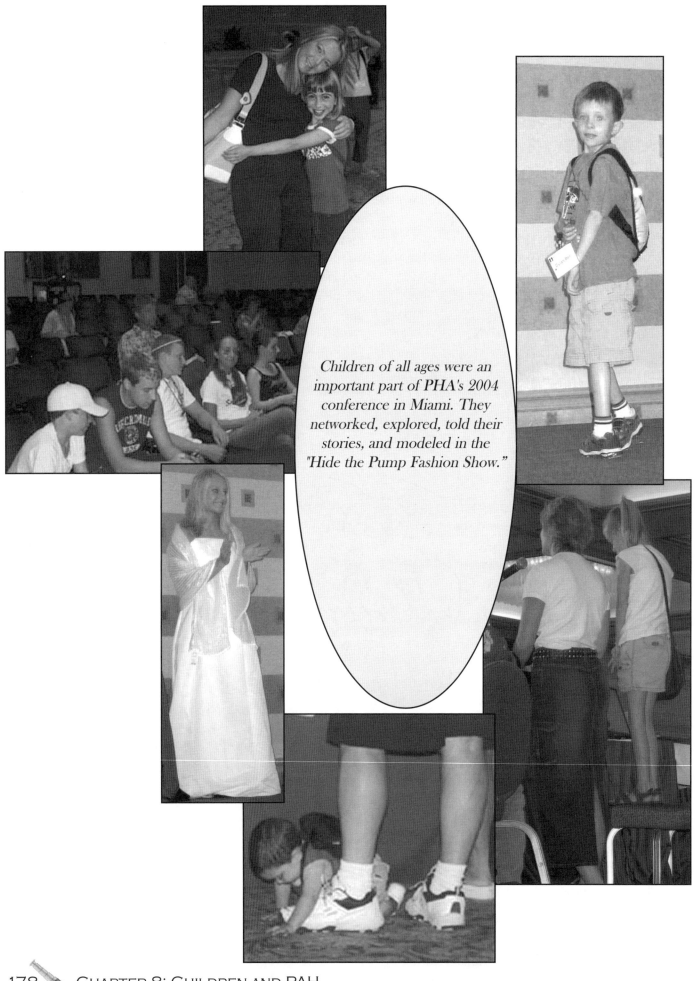

Children of all ages were an important part of PHA's 2004 conference in Miami. They networked, explored, told their stories, and modeled in the "Hide the Pump Fashion Show."

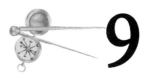

What to Eat When You Have PH

By Maureen Keane
Nutritionist, author, and PH patient

What is a good diet for someone with PH? Are there any special diets, foods, vitamins, or minerals that can substitute for traditional treatments? Unfortunately, there are not. The role of diet in PH is to help support your body while you are being treated for PH. A good diet can help you to keep your heart in good working order, maintain a desirable body weight, reduce edema, and give your stressed body the nutritional support it needs.

Macronutrients: the Big Three

Your body needs three kinds of nutrients: carbohydrate, fat, and protein. Carbohydrates are used for immediate energy needs. Fats store excess fat and provide energy in between meals when no carbohydrate is around. Protein (composed of amino acids) builds the soft tissues of the body. Together these three nutrients are called the macronutrients. Sugars (from carbohydrates), fatty acids (a simple form of fat), and amino acids (the building blocks of proteins) are also necessary for hormone, neurotransmitter, antibody, and enzyme formation.

Most foods are a mix of all three macronutrients. Contrary to some popular diet books, our digestive system was designed to digest all three at the same time. Digestion is not improved by eating foods in certain combinations.

Carbohydrates and protein provide about 4 calories per gram while fat provides 9 calories per gram. When the body needs energy, it first uses carbohydrates and then turns to the fatty acids stored in fat cells. If both are in short supply, the body burns the protein found in muscle cells. This reduces the amount of tissue in the muscles and heart, and produces nitrogen, which must be excreted by the kidneys. When protein intake is high it can stress the kidneys. This is one problem with today's popular high-protein, low-carb diets.

We All Need to Weigh In

Everyone with PH needs to watch their weight. Men and very active women burn around 2,500 calories/day and less active women around 2,000. When PH forces you to become sedentary, your daily needs can drop by about 500 calories. If you don't change the way you eat, those extra calories will be stored as fat and your weight will start to rise. Try to nip that weight gain in the bud by cutting back before you start to gain. Buy a scale and weigh yourself nude every morning before breakfast. Weighing yourself will also help you to recognize edema. A quick weight gain over a short period of time should be reported to your doctor.

It's no better to be *under*weight. It is impossible to get all the nutrients you need if you have only 1,400 calories coming in. It is quite possible to be skinny and have a terrible diet, just as it possible to be overweight and have a wonderful one.

Are you losing weight but not dieting? This should raise a red flag. It can be caused by the symptoms of PH or the side effects of PH treatments. If you are overweight, unintentional weight loss seems like a dream come true, but you must take care to minimize muscle tissue loss and maximize fat loss. Otherwise you end up harming the tissue in your muscle and heart. Even intentional weight loss that is too fast can cause this problem.

How Can I Lose Weight When I Can't Exercise?

One of the most common problems I hear from PH patients is that their doctor wants them to lose weight, but they wonder how they can do so if they can barely get to the bathroom without help. Exercise is important to weight loss, and you might be able to do more exercise than you think. It doesn't have to be the sweaty gym type exercise: running, weightlifting, aerobics and that kind of thing. Researchers have found that what they call an active lifestyle does wonders for weight loss. This means walking instead of driving, getting up to change the TV channel rather than using a remote, carrying your own bags in from the grocery stores, cooking and cleaning, and chasing a toddler around the house. It can involve as much exertion as using stairs or as little as brushing your teeth manually instead of using an electric toothbrush. It can involve walking briskly or sitting in a chair and lifting your arms up and down.

Many doctors recommended an exercise program called "10,000 Steps." It is part of the government's Shape Up America program. You use a pedometer (a small inexpensive gadget you hook to your belt) to record how many steps you make during the day. After setting a baseline, you add more steps each day with the ultimate goal of reaching 10,000, a level of exercise considered "active." This is a bit much for many PH patients, especially early in their treatment. Work with your doctor to set reasonable goals.

When you have a chronic disease, your exercise tolerance can differ from day to day. Try not to get discouraged if you have to miss several days or even a week of exercise. Make a pact with yourself, today, to do whatever you can, whenever you can, the best you can. Don't feel guilty for listening to your body. Ask your doctor to explain your limits. Is it safe for you to push your limits? Should you attempt aerobic exercise? Fast walking? Slow walking? Can you safely do some basic movement exercises while sitting? Your doctor may not want you lifting weights. If you are very overweight, you are lifting weights just by standing up. (See Chapter 13 for changing attitudes on exercise and PH.)

The Food Fight: Which Diet is Best?

Most fad weight loss diets are based on manipulating the three macronutrients (fat, protein and carbohydrates) in some way. High-fat low-carb, high-carb low-fat, and high-protein low-carb are the variations. *But no matter how the macronutrients are distributed, research shows people only lose weight when they reduce the amount of calories they eat.*

Which type of diet works best? Let's go to The National Weight Control Registry to answer that question. This database, of more than 3,000 people, was established in the U.S. in 1993. It is comprised of individuals who have a documented weight loss of at least 30 pounds and maintained that loss for at least one year. These successful dieters used the old fashioned high-carbohydrate, low-fat, and low-calorie diet to lose weight. The longer dieters kept the weight off, the greater was their chance of keeping it off permanently. It also got easier to control their appetite.

Some of you are going to protest: A high-carb diet? How can you say that when obesity in America has increased right along with our carbohydrate intake? Yes, but Americans are not just exchanging fat for carbohydrate; we are also eating *more* carbohydrate in the form of sugar. So while our fat intake is going down, our calorie count is heading up. According to the CDC, from 1971 to 2000, women increased their caloric intake by 22 percent, men by 7 percent. Cookies, pasta, and soda are among the villains. America is super-sizing itself to death. To repeat, to reduce your weight you *must* reduce the number of calories you eat.

A healthy diet isn't complicated. Eating shouldn't require a calculator or weird combinations of food. Most certainly it should not be determined by your blood type. The trick is to find a plan that controls your hunger. Some dieters find it easier to replace one meal a day with a low-cal shake. Others like the large quantity of food they can eat on vegan diets, or learn to avoid foods and situations that trigger impulsive eating. A good diet involves more than counting calories. You also need to give your body the vitamins and minerals and other nutrients it needs to function, plus antioxidants to protect against free-radical damage. This is especially important when you have a chronic disease like PH. Only a diet rich in fruit and vegetables, whole grains, legumes and nuts and seeds can provide this.

Many PH specialists do not like their patients to use the Atkins or other fad diets because of the stress they can put on your already stressed body. Fad diets can be very high in saturated fat, and there is an endless stack of research that shows this will damage your arteries.

Weight gain can be a sign of depression. It can also be a sign of edema caused by heart failure and a sign your PH is worsening. If you think your weight gain might be due to depression or edema, talk it over with your doctor, who may prescribe an antidepressant or diuretics.

No matter which low-calorie, high-carb diet you choose, your first step is to set a goal. Ask your doctor how much weight he or she wants you to lose; don't assume you know. It's sometimes unrealistic to expect you will be able to diet down to your "ideal" body weight, because your metabolism won't let you. Very often a weight loss of only 10 to 20 percent is all that is needed to reduce your risk of diabetes and heart disease. If this seems insignificant, try translating your potential loss into bowling ball equivalents!

Amy passed out at a Broncos game in Denver, and was diagnosed with PPH. Her doctor told her it would improve her chances for a transplant if she lost weight. "Everything was spinning out of control," Amy said, "but what I put in my mouth I had control over." She lost 75 pounds, using the Weight Watchers approach.

How to *Gain* Weight

It is as hard to gain weight as it is to lose it—honest. The most common reason for weight loss is eating fewer calories than you burn. There are several causes for this in PH patients: anorexia (loss of appetite); early satiety (you become full after a small amount of food); nausea; and diarrhea. Some of these symptoms can be side effects of PAH, and others can be side effects of medications such as epoprostenol (Flolan), treprostinil (Remodulin), the pain killer tramadol (Ultram), opiate pain meds including codeine, and antidepressants such as the serotonin reuptake inhibitors (SSRIs). While some patients have reported these symptoms with bosentan (Tracleer) and sildenafil (Viagra), in trials these symptoms did not appear to be any more common than in patients getting placeboes. If your PH is associated with another medical condition, the underlying medical problem might have an impact on your diet. Depression itself can also contribute to loss of appetite, with anorexia, as can the bloating caused by edema. Even if you are overweight, anorexia can be dangerous if it causes you to cut your caloric intake too much. A 5 percent weight loss is significant and you should tell your doctor about it. A weight loss of 10 percent or more is a sign that something serious may be wrong.

Other causes of weight loss are diarrhea or vomiting, which can be a side effect of some PH meds. If you vomit regularly or have diarrhea regularly, you need to inform your doctor. There are medicines that can help. See, too, the section at the end of this chapter on Nausea and Vomiting.

You could be losing weight and not know it; weight loss can be disguised by a water weight gain. If you are dieting and not losing weight, examine your body for signs of edema, and think about whether your sodium intake needs adjusting (see below).

A low-calorie diet can cause constipation if it is low in fiber. A fiber laxative such as regular Metamucil mixed with fresh juice is a good remedy. The ground psyllium seed can also lower high cholesterol levels. Apple, pear, and prune juice are also nutritious laxatives. Prune juice with pulp is a good source of fiber and iron. If you take fiber supplements, do not take them close to when you take your medications, because the high fiber content can prevent the absorption of the medicines.

No matter how good your diet is, when your intake of calories falls, so does your intake of protein, vitamins, minerals, fiber and antioxidants. Make sure you take a daily vitamin/mineral supplement.

Tips for caregivers cooking for a patient who needs to gain weight. Although this section is addressed to caregivers, patients can learn from it, too. Cooking and feeding someone with a chronic disease can be frustrating. Accept right now that you cannot control your patient's appetite no matter how much you nag, hassle, and tease. Accept that his or her choices are not your responsibility. If a patient wants to eat one food all day and that prevents weight loss, so be it. Any nutritional deficiencies in the meal can be countered with multivitamin and mineral supplements. Bite your tongue when you feel the need to nag and don't give a patient nutritional advice you picked up at the beauty shop or from Aunt Ethel's second cousin who sells vitamins.

If the patient you care for is very sick, a loss of appetite can be the natural prelude to dying. Don't worry that he or she is starving; they do not feel hunger because their body is shutting down. You might be tempted to try to force food and water at this time, but that can just make your patient more uncomfortable. Ask your doctor for guidance and listen to it carefully. Here are some other tips:

- Praise good eating habits and ignore the bad.
- Serve smaller meals more frequently. Offer food whenever your patient asks. Large meals can push the diaphragm upward, displacing the heart and further restricting breathing.
- Serve smaller meals on a smaller plate. If you have a small appetite, the sight of a mountain of food can nauseate you.
- The more varied the meal, the more your patient will probably eat. Instead of serving a whole sandwich, cut a half sandwich into two squares and serve it with a few apple wedges and a very small salad or half cup of soup. Don't comment on any leftovers but take note of any favorites.

- Vary the textures and flavors in the meal. Serve savory foods with sweet, bland foods with spicy, hot with cold, and crispy with creamy.
- Serve your patient's comfort foods frequently.

How to add fat to your diet. If you have lost a lot of weight, your physician may ask you to increase the amounts of fats in your diet. This is because fats contribute more than double the energy of other calorie sources. Fats are also easily stored in the body, providing you with a back-up source of energy for times when you cannot eat.

High-fat diets, even those with "good" fat, may increase the risk of heart attack and stroke, so always ask your doctor before making any major changes in your diet. It's true that some fats are better than others. While whole dairy products are excellent sources of fat and calories, they are also excellent sources of saturated fat that can damage your arteries. A much better choice is foods and fats high in the monounsaturated fatty acids or those high in omega three fatty acids (fish oil). The high-fat foods below will not only increase your calorie intake, but will also aid in lowering your cholesterol levels. Each serving contains 5 grams of fat (45 calories). By adding four servings to your diet, you will gain 180 calories.

2 whole walnuts or pecans
20 small peanuts
2-3 whole macadamia nuts
2 teaspoons peanut butter
2 teaspoons tahini (sesame seed butter)
1 tablespoon sunflower seeds
10 small or 5 large olives
1 tablespoon pine nuts or cashews
2 teaspoons pumpkin seeds
2 teaspoons canola mayonnaise

1 teaspoon olive, canola, or fish oil
2 tablespoons salad dressings
2 tablespoons shredded coconut
1/4 cup humus with olive oil
2 (1000 gram) fish oil capsules
2 1/2 teaspoons coconut milk
1/8 medium avocado
1 egg
1 ounce cooked pacific herring
1 ounce cooked Atlantic mackerel
1 ounce cooked sablefish
1 ounce cooked American shad

Nuts and seeds score a triple run – they are rich in heart-healthy oils, fiber, and protein. Choose the kind that are unsalted and roasted (instead of fried).

Avoid saturated fat by using only low-fat dairy products and substituting one of these:
- Extra-virgin olive oil
- Cold-pressed canola oil
- High-oleic safflower oil
- Salad dressings made with one of the above
- Mayonnaise made with one of the above

More Tips to Increase Calories:
- Some people can eat sweet foods even when they can no longer stomach savory ones. So find what appeals to you and take advantage of it. If you can eat sweets, drink healthy smoothies, sweetened cereals, puddings etc.
- If you find liquid meals more appetizing, try drinking low-fat vegetable soups (you will be able to drink more low-fat soup than high-fat). Vegetables can be pureed and added to soups. Meal shakes intended for dieters make good meal supplements. So do those marketed to seniors, such as Ensure.

- Avoid foods that cause gas and bloating. If you enjoy foods in the cabbage family or beans, you should use an enzyme supplement with the unfortunate name of Beano. Do not drink carbonated beverages. The gas that makes them fizzy will fill your stomach and blunt your appetite. Sometimes they can cause nausea.
- Eat the protein foods first and then the carbohydrates. If you eat the fatty foods first, they can blunt your appetite.
- Do not drink no-cal or low-cal liquids with meals. They will fill up your stomach. Instead, sip small amounts of water if you must drink.
- Reduce the amount of raw food you eat. The fiber can fill you up leaving less room for protein and calorie-rich carbohydrates. Substitute fresh or canned vegetable juice.
- Exercise can increase appetite, so take a walk before meals if you are able to.
- A teaspoon of lemon juice in a glass of cool water is an old remedy for stimulating the appetite. Sip on it half an hour before meals.

Protein and Weight Loss

Anytime you restrict your intake of food, you risk protein deficiency. Therefore, protein is a concern both for those needing to lose weight and those who need to gain it. A diet that is low in protein, or too low in calories, results in a kind of tissue wasting or destruction. If not enough protein is provided in the diet, the body will break down proteins in muscles, blood, and enzyme pools. Of concern for PH patients, the strength of the diaphragm and of the respiratory muscles can be reduced, which in turn reduces your ability to breathe well. Ultimately, the mass of the heart can also be affected.

The body cannot make protein from the other macronutrients; it must be supplied by your diet. You need at least 55-70 grams of protein each day to maintain your bodies' requirement of 0.8 grams per kg per day. If you are underweight and need to regain a significant amount of muscle tissue, your protein needs may be double this. In this case, a high-protein diet won't stress your body, because you are eating so few calories.

Some researchers think that by adding a bit more protein to a high-carb diet you can help minimize the loss of muscle tissue that is unavoidable when losing weight for any reason. However, you should not get above 20 percent of your calories from protein when weight loss is your goal. To put this number into perspective, the Zone and other high-protein diets call for getting 30 percent of your calories from protein, and the FDA's recommendation is to get 15 percent of your calories from protein.

Protein is found in almost all foods. The richest source is muscle meat. Although we tend to think of animal protein as superior to plant protein, this is not true. Animal protein comes packaged with lots of fat, few vitamins and minerals, and no fiber, while plant protein is accompanied by lots of vitamins, minerals, and fiber. If you are a vegetarian, as long as you are getting enough calories you are probably eating enough protein. Much of that protein will come from grains such as bread and rice, and legumes such as split peas, peanuts, and beans. Nuts and seeds are also good protein sources.

Ways to increase protein:
- Drink a protein supplement. Both soy and whey protein are good choices and they can be added to a wide variety of liquids including juice, milk, soymilk, and yogurt. Add full-fat coconut milk for an energy boost.

- Keep thinly sliced low-fat, low-salt deli meat in the fridge and snack on a slice.
- Snack on protein-rich, crunchy, unsalted soy nuts.
- Munch on meal replacement bars between meals. High protein bars made for the Zone dieters are a good choice.

ROUGH APPROXIMATIONS OF PROTEIN CONTENT OF FOODS

FOOD	PROTEIN	SERVING SIZE
Meat, fish, legumes, cheese	7 grams	1 oz. (a pork chop is about 3 oz.) or 1/2 cup legumes
Milk	4 grams	1/2 cup
Cereals, grains, potatoes	2 grams	1/2 cup or one slice
Vegetables	1 gram	1/2 cup
Fruit	0.5 gram	1/2 cup

One gram of protein always equals 4 calories. Let's say you eat 1/2 cup of oatmeal. It has 5 grams of protein according to the Quaker Oats box.* Multiply 5 grams X 4 (the number of calories in each gram or protein) = 20 calories. The Quaker box says there are 150 calories in 1/2 cup. So the percent of calories from protein is 20 divided by 150, or 13 percent.

*(The grams given above are approximations for purposes of comparison—use the more accurate product labels, where available. Breakfast cereals range from lightweight Cocoa Puffs at 1.2 grams, to Raisin Nut Bran, which weighs in at 5.16 grams of protein.)

Heart Failure and Diet

Most PH patients have heart failure to some degree. Heart failure causes shortness of breath, and you may find yourself breathing through the mouth. This makes eating difficult as you try to swallow food in between breaths. If you have difficulty breathing and chewing at the same time try these suggestions:

- Soft or liquid food is easiest to eat. Add healthy smoothies to your diet. Toss frozen or fresh fruit, a scoop of soy protein, and nonfat milk into your blender. Moisten dry foods with sauces and gravies.
- Put only a small amount of food in your mouth at one time.
- Avoid hard, dry, or chewy food.
- Eat four or five small meals rather than three large ones. Large meals can push the diaphragm upward, displacing the heart and restricting your breathing even more.
- Avoid foods that cause gas or use an enzyme product called Beano that prevents gas formation and flatulence.

Health Store Nutrients That May Help Support a Failing Heart

An overworked enlarged heart needs more energy and nutrients and the rest of the body needs more oxygen. The nutrients most often recommended to support a failing heart include Coenzyme Q10, carnitine, and taurine.

Coenzyme Q10, (CoQ10) is an antioxidant, vitamin-like substance made by our bodies and found in many foods. Wild, unproven claims have been made for it as an anti-aging and cancer remedy. There's a bit more reason to think that it might help treat congestive heart failure. Still, there is little scientific evidence to support its effectiveness for this, either. The American Heart Association, in their recent "Guidelines for the Evaluation and Management of Chronic Heart Failure in the Adult," reviewed the research on Coenzyme Q10 and concluded they could not yet recommend it as a sole therapy for heart failure. It should not replace conventional treatment.

Some populations have been shown to have lower levels of CoQ10. This includes type 2 diabetics and persons taking certain drugs. The cholesterol-lowering statins such as simvastatin (Zocor) and lovastatin (Mevacor, Altocor) can decrease CoQ10. In 34 patients taking 20 mg of simvastatin this was prevented by taking 100 mg of CoQ10. Other drugs that decrease CoQ10 levels include gemfibrozil, certain blood pressure lowering drugs such as atenolol and propranolol, tricyclic antidepressants such as amitriptyline, doxepin and imipramine, and beta blockers. No one yet knows if supplementation is more effective in populations that have low levels of this nutrient.

CoQ10 is chemically similar to vitamin K, which may explain why there are reports that it counteracts the effect of warfarin (Coumadin). If you take both, the amount of Coumadin needed to thin your blood might be greater. It is very important that you talk with your doctor before starting this supplement and that, once started, you don't discontinue its use without being carefully monitored.

Some small studies have suggested that another nutrient, carnitine, might be effective for a variety of cardiovascular disorders. Theoretically, it might be helpful in the treatment of heart failure, but when researchers have given heart failure patients carnitine under controlled conditions, the results have been mixed. If you wish to try carnitine supplements, ask your PH doctor first. The dose utilized in clinical studies was 600 mg three times a day. Side effects included nausea, vomiting, diarrhea, rashes, and headache. An alternative is to help your own body make carnitine by having enough of its raw materials always around. It is made from the amino acid lysine with the help of vitamin C, pyridoxine (B6), niacin, iron, and the amino acid methionine.

Taurine, another nutrient, improves the ability of the heart muscle to contract, protects the heart from calcium imbalances that can cause cell death, and is a powerful antioxidant that protects heart cells from free radical damage. Taurine also reduces platelet aggregation and high cholesterol, and may help to lower blood pressure. The usual dosage used in clinical studies has ranged from 500 mg/day to 3 g/day taken in two doses. Like all amino acids, it is best taken on an empty stomach. No significant side effects have been reported, but as with all supplements, check with your doctor first.

Sodium, Salt, and Edema

Sodium helps regulate the balance of fluids in your body. When water builds up in your tissues, one of the most effective ways of getting rid of it is to reduce the amount of salt or sodium in your diet. Doing so can reduce the amount of fluid in tissues, which in turn reduces the volume of blood your heart has to pump. Avoiding salt in your diet reduces the amount of *sodium chloride* in your food. If the edema is severe or if it doesn't respond to a low-*salt* diet, your doctor may recommend a low-*sodium* diet. A diet that is low in salt is not necessarily also low in sodium. Research has shown that a low-salt diet will have a greater impact on your health if it is coupled with a diet rich in calcium, magnesium, potassium, and phosphorous.

Your taste for salt will decrease over time. Therefore, if you decrease your salt intake in steps, you will hardly notice its absence. You will notice how much more flavorful your food tastes.

Here are some ways to cut back on salt:

♦ Most salt enters the diet with prepared and packaged foods. Read the labels of all prepared foods and look for low-salt versions.

♦ Don't salt your food automatically.

♦ Don't add salt during cooking; let your family season to taste on their own plates.

♦ Put the tip of a toothpick into two holes in your saltshaker and break them off. Now when you use your shaker you will be getting less salt. Each day close off two more holes.

Here are some salty foods to avoid:

♦ Those preserved in brine or pickled, such as olives, sauerkraut, pickles, pickled herring and pickled eggs

♦ Salted condiments such as relish, catsup, soy sauce, and Worcestershire sauce

♦ Prepared meat products such as hot dogs, sausage, salami, dried beef, smoked meats, cooked chicken breasts and rolls, cold cuts, and canned meats

♦ Breaded or battered foods, both fresh and frozen

♦ Seasonings containing salt, such as coating and baking mixes for meat and celery salt

♦ Packaged/bottled sauces such as clam sauce, red spaghetti sauce, and curry sauce

♦ Salted snack foods such as potato chips, corn chips, pretzels, crackers, and salted nuts

♦ Buttermilk

♦ Some instant breakfast drinks

♦ Most packaged and canned soups, stews, vegetables, and pasta dinners

♦ Pre-seasoned frozen vegetables

Instead of seasoning your food with salt, try these substitutes:

♦ Fresh or frozen lemon juice: it doesn't make food sour, but "brightens" the taste, pepping up everything from vegetables to chicken and fish

♦ Peppers: bell peppers, hot peppers, and freshly grated peppercorns

♦ Garlic: fresh chopped garlic, dried garlic flakes, bottled garlic puree

♦ Fresh herbs: these are far superior to the store-bought variety and can grow in a window-sill garden

♦ Potassium-containing salts (not potassium chloride, which is dangerous): available in most supermarkets, and have the benefit of acting as a potassium supplement, which may help you if your blood potassium levels are sometimes low

A pot of fresh herbs can please the eye, the nose, and the palate.

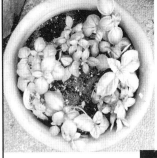

◄*Three kinds of basil.*

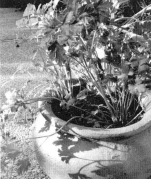

Parsley ►

To decrease your *sodium* intake:

- Read the labels of *all* prepared foods. Most of the sodium in your diet will come hidden in prepared foods. Many foods now have low sodium versions. Don't be misled by "light" or "reduced sodium" labels. "Light" soy sauce has over 500 mg of sodium per tablespoon!
- Check the serving size on processed foods when adding up your sodium intake.
- Ask your physician about the sodium content of your prescriptions. Most medicines contain less than 5 mg of sodium per dose, but some contain up to 120 mg per dose.
- Do not use celery flakes or parsley flakes—they are really high in sodium.

Hidden Sources of Sodium:

- Some chewable antacid tablets
- Aspirin (50 mg/tablet)
- Celery flakes
- Parsley flakes
- Some prescription drugs   (ask your pharmacist)
- Laxatives
- Mouthwashes
- Toothpastes
- Sauerkraut
- Canned tomato juice
- Canned vegetables with added salt
- Olives
- Cheese
- Milk
- Cold cuts
- Frankfurters
- Any salted crackers, chips

Sodium levels in salt. The American Heart Association (AHA) recommends that healthy adults reduce their sodium intake to no more than 2,400 milligrams per day. This is about 1 and 1/4 teaspoon of sodium chloride (salt). They further recommend that if you have heart failure, you reduce your sodium to 2000 mg. Some doctors advise PAH patients to follow the AHA guidelines. Listings of the sodium content of various foods and other guidelines can be found on the AHA's website (www.americanheart.org).

1/4 teaspoon salt	=	500 mg sodium
1/2 teaspoon salt	=	1,000 mg sodium
3/4 teaspoon salt	=	1,500 mg sodium
1 teaspoon salt	=	2,000 mg sodium
1 tsp baking soda	=	1,000 mg sodium

How to interpret sodium descriptions. Prepared foods must follow these FDA set guidelines when making claims on their labels. The amounts given below are for one serving, so you must read the label to determine the serving size.

- **Sodium-free** means less than 5 milligrams of sodium *per serving*
- **Very low-sodium** means 35 milligrams or less *per serving*
- **Low-sodium** means 140 milligrams or less *per serving*
- **Unsalted, no salt added** or **without added salt** mean exactly what they say: no salt is added to the food. These foods are not necessarily low in sodium, because some sodium may naturally be present in the ingredients.
- **Healthy** means less than 360 mg sodium *per serving*, or no more than 480 mg *per meal* for meal-type products.

Diuretics and Diet

Diuretics can deplete levels of calcium, magnesium, phosphorus, potassium, vitamin C, pyridoxine (vitamin B-6), and thiamine (vitamin B-1). Low levels of these minerals can lead to bone loss (osteoporosis), muscle cramping, muscle weakness, irregular heartbeat, high blood pressure, anorexia (loss of appetite), and nausea. Low levels of the vitamins can cause confusion, memory loss, insomnia, fluid retention and fatigue. Thiazide diuretics can raise calcium levels in the blood, but deplete magnesium, zinc, potassium, and CoQ10.

Some foods act as natural diuretics. They include asparagus, parsley, beets, grapes, green beans, leafy greens, pineapple, pumpkin, onion, leeks, and garlic. They should not replace diuretic drugs, but are worth a try if your edema is mild. Couple these foods with a low-salt diet.

Vitamin B6 has diuretic properties. For this reason, some call it "vitamin P." It's found in fortified cereals, oatmeal, potatoes, beans, meat, poultry, fish, bananas, and some other fruits and vegetables. You need B6 to make the hemoglobin inside red blood cells that carries oxygen to tissues: B6 helps load up those cells with oxygen. Too little B6 can cause a form of anemia.

Other Nutrients of Interest

Vitamins in General

Vitamins are not benign substances; you can harm yourself by overloading on them and taking more then the RDI (Recommended Dietary Intake, which replaced the RDA, the Recommended Daily Allowance). When several supplements are combined, it is easy to overdose and not realize it. Minerals (often included in one-a-day type pills) interact with one another and an overdose of one will cause imbalances with the others. It is very important that you make a list of every type of food supplement you take and give a copy to each of your doctors and your pharmacist. This is to help avoid drug interactions.

Once you start on a supplement regime, follow it consistently so it will not affect your INR. We've already discussed how Vitamin K can block the beneficial effect of warfarin. As a general rule, it's more dangerous to take too much of the fat-soluble vitamins (A, D, K, and E) than the water-soluble ones (the Bs and C).

Take all your vitamins and minerals with a meal. This is especially important for fat-soluble vitamins, which need fat to be absorbed. Read labels and avoid multivitamins with megadoses (in the thousands of percents of RDI or RDA of any one vitamin).

Vitamin E

Vitamin E is what are collectively called the tocopherols—a family of eight related fat-soluble nutrients. They are powerful antioxidants that protect your cell membranes and genetic material from free radical damage. Vitamin E is necessary for proper immune functioning and can prevent the formation of certain cancers. In your blood vessels, it can help protect your endothelium from inflammation. Surveys show that 70 percent of Americans do not get the recommended amount of this nutrient from diet alone, so chances are that you don't either.

The most expensive and probably the most effective supplement contains a mixture of all eight tocopherols. The most common tocopherol found in supplements is alpha tocopherol. The natural form (d-alpha tocopherol or RRR-alpha tocopherol) is more active than the synthetic and cheaper form (dl-alpha tocopherol or all-rac-alpha tocopherol). That is why vitamin E is measured in international units (IUs) instead of grams; IUs take the difference in activity into consideration so you don't have to worry about it.

As already mentioned, vitamin E boosts the effect of warfarin, so it will make you more likely to bleed if you take high doses. In really high doses (over 1000 IU) it has been shown to be bad for you if you have heart failure. As long as you take no more than 400 IUs of vitamin E or mixed tocopherols, and keep your intake constant, vitamin E supplements will not hurt you and will probably help. Check your multivitamin: it probably contains all the supplemental vitamin E you need.

Magnesium

Magnesium and calcium are responsible for muscle tone in blood vessel walls, which makes these minerals of particular interest to PH patients. Calcium stimulates smooth muscle, while magnesium relaxes it. Magnesium increases the amount of blood that flows through the heart with each beat, and helps prevent the formation of blood clots by preventing platelet aggregation. Diuretics increase the loss of both minerals to the urine. Since digoxin (a drug taken to regulate the heartbeat) reacts with both magnesium and calcium, your physician will monitor your blood levels of these minerals and may ask you to take supplements.

In addition to its ability to relax the muscle cells in blood vessel walls, magnesium can correct heart arrhythmias, relieve muscle cramps, improve sleep, and reduce anxiety, depression, and the effects of stress.

The typical American diet is high in refined grains, salt, sugar, caffeine, and alcohol—all of which increase the loss of magnesium in the urine. Magnesium has the tendency to sneak out of the body along with bodily fluids. If you have diarrhea from epoprostenol or treprostinil, or vomit a lot, magnesium will be lost in those fluids, too.

Digoxin can increase the loss of magnesium in the urine. Side effects of digoxin are magnified if you have a magnesium deficiency, so it is important to maintain normal levels of this mineral during treatment. Type 2 diabetes patients also have to watch their magnesium—25 to 38 percent are deficient in magnesium. Magnesium deficiency is also associated with heart disease, kidney malfunction, and any stomach and bowel disorder.

To maximize the amount of magnesium you get from food, eat only whole grains. Whole-wheat bread, for example, has twice as much magnesium as white bread. Other rich sources are oatmeal, tofu, and soybean flour; Brazil nuts, almonds, cashews, black walnuts, pistachio nuts, and pine nuts; pumpkin and squash seeds; peanuts and other legumes; green leafy vegetables; and blackstrap molasses.

Well-absorbed forms of magnesium are magnesium citrate, magnesium gluconate, magnesium malate, and magnesium lactate. Think twice before buying a cheap magnesium supplement (such as magnesium oxide or magnesium hydroxide) that is not well absorbed; the magnesium that reaches your large colon will attract water and the result is loose stools or diarrhea.

Calcium

Calcium is needed to regulate the heartbeat and for proper blood clotting. It influences the release of neurotransmitters, and the release and activation of enzymes, and is required for muscle contraction and nerve transmission. Best known for preventing osteoporosis and making strong teeth and bones, calcium can also keep your heart regular, lower high blood pressure, reduce irritability, insomnia, depression, and headaches during menopause, reduce cramps and moodiness from premenstrual syndrome, and prevent colon and rectal cancer. Recent studies indicate that dietary calcium may help you to lose weight. The more calcium-rich foods you eat, the less likely you are to be obese.

Calcium interacts with the same drugs as magnesium. Too much calcium may increase your chance of having a toxic reaction to digoxin. On the other hand, if you get too little calcium your digoxin might not be effective. Diuretics can cause this mineral to be lost in the urine.

A diet that contains a lot of soft drinks, sodium, sugar, saturated fat, caffeine, and alcohol can increase the loss of calcium in the urine. As we get older it gets harder for our bodies to absorb calcium. Dairy products are the richest sources of calcium, but other good sources include nuts (almonds, Brazil nuts, and hazelnuts), greens (collards, dandelion, turnip and mustard), green vegetables (broccoli, bok choy, kale, and cabbage), soybean flour, dried figs, and oysters.

If you take a calcium supplement, there are several choices. Calcium carbonate is the cheapest form of calcium. It needs acid to be absorbed, so you must take it during meals when you stomach acid is highest. Rolaids and Tums contain calcium carbonate. Calcium citrate is another option. Unlike calcium carbonate it does not need stomach acid for absorption, so you can take it any time of the day. Avoid natural sources of calcium; they are more likely to be contaminated with lead from the environment. Natural sources include oyster shells, limestone, coral, bone meal, and Dolomite. Vitamin D enhances the absorption of calcium, but they do not have to be taken together. If your multivitamin contains vitamin D, you do not have to buy a calcium supplement with it.

Adults aged 19 to 50 should take 1,000 mg of calcium each day. Those over 50 need at least 1,200 mg each day. When deciding how much calcium to take, remember that you will also be getting some from your diet. If you eat a lot of dairy products, you may want to take less calcium. Take your calcium supplement twice a day; your body cannot absorb a whole day's worth of calcium at once. If you can, take it apart from other mineral supplements.

Potassium

Potassium is one of the electrolytes, the others being sodium and chloride. Electrolytes are important because they carry the electrical currents for all the cells of the body. They are necessary for heart functioning, brain activity, and muscle movement, and they regulate blood pressure.

So much potassium can be lost during vomiting, diarrhea, or the use of loop diuretics (such as furosemide and bumetanide), that the losses can be life threatening. In addition to diuretics, other drugs that can decrease your potassium level include NSAIDs (such as aspirin and ibuprofen), beta-blockers (such as metoprolol and propranolol), Thiazide (such as hydrochlorothiazide), and overuse of antacids. Low potassium levels can increase the likelihood of toxic effects from digoxin.

Supplements come in tablets and capsules of various sizes and shapes; the small capsules are easiest to swallow.

You get potassium from unprocessed fruits, vegetables, and grains. Particularly rich sources include: salt substitute (potassium chloride); beet greens; chard; and spinach. Good sources include melons, citrus and vegetable juices, prune juice, bananas, figs, peaches, yogurt, tofu, and sunflower seeds. Adults need 3,500 mg/day.

Herbals: Which Are Safe for Us?

Be really cautious using herbal medicines. Don't assume herbs are safe because they are "natural." Poison darts are natural, and so are Death Cap mushrooms. Many herbs are powerful medicines, and the FDA does not regulate their potency and freedom from contamination. Time after time, studies have found that "food supplements" do not contain what they claim to, are erratic in dosage, or contain dangerous chemicals that are not on the label. Contaminated herbal remedies have *given* people PH! The National Institutes of Health has set up a National Center for Complimentary and Alternative Medicine, which has a somewhat useful website (http://nccam.nih.gov). Before taking any herbals, check with your doc. Also tell the anesthesiologist what you take if you are planning surgery.

Keeping these warnings in mind, some research papers suggest that some types of ginseng may help endothelial cells make more nitric oxide (and perhaps less endothelin). Nitric oxide causes the little pulmonary arteries to relax, which is a good thing for PH patients; endothelin makes the little arteries tighten up. A warning, however: Asian ginseng interacts with warfarin.

One herb recently banned in the U.S. can be particularly dangerous for us: ephedra (a.k.a. ma huang, desert tea, Mormon tea). Ephedra contains ephedrine, which mimics the effects of adrenaline and decongestants (ephedrine, fenfluramine, and amphetamine have similar chemical structures). Ephedra is found in products like Metabolife, Stacker 2, Ripped Fuel, Xenadrine, YellowSubs, TrimSpa, Thermo-Tek and Up Your Gas. Ephedrine can cause arrhythmias like supraventricular tachycardia and atrial fibrillation, which are not well tolerated by PH patients. If you have any products around containing ephedrine, toss them.

Diet products are now advertising that they are "ephedra-free." That doesn't mean they are safe for you. Many use bitter orange (*Citrus aurantium*) or/and green tea extract, and maybe a pinch of caffeine as well. All are stimulants, and in combination may be dangerous. The synephrine in bitter orange acts a lot like ephedra, and like ephedra is associated with deaths and other "adverse reactions." Bitter orange is found in Stacker 2 Ephedra Free, Twinlab's Diet Fuel Ephedra Free, and Mind-FX's Maxx Impulse Terminal Velocity Energy Formula (no kidding, that's its name). There is no evidence that any of these products help you shed pounds.

A component of grapefruit juice called bergamottin interacts with the immuno-suppressive drug cyclosporine, possibly increasing its effect to toxic levels, so avoid grapefruit juice if you have had a transplant. (Transplant patients are also supposed to avoid overly ripe Mediterranean oranges and limes for the same reason.) The beverages Sun Drop and Fresca also contain bergamottin.

Green tea contains antioxidants that help fight disease. It also contains caffeine and catechins. The latter boost the effects of synephrine, ephedra, and similar compounds. So avoid green tea when it is used in combinations. The technicians who check patients' INRs at the University of Washington swear that even clear green tea with no leaves in it still has enough vitamin K in it to mess up INRs, and that they have personally observed this. (Vitamin K is fat-soluble, not water-soluble, so this seems illogical.) To be safe, if you use warfarin, keep an eye on your green tea consumption and be consistent about how much green tea you drink.

Everyone knows caffeine is in coffee and tea. But caffeine has a few disguises to watch out for: guarana, kola nut, maté, paullinia cupana, and tea extracts. Caffeine is often found in soft drinks. Many PH patients drink beverages containing some caffeine, but you don't want to overload on it.

Liver damage has been found in some patients using kava, echinacea, and valerian. If you take bosentan, you might want to avoid these until more is known about the safety of combining bosentan with these supplements.

If your doctor approves your use of herbs, avoid combination formulas; very often they are less effective and are almost always more expensive. Each individual herb already contains a group of synergistic compounds. *Beware: just because your favorite natural remedy isn't listed below doesn't mean it's safe.* Finally, don't buy herbs made in China—some are contaminated with prescription drugs. Stick to well-known brands.

"NATURAL REMEDIES" THAT MAY HARM SOME PH PATIENTS		
DON'T MIX:	**WITH:**	**BECAUSE:**
Dong quai Dang gui (angelica) Danshen	Warfarin	You may bleed excessively
Ephedra (ma huang)	No PH patient should use	Can increase heart rate and blood pressure
Feverfew	Warfarin	You may bleed excessively
Garlic (as a supplement; it's okay in seasoning amounts)	Warfarin	You may bleed excessively
Ginko biloba	Warfarin	You may bleed excessively
Ginger (as a supplement; it's okay in seasoning amounts)	Warfarin	You may bleed excessively
Ginseng	Digoxin	Affects strength of the medicine
Licorice root	Digoxin, diuretics	May cause excessive potassium loss
Omega 3 fatty acids (fish oils)	Warfarin	You may bleed excessively
Papaya extract	Warfarin	You may bleed excessively
Saint John's wort (hypernica)	Antidepressants CCBs Irinotecan (Camptosar) Oral contraceptives Digoxin (Lanoxin) Immunosuppressants	Exacerbates their effects Increases or decreases action Reduces effectiveness Decreases effectiveness Reduces effectiveness Interferes with
Vitamins A and E	Warfarin	You may bleed excessively if you don't take consistent amounts
Vitamin K	Warfarin	Decreases effectiveness

Nausea and Vomiting

Nausea and vomiting can be a side effect of drugs like epoprostenol, treprostinil, and bosentan. They can also be caused by the heart failure common in PH. Vomiting is how our body gets rid of food it thinks should not be in the stomach. It is stimulated by sensory receptors in the wall of the stomach including stretch receptors that indicate when the stomach is too full, and chemoreceptors that detect possible toxins and poisons. The emetic center in the brain responds by causing a wave of reverse peristalsis in the stomach muscles, expelling the contents.

While vomiting is unpleasant, it is only dangerous when it is severe or prolonged. The main danger is loss of fluids and minerals (magnesium, calcium and potassium). This can cause dehydration, weight loss, and an electrolyte imbalance. If too much fluid is lost, the situation can become dangerous and intravenous fluids and electrolytes may be needed to reverse the imbalances. If you have prolonged nausea or vomiting, contact your doctor.

Here are ways to avoid nausea:

- Don't eat large meals that fill your stomach, drink large amounts of liquids with meals, or drink too many carbonated beverages.
- Avoid greasy and fatty foods: fat causes food to remain in the stomach longer, increasing the chance you may vomit.
- When you feel nauseated, nibble on high-carb foods such as crackers, pretzels, dry toast, and soft bread.
- Cold non-acidic liquids often help to settle a stomach (try small sips of ice water, ice chips, iced herbal teas, ice tea, and small tastes of fruit sorbets).
- Sit up when you eat and don't lie down immediately after eating.
- Avoid any food that you know causes gas or "repeats" on you (makes you burp).
- Place an ice pack on the back of your neck. The gel pacs used to cool Flolan work well.
- Open windows and let in fresh, cool air. Stale or smoky air makes nausea worse.
- Keep you teeth and tongue brushed, your teeth flossed, and your mouth rinsed. This will help keep bad flavors and odors from developing.

10

Dealing with Emergencies, Doctors, Colds, and Flu

Help! Is This an Emergency?

If you have a programmable telephone, go to it right now and program in your doctor's emergency telephone number. Psychologically, it might make it easier for you to call him or her when you should. (Or make it easier for a child or neighbor to call should you be unable to reach the phone yourself.) Because PH can rapidly get worse, it's best to err on the side of caution. Most physicians carry a beeper so they are in round-the-clock contact with the nurse on call. If you are uncertain, ask the nurse if your situation merits paging the doctor. Most doctors would rather have you call them in an ambiguous situation than have you "wait to see if the problem goes away."

If you experience any of these—and they are not situations that you and your doctor have already discussed how to handle—go to your local ER and call your doctor from there (or call from your cell if someone else is driving you):

- Chest pain
- Rapid or irregular heartbeats
- Fainting or near-fainting
- A high or prolonged fever (especially if using epoprostenol)
- Coughing up blood
- Coughing up colored mucus
- Bronchitis or chest congestion
- Unusual (for you) shortness of breath
- Unusual (for you) fluid retention

If you are having epoprostenol (Flolan) problems, call your PH specialist or health service company, whichever one your doctor has instructed you to call. (The Accredo Therapeutics' National Customer Support Center (NCSC) at 1-866-344-4874 (1-866-FIGHT PH); TheraCom at 1-877-FLOLAN-4.) Also see Nurse Cathy's Flolan emergency chart on pages 280-281 at the back of this book. You may need to call 911.

If you are having treprostinil (Remodulin) problems, call your PH specialist or health service company, whichever one your doctor has instructed you to call. (The Accredo Therapeutics' National Customer Support Center (NCSC) at 1-866-344-4874 (1-866-FIGHT PH); CVS Caremark at 1-866-879-2348; and Curascript at 1-888-773-7376.

If you take an anticoagulant, see the list of side effects to report to your doctor under Anticoagulants, Chapter 4.

Also call your PH specialist during regular business hours, please, when these nonemergency situations arise:

- Pregnancy
- Diarrhea (it may affect your meds)
- If you see signs that your PH is getting worse
- If your oxygen sat drops from, say, 94 to 89 or 90

- If you make changes in your medications (including over-the-counter drugs and vitamins), or see that in a couple weeks you will need a prescription refill
- If you plan to undergo dental or other surgery

If you are going to have surgery, ask your PH specialist about the need for prophylactic antibiotics to help prevent endocarditis (a bacterial infection of a heart valve, or of the lining of the heart or aorta). Ask, too, if you will need to substitute heparin for warfarin for a while before the surgery. (Heparin is administered by injection. Its anticoagulant action is more easily reversed than that of warfarin, and it remains in the bloodstream for a shorter time.)

Help ("panic") buttons. If you often feel as if you might pass out, consider getting a "send help" button that you can wear on your person (even in the shower or swimming pool), in case you cannot make it to a phone. A help button can take some of the stress off both you and family members who feel responsible for your well-being.

The social worker at your hospital can tell you about local companies that provide such services. Lifeline Services is available through over 200 hospitals and health care providers in the U.S. and Canada. Their button is on either a necklace or bracelet and activates a small, sensitive, two-way speakerphone that allows you to talk to a Lifeline staff member from almost any room in your house and ask for the type of help you need. If you press the button but are unable to speak, Lifeline will immediately send the medics. Lifeline is affordable and you can cancel the service at any time. Phone 1-800-380-3111 to learn more, or go to www.lifelinesys.com. Home alarm companies also offer help buttons.

Avoiding Disaster at the Emergency Room

Patients on drugs that are continuously administered through a central line have more than their share of dramatic medical moments, but except for the advice on pumps, the information in this section applies to anybody with PH. Because PH is uncommon, and its care is changing quickly, many ER teams will not be familiar with epoprostenol or treprostinil or the possible danger from stopping it, so you will need to accept the responsibility to help them learn.

Keep your pump pumping. *Epoprostenol and treprostinil are unique types of continuous infusion drugs. Epoprostenol and treprostinil cannot be interrupted.* It is possible to give epoprostenol through a peripheral line, although high doses can cause phlebitis. If you're having trouble with your catheter and are taken to an emergency room, the doctor or nurse might refuse to connect the IV to your pump because they want to use their *own* pump. *Don't let them!* Standard pumps will not work with epoprostenol, because they are not calibrated to the right infusion rates to accommodate epoprostenol and treprostinil when they are mixed in the standard way. Changing the dilution is tricky and they should not try it. Make it clear that turning off your CADD may kill you, so you cannot allow anyone to do that. Get your PH center on the phone (keep their number on your pump, along with your health service company's). In a pinch, show the ER staff this page of this book! Hospital policies vary; some might require a family member to stay with you 24/7 if you use your own pump. (See the section below on contacting emergency rooms before you need them.)

Carry written emergency instructions. Get written emergency instructions from your doctor or health service company that include information on the PH drug(s) you use, on how it's administered, on your pump (if you use one), and on what to do in emergencies. Carry a pump/catheter repair kit with you. Ask your PH center for an IV that will fit your Hickman, if you don't already have one to carry with you.

Pump problems also arise when you are a patient in a hospital, because hospitals want to use their own equipment and drugs and take yours away from you. Get your health care provider or your PH specialist to convince them to let you keep your own pump and meds (PH specialists are used to having to do this).

Involve your PH specialist. Any PH patient who goes to an emergency room because of chest pain or passing out should tell the emergency room doctor to call their PH specialist stat. This is hard to do if you are unconscious, so see the section on "MedicAlert bracelets," below.

Getting the most from 911. Call 911 and say, "This is a test. If I dial 911, where will the ambulance come from that is dispatched to my home (or workplace, or school)?" Write down the answers. Then ask if you can give them information to put on file that will appear on their screen whenever someone dials 911 from your house. They can often keep a record of things like the medications you take, what your doctor says to do if you are found unconscious, your doctor's name and telephone number, and maybe even a previous EKG and the address of a neighbor who has a key to your house.

For added safety, you can visit the fire station/EMTs or other place that will send the ambulance to your house and explain your pump and medical conditions in person.

In Southern California and some other areas, callers to 911 are sometimes put on hold for long periods. So get the full, seven-digit, direct emergency number for your area

and program that into your telephone, rather than risk delays by using the 911 system.

Remember that if you call 911 from a cell phone, the person who answers may not know where you are physically located, so you may have to tell them. Newer phones can pinpoint your location—sometimes. But even if your phone is so equipped, the system might not work, so tell them immediately where you are. When driving, make it a habit to mentally note landmarks, exit signs you pass on a freeway, or highway mileage markers. (It comes in handy, too, if your car breaks down and you have to call AAA.)

Contact emergency rooms before you need them. At the 2000 PHA conference, here is how a PH specialist described what goes through the head of Doc Pooped-Out at Pus Pocket Memorial Hospital when you arrive with problems:

1. She looks okay, although her blood pressure is a little low.
2. What the heck is "Flolan?" Gee, I've never had a patient on one of these weird pumps.
3. Oh, Flolan's a vasodilator. Well, her blood pressure's low, so I guess we should stop that Flolan stuff.
4. I've never heard of pulmonary hypertension and don't want to learn now; my shift ends in three hours and I'm outta here.
5. Anything I do, I could be sued.
6. So I'm gonna punt.

If this happens to you, refuse to leave the emergency room until care is provided. Don't sign any discharge papers until you are satisfied. If an emergency room tries to turn you away, demand to see the person in charge (there is always an "administrator on call"). Remind them that they have a legal duty to help you. Use the oxygen analogy: if I needed supplemental oxygen and ran out, would you send me home to suffocate? If you have to, say you will go to the state board. If you have to, get yourself helicoptered to your PH center.

Try to avoid this all-too-real scenario by planning ahead. Call your emergency room and ask for the triage desk, the head nurse, or the medical director. Explain about your condition and the continuous infusion pump. There are three shifts of personnel; Phil called them all, at his hospital, to be sure everyone knew about his condition. They may ask for a letter from your doctor or for other emergency instructions to keep on file (you will probably have to remind them it's on file, should it ever be needed).

Unfortunately, the Emergency Medical Treatment and Labor Act of 1986 (the "anti-dumping statute") may be weakened by a regulation effective in late 2003 that eases requirements for on-call specialists. You might want to check with your local emergency room to see what the situation is there.

MedicAlert bracelets. Get one of these (see Chapter 14) and/or carry a wallet card with your medical information. On the bracelet are your personal ID number, primary medical condition(s), and the 24-hour phone number of MedicAlert's emergency response center. If you can fit it on, and it applies, say, "Don't stop the pump!" or "Takes Coumadin." Emergency personnel can call the MedicAlert number toll free and learn more about your condition, your medications, medical devices you use, your allergies and insurance information, the names and telephone numbers of your doctors, family members, and health service company (Accredo Therapeutics or TheraCom, if you use Flolan). In the instructions, say that your medicine cannot be interrupted or you might die. Keep the information up to date.

Does taking these precautions really do any good? Dr. Lewis Rubin reports that he has, indeed, received calls from ER rooms that got his number off his patients' bracelets.

Picking a Hospital

Many hospitals in the U.S. today are dangerously short of well-trained nurses. If you have a choice of hospitals, do some research before deciding which to use. *The quality of the nursing staff is just as important as the quality of the doctors.* California was the first state to implement laws (which went into effect January 2002) requiring a certain ratio of nurses to patients in given situations. Many nurses do not think that California has gone far enough to protect the safety of patients. In many places, the situation has gotten so bad that even nurses advise those who are seriously ill, and fortunate enough to afford it, to hire a skilled private nurse to be with them at all times in a hospital. If this isn't possible for you, a family member or friend can hang around to make notes about medication changes, watch that transitions go smoothly as shifts change or you are moved from one level of care to another, and help you in some ways when the staff is busy. Your companion can also make demands on your behalf when, for example, your dinner is three hours late or your pain medicine is insufficient.

Consumers Reports magazine did a special report on "How Safe is Your Hospital?" that is worth reading. Published in the January 2003 issue, it suggests ways to get information on hospitals and other things to consider. You can also get this information on the magazine's website: www.ConsumerReports.org.

When you are to be admitted to a hospital, pack a list of all your medications and dosages, your doctors' telephone numbers, the number of your health service company (if one provides your PH drugs), insurance information, and a summary of your medical history. Also pack a notebook, in which you can keep your own record of your hospital stay, as well as your post-hospital care instructions. Mary took along a framed photo of herself and her husband playing golf, so her medical team could see how different she looks when she's well. It reminds the staff that she is a person with a life, not just a body in a bed. It also cheers her up to look at the photo.

How to Manage Your Doctor

Developing a good relationship with both a PH specialist and a primary care physician is crucial to your survival. You need regularly scheduled visits with both, to catch problems before they get out of hand. It is equally important to develop good relationships with the RNs or physician's assistants who work with your doctors; remember their names and treat them with the same respect you show your doctor. They are highly trained (underpaid) professionals, and can answer many questions. They also know a lot of "insider"

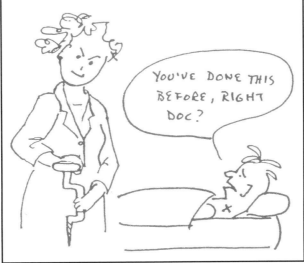

information. If a nurse even vaguely hints that you might want to consider a different doctor or treatment, look into it.

A good place to get to know medical professionals is at support group meetings and PHA conferences. To quote Christie, who was attending her third PHA conference, "I enjoy getting to know my doctors and nurses on a more personal level as well as being able to put a face with the researchers and specialists that are cited in the *Pathlight* articles."

It often helps to make an effort to break out of the pattern where the doctor asks all the questions and you give "just the facts, ma'am" answers. By doing some things that help equalize the imbalance inherent in the

doctor-patient relationship, you will get more satisfaction out of your visits. To be assertive without being confrontational, you might use rhetorical questions and anecdotes as a way to let the doctor know what you are thinking and feeling. In other words, have a friendly conversation. Demonstrate and expect respect. Discuss health-related issues that are important to you even if they aren't the reason you made the appointment. A study of over 500 patients by Dr. Klea Bertakis at UC Davis found that improvements in patients' health were directly related to how well the patients were able to talk to their doctor about their current emotional state and family relationships.

Here's an example of claiming power suggested by Bonnie Dukart, a past president of PHA (Bonnie died of PAH in 2001): rather than directly challenge your PH specialist's knowledge or judgment, ask your doctor why he or she made a particular decision. If your doctor says, "Because I'm the expert," you say, "I'm here because you're the expert. But could you tell me a little more about your reasoning?" It is also okay to politely ask your health care providers how much experience they have had treating PH patients.

Practicing medicine is not like reading a cookbook—if it were, we could diagnose ourselves with a computer program. Some of the decisions doctors make don't have a firm scientific basis. This is why doctors disagree about things like the ideal INR. (It takes oodles of resources to do a randomized clinical trial, so a lot of interesting medical questions are never going to be answered.)

Another reason you can't totally turn over responsibility for your own health to another person is that far, far too many Americans die each year because of mistakes made by their health care providers. The Institute of Medicine (a division of the National Academy of Sciences) says that such mistakes account for up to 98,000 deaths a year!

Arrive prepared. Think through your symptoms before your appointment and jot down any questions (leaving space between them for the doctor's answers). It's also helpful to arrive with a current, complete list of all the medicines (over-the-counter as well as prescription), food supplements, and vitamins that you take. Joyce (a scleroderma / PAH patient) has prepared an amazing information sheet she hands to her doctor at each visit. Here is just some of the information on that sheet: the current date, her name, birth date, and SSN. Then, in red, her allergies. She notes her vaccinations and the dates she got them, and her key diagnoses. All of her 24 prescription medicines (identified by both their generic and trade names) and the 9 supplements she takes are listed, along with their dosage, the time of day she takes each, and the reason she is taking each. She finds space for the names and telephone numbers of her doctors, insurance information, and major "turning points" in her medical care. Joyce fits all this on one page! She uses a spreadsheet to do it. She makes the information more readily accessible by using three colors: red (for allergies, recent complications, emergency contacts); blue (for billing matters like insurance companies, religious preference, and the fact she has an advance directive); and green (for information on her family doctor and nonemergency ways to contact her PH and other specialists by fax and phone). Wow! You might be shaking your head, but keeping yourself and your doctors

organized is a good thing. Doctors see hundreds of patients, and it would be impossible for them to remember everything important about every patient. Few clinics are yet fully computerized, and critical information is buried in our thick, thick files. Joyce takes several copies of her rap sheet with her to each appointment (color doesn't copy well on many doctor's office copiers) and reports that they are greatly appreciated.

Most of us PH patients have HUGE medical files that nobody likes digging through for information. So you should at least keep a few of your own notes on major medical incidents, when you change meds or dosages, important test results, and whatever else you think may be useful. If you've forgotten some important facts, you can look them up in your old medical files, which you now have a legal right to see and copy.

This is the age of mining the Internet for medical information, and many of us arrive at the clinic waving printouts. By educating yourself, you save your doctor loads of time trying to explain things. On the other hand, it's hard for doctors to immediately sort through all the stuff we ask them about, especially if we forgot to jot down the source / authority. Some medical websites are full of garbage, not gold nuggets.

Consider taking somebody with you. If your visit is a really important one, or if you're feeling weak and nonassertive, consider taking along a family member or friend as an advocate and/or note taker. It's even better if your advocate is dressed like a busy person who has many important things to do, but has put this visit at the top of his/her list. The doctor might try just a bit harder, with two pairs of eyes turned on him, and may see you more as a person in a social context and not just as "the 2:45 patient who's been waiting an hour." If you can't find a pal to accompany you, consider taking along a microcassette tape recorder (ask your doctor if it is okay to record your conversation before turning it on). It's hard to listen well when you are upset; you can re-listen to the conversation later, and make notes.

Dealing with hackers. When you arrive at a doctor's office or an emergency room, if the waiting room is full of coughing people, tell the person at the desk that you have a life-threatening pulmonary disease and that catching a cold can be a serious problem for you. Ask them to please ask the coughers to wear facemasks. Many waiting rooms now have a stack of masks handy, and a sign asking coughers to use them. As a last resort, you can put one on yourself, although it won't do as much good.

Remind the doc to check your thyroid. "PPH" is associated with an unusually high incidence of hypothyroidism. It is wise to do a blood test for this disorder, especially if your symptoms unexpectedly change or you have fluid in your heart cavity (pericardial effusion). Hypothyroidism is much more common among women than among men; older women are particularly prone to it. To check for thyroid deficiency, a blood test for thyroid-stimulating hormone (TSH) is used (the hormone tells the thyroid to work harder, because there aren't enough thyroid hormones in your blood). A high TSH level indicates an underactive thyroid. It used to be that doctors called levels up to about 5 milliunits/liter normal, but most healthy people have fewer than 2 milliunits, and many docs now think readings above 2.5 or 3 should be treated.

The symptoms of hypothyroidism are common to many disorders: fatigue, depression, trouble remembering things, dry skin, constipation, heavy menstrual bleeding, weight gain, hair loss, trouble sleeping, trouble swallowing, not tolerating cold well, a lump in the neck (a goiter), high cholesterol levels,

etc., etc., etc. We ALL have some of these symptoms, so listing them is not much help. Furthermore, if your levels are only a little low, you might not have symptoms. That's why you need to ask your doctor to do the inexpensive blood test. If your thyroid turns out to be sluggish, your doctor will prescribe oral medication to correct your hormone levels.

Some PH patients have the opposite problem, *hyper*thyroidism, or too much of the hormone. It, too, can be handled with a pill. The symptoms are weight loss, hand tremors, increased pulse rate, diarrhea, fatigue, protruding eyes, and irritability. For what it's worth, the author has run into quite a few patients on epoprostenol who have Grave's disease, which is associated with hyperthyroidism with diffuse goiter, diseases of the eyes, and areas of raised and thickened skin (sort of pebbly and orange, and maybe itchy) over the backs of the hands and feet.

Some things it's okay to do:
+ To ask when you can expect to hear back from your nurse or doctor. Or to say, "I need to hear back today," or "I need to know by (date)."
+ To call back later if your problem does not go away by the time your doctor thinks it should.
+ To ask what constitutes an emergency when you should call your doctor rather than waiting for a call back.
+ To ask if it is okay to communicate by e-mail in nonemergency situations. Many institutions don't do this; they say it isn't as secure or confidential.

The BIG talk. If you need to talk to your doctor about those industrial strength issues— like whether you are likely to die soon, or is it time to get worked up for a transplant, or should you donate a lung lobe to your child who has PH—you should set up a separate appointment. Call and say, "I need to talk to you about x." Your spouse and/or the nurse may or may not be included, as you wish. If you would rather talk to the doctor in his or her office than in an exam room, say so. By planning it this way your busy doctor will have time blocked out for the talk, and you will both be more comfortable. Doctors will seldom be able to answer those big questions for you with any accuracy. There is just too much variation among patients to predict, for example, if and when you will die from PH. They can, however, tell you about where you are in the course of the disease and give you some averages. They can also lay out the pros and cons of transplantation.

No matter how charming you are, you will be a bit of a nuisance patient. On top of all the usual paperwork, your doc will have to spend extra time explaining your condition to insurance companies and filling out forms for Medicare, Medicaid, and disability insurance companies. Medical insurance sometimes does not fully cover the costs of treating a PH patient; in other words, your doctor may not exactly view you as a profit center.

On the other hand, you are an interesting patient, and may help your primary care doctor learn more about the disease and how to spot the symptoms of PH. Doing so may help save somebody else's life. If your doctor is a PH researcher, your cooperation may help him/her do good research, publish a good paper, and advance career-wise.

When To Get a Second Opinion. If you have read this far, you know more about PH than most doctors. So if you think a second opinion is in order, you are probably right. At the PHA 2000 conference we heard over and over, from the docs themselves, that as PH patients we must be proactive and assertive. On the other hand, once you find a PH specialist who knows his/her stuff, listen well to the advice you get. Without going to medical schools ourselves, there is no way we can acquire the rounded knowledge needed to make wise decisions.

Dr. Jerome Groopman, author of the book *Second Opinion*, says that a second opinion should be sought when you are dealing with a life-threatening illness, when the diagnosis is unclear, when the treatment is risky or toxic, or when you sense you are not really being listened to and taken seriously. As Dr. Groopman says, no one knows your body as well as you do. If your HMO is reluctant, go to their patient advocate and demand a second opinion.

Although a doctor's ego may sometimes be bruised when a second opinion is sought, a wise doctor knows that a timely second opinion makes it less likely he/she will be sued for malpractice.

What do you do if you get several expert opinions and they differ? Try to get the doctors to talk to each other: some will, some won't. Some docs view it as an opportunity to expand their knowledge, others believe that many conflicts just can't be reconciled. Sometimes (when it's something really important, like is the time right to get a transplant) it is possible to get a third doctor to mediate a dispute.

Colds and Flu: What to Do

Cold Comforts

Getting a cold can be real misery for us because stuffy noses deplete our oxygen, we tire even more quickly, and we aren't supposed to take most medicines used to alleviate cold symptoms. The best remedy is to try to avoid catching colds—wash your hands before touching your eyes, mouth, nose, or food. Using an alcohol-based gel (like Purell, although the generics work fine, too) to clean your hands might be easier than washing, washing, washing. It might also kill more germs, according to the CDC. Unlike soap, the alcohol-based gels damage the structures of bacteria, fungi, and some viruses. Teach family members to cough into their hankies or elbows, not into their hands. Talk your spouse into caring for an infectious child (do something nice for your spouse in return). Unfortunately, during colds season (fall through spring, whether you live in the desert or on an iceberg), the average American adult will catch two to four colds; the average child will catch six to eight. Someone with a cold most likely has germs all over their hands and face, which they will transfer to anything they touch. Cold viruses can survive for hours on most fabrics and surfaces, including skin. They don't live long, however, on facial tissue or cotton hankies. You might have a little luck by using antiseptic skin cleansers that contain pyroglutamic acid or salicylic acid, which will kill cold viruses for hours. Pyroglutamic acid is often found in skin moisturizers; salicylic acid in over-the-counter acne treatments.

NSAIDs (pronounced EN-seds) are nonsteroidal anti-inflammatory drugs like aspirin, ibuprofen (Advil, Motrin), naproxen sodium (Aleve), and ketoprofen (Actron, Orudis KT). As mentioned earlier, they can mess with your warfarin and make you too likely to bleed. (Sometimes a doctor may allow short supervised courses of these drugs; because of the risk of Reyes' syndrome, children should almost never take aspirin, not even "baby" aspirin.)

Decongestants can be dangerous for us, because they are vasoconstrictors. PH patients who are already feeling borderline may find themselves quickly made worse by these drugs. Decongestants include phenylephrine (found in many cold medicines), and, until recently, phenylpropanolamine (PPA). PPA and phenylephrine are closely related, chemically, to amphetamines. As mentioned earlier, PPA was removed from the market in November 2000, but you may still have it in your medicine cabinet. A vasoconstrictor, it was found in decongestants like Alka-Seltzer Plus Night-Time Cold Medicine, Contac 12 Hour Capsules, Triaminic, Dimetapp Cold and Flu Caplets, Robitussin CF, and Tylenol Cold Effervescent Tablets. Acutrim, Dexa-trim, and Stay Trim also contained PPA. Sudafed contains pseudoephedrine, another vasoconstrictor. Decongestants often also contain quite a lot of caffeine, a stimulant that can cause palpitations and irregular heart rhythms. It makes no difference if these drugs come in tablets, caplets, liquids, liqui-gels, or nasal sprays—avoid them.

Antibiotics aren't helpful against cold viruses. Really.

So what *can* you do to treat cold symptoms? Get extra rest and drink warm liquids. Acetaminophen (Tylenol, Panadol) can help with mild aches and pains that aren't associated with inflammation. Buy generic acetaminophen; it's cheaper and works as well. A note of caution, however: *big* doses of acetaminophen may damage your liver and interact with warfarin. Doctors don't know yet if taking acetaminophen increases the chance of liver damage if you take bosentan.

Antihistamines (e.g., diphenhydramine, Benadryl, Claritin) are usually okay (drink extra water, because they thicken your secretions). Corticosteroid-containing nasal sprays (such as Flonase and Nasonex) are usually safe, as are plain saline nasal sprays. Some of us have used Afrin nasal spray for no more than 3 days without problems (if you use it longer you get rebound congestion) even though it does get from the nose into the rest of the body. Plain Robitussin may help loosen secretions if your cold gets into your chest.

A couple of controlled studies have suggested that echinacea may shorten (but not prevent) colds and lessen their symptoms if you take it as soon as the cold starts (on day one, when your throat is a bit itchy and scratchy, but before your nose and sinus membranes are thickened). But there are three species of echinacea and various ways of getting it into pills, so who knows if you will get the right stuff or the right dosage of active ingredients. If you take it for more than 4 weeks in a row, it might depress your immune system.

Vitamin C and zinc lozenges (used at the onset of a cold) have their supporters, but the evidence is murky, at best. Vitamin C might modestly reduce symptoms; the only thing known for certain about zinc is that it tastes bad. If you take zinc in high doses over an extended period it may weaken your immune system.

That leaves chicken soup, which is, of course, the best medicine, especially if it's made by Mom and she doesn't add salt. We're not joking about this. A study included in the October 2000 issue of *Chest* found that a traditional Jewish-style chicken soup reduced cold symptoms, maybe because it had a mild anti-inflammatory effect. The soup included chicken, onions, parsnips, turnips, and other vegetables. Fat was skimmed off. Matzo balls were not essential. Commercial chicken soups, however, varied greatly in their beneficial effect and are often high in sodium.

Flu Busters

Flu vaccine. Get a flu shot every year, early in the flu season if possible (around October/ November). Don't even think of boarding that crowded Thanksgiving Eve airplane unless you've had your vaccine! And be sure everyone in your house gets flu vaccine, too, because they are likely to catch the virus at work or school and bring it home. The vaccine's effectiveness wears off, as months pass, and it doesn't give complete immunity.

New anti-viral meds. If you do get the flu, or if somebody in your house gets it and you don't want to catch it, ask your doctor if you should try one of the new prescription drugs, like zanamivir (Relenza), oseltamivir (Tamiflu), amantadine (Symmetrel), or rimantadine (Flumadiine). A study paid for by the drug company that sells it showed that Relenza reduces your chances of catching the flu from a relative by about 79 percent. It also cuts the duration of an episode of flu by a day or two. Relenza is inhaled through the mouth. Tamiflu comes in pill form. You have to begin taking these medicines within a day or two of the time your illness starts for them to do any good. They may reduce your chances of getting bronchitis along with the flu. Side effects may include throat discomfort, headache, or an upset stomach. Heaven forbid that avian flu starts spreading among humans, but if it does, it is believed susceptible to the most expensive flu drugs, the neuraminidase inhibitors such as Tamiflu.

11

You're Not the Only One with the Blues

Coping with Depression, Guilt, & Stress

This is how one woman felt when she learned she had PH: "It's like the whole world crashed down on my head....One fell swoop, and BOOM I couldn't have kids. BOOM I had this fatal illness."

Depression often comes hand-in-hand with the illness; fatigue, lack of oxygen, anger turned inward, some medications, and a lot of other things can trigger depression. Many (perhaps most) PH patients struggle with depression, and many of us use medicines to treat it. The coordinator at one PH center says that for PH patients to use antidepressants is the rule, not the exception. It is possible that some of the drugs that we take to treat our PH may affect our moods. For example, nervousness and jitteriness are listed as possible side effects of Procardia XL.

Depression is bad for your body. A link has been found between depression and heart attacks. Some of the new antidepressants affect serotonin levels (which are linked to your mood), as did the diet drugs (Redux and fen-phen) that triggered PH. But despite this fact, drugs like Prozac, Zoloft, and Effexor are presently thought to be safe for us. Many patients say these medicines have helped them a lot. By improving our moods, anti-depressants might—theoretically—even reduce our pulmonary pressures. Being under stress also puts you at greater risk for developing colds and flu.

Intriguing research done at the University of Wisconsin and reported in *The Proceedings of the National Academy of Sciences* offered some evidence that your mood can affect your health. A group of women were asked to think of, and then write about, a time of intense happiness or joy in their lives. They were also asked to think of a time of intense sadness, fear, or anger. Negative emotions are associated with a lot of activity in the right prefrontal cortex of the brain. The women who had the greatest amount of this activity during and right after the second exercise showed the weakest response to a flu vaccine (i.e. they got less benefit from it) when antibody levels were measured 6 months later. Presumably, these women would also be more vulnerable to infections of various sorts. Fascinating as this study is, don't read too much into it: your mental attitude did not cause your PH, and if it plays a role in your response to treatment, it is only one factor (and almost certainly not the most important one) among a host of factors. Still, why not do what you can to improve your mood?

Most every PH patient feels guilty about something, whether it is about not being able to financially support his or her family, for taking the cursed diet pills, for not being able to do a full share of work around the house, for not feeling up to social events, for being a burden, for still being alive when friends die of PH, or for being able to run 5 kilometers when a PH pal who also has PH needs continuous oxygen. Try to stop blaming yourself; you sure didn't want this illness, you didn't wish it on anybody else, and you are doing all you can to feel well.

Some of what you're feeling might be stress, not guilt, because you think others think you're shirking. If so, here are some ideas:

- Ask a health care professional to explain to your family what you physically should and shouldn't do. It's important to resolve this issue with your friends and family so that they understand your illness better, and so that you *know* they understand.
- Send a doubting friend or family member a copy of this book, a subscription to *Pathlight*, or refer them to PHA's website.
- Some patients find it helpful to visualize packing all the worries they can do nothing about into a trunk, and sending the trunk way out to the horizon where it is just a tiny dot. Then they have room in their mind to focus on ways to make today as good as it can be.
- You can always fall back on that old adage about living one day or even one hour at a time. For some of us, it actually works.

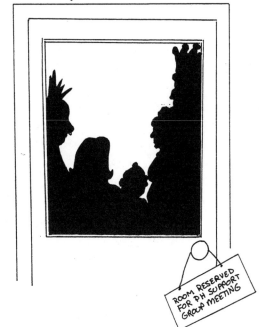

Find someone appropriate to talk to. One cause of depression is anger turned inward, on the self. Of course you're angry! It's NOT fair that you got PH, and no, you didn't deserve it. You try not to take it out on your family and friends, but may end up taking it out on yourself. It is a very, very good idea for a new PH patient and her/his caretaker to get some counseling, either together or separately. There is no shame in it. Think of it as a way to take some of the load off your family. A counselor can help you face the changes in your life and suggest methods and medicines to help you cope. Our illness frightens many of our friends (they think, yikes, I might be mortal, too!) and they might try to deny it or even avoid us. Some old friends might not want to hear the details. But talking out our worries and anger is very important. A counselor is somebody appropriate to talk to.

Another good place to talk things out is in a PH support group (see below).

"But you don't *look* sick." Do you get tired of hearing this? It's helpful to mentally rehearse a response to this comment. Sometimes it's a genuine compliment. But sometimes the tone or expression of the person saying it implies that you're faking your illness, and that wakes up your irrational guilt. When you hear, "But you look so good," the best response is probably just to smile and say, "Why, thank you!" My gosh we're lucky, compared to those with visible disabilities, people who can never blend in. Our PH friends who carry around portable oxygen or use wheelchairs wish they had this complaint.

There truly is a bright side. The emotional fallout from PH isn't all negative. "I feel somewhat blessed," says Lily, a PH patient. "PH made me slow my life down and appreciate every day. As a family we've grown closer. I think my children will be better adults because they have learned what it is like to live with a serious illness." Several dads with PH have said their illness has made them realize that their families are what is most important to them, and they relish every moment they spend at a child's ballgame or helping kids with homework. One PH specialist often tells the newly diagnosed and their families to think of it as the first day of their life. A diagnosis of PH is a time to reflect on all the things you've always wanted to do, but put off. Make definite plans to actually do the enjoyable things you can still do. This is probably good advice for everyone. As the specialist says, "No one knows their own destiny."

How the #!#?X*! Can I Relax If I Know I've Got PH?

You can do it because you have serious motivation: stress can significantly aggravate PH symptoms. Adrenalin causes a surge of blood pressure in the lungs and the rest of the body, which can damage arterial linings. When under stress, your heart speeds up, breathing becomes quick and shallow, blood sugar goes up, pain may get worse, and you may have trouble concentrating, remembering things, controlling your temper, and sleeping, or getting up in the morning.

A small study done in Switzerland of seven patients with severe PH found that when they were given a 10-minute moderate mental stress test, their pulmonary artery pressure increased and their cardiac output fell. Because their pulmonary vascular resistance increased, so did the physical stress on their right ventricle. In other words, even moderate short-term stress may worsen our symptoms.

An initial study at Duke University Medical Center on the effect of stress on heart patients found that teaching patients how to avoid stressful situations or to respond to them differently, along with biofeedback and group support, reduced their risk of heart attacks or heart surgery by a whopping 74 percent. (See the October 1997 issue of the AMA's Archives of Internal Medicine.) In 2002, a study published in *Circulation* by Dr. H. Iso and others reported on 73,424 Japanese men and women who were followed from 1988 to 1990. The researchers found that perceived mental stress was associated with increased mortality from stroke and with cardiovascular disease for women, and with coronary heart disease in both men and women. This study is of special interest because previous studies have focused on white men.

What is meant by "stress"? Anxiety is a form of stress, of course, and so is hostility in the form of anger, aggression, and cynicism. The last three emotions seem particularly bad on hearts.

Meditation, biofeedback, yoga, prayer, progressive muscle relaxation, hypnosis, guided imagery, "cognitive restructuring," and massages can all be good stress reducers. What they seem to have in common is that they return you to a point of concentration when your mind wanders.

Hundreds of self-help books have been written on stress and/or depression. A scientifically- based, but easy-to-read, book is David G. Myers' *The Pursuit of Happiness.* He reports that your health (especially in older adults) relates directly to your happiness—no surprise there. On the other hand, your age, how much money you have, and your gender are all pretty irrelevant. The author tells what things in addition to health really relate to happiness. He suggests changes to make in the parts of your life over which you have control.

You might also want to get the tape of one of Jon Seskevich's sessions on stress management (PHA 2000 conference, tape PHA033, available for purchase from AVEN; see the section on PHA in Chapter 14). Jon explains effective and ineffective ways to cope, relaxation techniques (he talks you right through one), learning to say no, how to be an assertive (but not passive or aggressive) communicator, and how to give one heck of a fine neck and shoulder massage.

Support Groups

Many PH patients and their family members and caregivers have found that joining a support group reduces their anxiety and sense of loneliness; it also provides them with a lot of useful information. Support groups can be an appropriate place to vent all that anger and guilt and fear.

PHA has helped to set up over 150 groups across the United States and elsewhere. Call PHA's toll-free number (1-800-748-7274) to learn if a group already exists in your area, or if there are others who might like to join you in setting up a group. If no other PH patients live near you, but you have a computer with a modem, you can at least join the lively dialogue on the message board on PHA's website (www.phassociation.org), where you can sometimes even find sleepless soul mates in the wee hours of the morning. The PHA website also hosts half a dozen weekly on-line chat rooms.

Any two people can start a support group. PHA has a volunteer (in 2004 it's Betty Lou Wojciechowski) who specializes in support groups and who can provide information on how to start a group and make it a success. She can also suggest program topics and resources. PHA will send out flyers, reimburse some postage and photocopying expenses, and provide a Support Group Leader's Manual. You might also ask your health service company (e.g., Accredo Therapeutics or TheraCom) if they can help you get a group started (by sending a mailing to their local clients, for example).

People in support groups come from all walks of life, from all ethnic backgrounds, and are of all ages. Many people who join a group relish this opportunity to get to know people they wouldn't ordinarily meet. An astrophysicist might sit next to a teenage mom, a fisherman next to a flight attendant. It is another way in which you begin to feel less isolated.

Caring for the Caregiver

Talk about stress! Your partner gets PH and drops out of the work market, leaving you the sole breadwinner. You need to do more of the shopping, child-rearing, and housework. And it's your partner who is getting all the sympathy and attention!

There's a Japanese expression, wagamama, which translates as "it's all about me." Well, PH isn't only about the patient. If we patients are too wagamama we stand to lose a lot. Even remembering to say "thank you" to our caregivers can go a long way. Every conversation shouldn't be about our disease and us. Ask about your caregiver's day and talk about current events, the kids, the grandkids. If your caregiver has had to take over some of your tasks, maybe you can take over some of the sedentary things that he/she does, like paying the bills, doing the taxes, or addressing the holiday cards.

In a few states there may be some help available for caregivers in the form of tax breaks, visiting nurses, adult day care, home health care, etc. It may take a lot of digging to uncover such help, but it's worth trying. Search on the state, county, and city levels.

An article by Peter T. Kilborn appeared in *The New York Times* (5-31-99), "Disabled Spouses Increasingly Face a Life Alone and a Loss of Income." Kilborn wrote about how, as modern drugs and medicine are helping people live longer with chronic diseases, more and more of them are finding themselves divorced. A survey by Louis Harris & Associates found 13 percent of the disabled were divorced in 1998, compared to 9 percent in 1984. Similarly, the 1994 Government's National Health Interview Survey found 20.7 percent of disabled adults were divorced or separated, compared to 13.1 percent of healthy adults. Men leave their wives more often than wives leave their husbands.

Why does this happen? The stress on the health of the partner and worries about money are two big reasons relationships break apart. Furthermore, a sick person may withdraw or become moody or angry or depressed. He or she may not be available as a social, travel, or sexual partner. There is also less stigma attached to divorce today than there was in the past. Finally, couples may need to legally separate so that one of them may become "destitute" and qualify for government help. Here's a horror story about what happened to Merle and Thomas, who for a quarter century were a happily married couple. When Merle was diagnosed with PPH, her doctor said she needed epoprostenol to live. The drug would cost her between $100,000 and $125,000 a year. Her insurance company refused to pay because epoprostenol is an infusion-type medicine and because the couple earned $1,200 too much in a year. The only solution was to qualify for public assistance. So Merle and Thomas, who still loved each other, had to legally separate, and Merle had to move out of their home and live somewhere else. Thomas couldn't even stay overnight with her. Here's the catch: if the epoprostenol improves Merle's health to the point that she can work again, she will lose her public assistance. Which means she loses her epoprostenol. Which means she will get deathly ill again. Which means she will re-qualify for public assistance (if she is still alive)! Crazy, eh? Merle works out her anger in her support group, which is helping her lobby for federal legislation to fund PH research.

There are stories of marriages breaking up for other reasons, soon after PH is diagnosed in one partner. In the state of Washington, a man was said to have walked out on his wife the week she was diagnosed saying, "I can't deal with sick people." She didn't have the strength to haggle with her insurance company about getting the medical help she needed, so she died. (She didn't know about ACCESS and their free legal help.) That pitiful ex-husband of hers is, fortunately, the rare exception. Those of us with PH are deeply grateful that most of our partners turn out to be amazingly adaptable and strong.

There are things patients and caregivers can do to help protect their marriages. A first step is to realize that caregivers need to take care of themselves first. It's like on an airline when the oxygen masks drop; the instructions say to put your own mask on first before turning to help a child or someone else. A study in the *Journal of the American Medical Association* found that if a caregiver is under mental or emotional strain they are at an increased risk for illness and premature death themselves. If your caregiver says to you, "I need a break for a few days," don't get angry or overwhelmed with guilt at being such a burden. Instead, say, "Thank you for telling me. Let's see how we can work that out."

So what can caregivers do to help themselves? First, try to maintain a balanced life. Even if you have to modify some activities that are important to you, don't give them up entirely. Fire up the Harley hog if it's your big love (but please wear your helmet). One woman with PH made her husband promise to take a full weekend day off every two weeks—a day for him to go fishing or to the ball game and do other things that recharged his batteries. This wonderful idea was heartily endorsed by those who learned of it during the PHA 2000 conference session on caring for the caregiver.

Here are a few other suggestions for caregivers that emerged from that session:

- Have a backup caregiver lined up for times you are sick yourself or away from home or just need a break. It's also good to carry around the number of a neighbor who is home during the day and who could respond to an emergency if you are, say, stuck in a traffic jam. If this isn't possible, you can get your partner a "send help" button.
- Counseling and a good support group can help you as much as they can help your sick partner.
- Make use of the message board for caregivers and the caregivers' listserv on the PHA website (www.phassociation.org).
- It's okay to say, "Right now it's just too much for me to do (whatever). Let's put it off until (a time or date)."
- Train your kids to help out around the house. You are setting an example as to how they should treat you if you get sick or (surprise!) old.
- If you can afford it, hire a house-keeper. Check with your church, etc.— there may be someone who will do this for you for free.
- Order groceries on the web; they are delivered right to your kitchen counter.
- If the patient is able to, he/she should mix their own epoprostenol, fill their own pillbox, and keep their own medicine-related calendar.
- Learn about PH and talk to your partner's PH doctor about what he/she should or should not do.
- Be positive: when epoprostenol came along, many caregivers suddenly had partners who were able to resume much of their old lives. The future will see more advances in treatments, and probably even a cure.

- Prioritize and accept the fact that some things just won't get done.
- If you can afford it, and your partner needs more care than you can give without getting burned out, hire a professional caregiver. Decide on the sort of help you need before starting your search. Some caregivers are merely companions, some do housekeeping, and some perform health and personal care services under the supervision of a licensed nurse. Check references. Look for somebody whose questions during the interview focus on the patient and the patient's needs, not on the professional caregiver's.

Here are some resources for caregivers:

- NFCA (the National Family Caregivers Association) is a charitable group dedicated to making life better for the 25 million caregivers in the U.S. Their sensible "10 Tips for Family Caregivers" are posted on their website (www.nfcacares.org. or call 800-896-3650).
- The Well Spouse Foundation (www.wellspouse.org or call 800-838-0879).
- Half the Planet is a disability resource network. (www.halftheplanet.com, or call 202-429-6810.)

We feel happier when we compare our situation to those who are coping with even more, so here's a true story for you caregivers. Cindy (not her real name) is the primary caregiver for her daughter-in-law, who is on epoprostenol (Cindy's son is a long-haul trucker). Cindy also lives with her legally blind brother, helping him in his business. About all of this, Cindy is upbeat. But what does irk her is when her mom, who is 83, tries to get sick to get attention!

Laughing through Our Tears

Hide-the-pump fashion shows. About 200 women squeezed into a room at PHA's 2000 conference in Itasca, Illinois, to watch a fashion show and guess where the models (real-life prostacyclin users) had hidden their pumps. (Sorry we had to exclude the men, but women were showing all.) The show was so popular we repeated it at the next conference. You already know about using backpacks, fanny packs, and classy little Coach purses to carry pumps. The small treprostinil pumps can sometimes be tucked into a bra or the waist of stretch jeans. The atmosphere in the room was joyful. Laughter and applause greeted each model. Here are some other winning ideas:

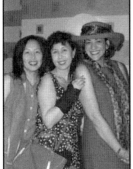

* A trial attorney hides her epoprostenol pump from jurors – she bought a cheap sports bra from K-Mart and sewed a little pocket for the pump inside it, under her arm.
* To swing her golf club freely, another woman sewed a pocket inside a tight T-shirt.
* A pump pocket can be sewn into jogging pants.
* Samantha, 11, hid her pump under the bike shorts she wore under a pretty party dress.

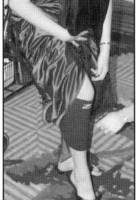

* A model wearing a clingy strapless top and slinky skirt had us all baffled: her pump was held against the inside of her leg by an ACE bandage.
* Some carry their pumps in a fashion (beaded, etc.) handbag.

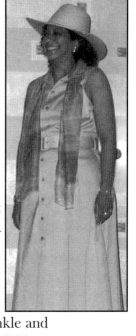

* A treprostinil pump can go inside biking shorts under a sundress, or in a passport holder worn under a sweater.

Most people aren't as observant or interested in us as we think they are. Men using epoprostenol seem less concerned than women do about carrying the pump. "People just think it's a tool belt or a merchandise reader from Wal-Mart," one man says. The smaller treprostiil pump can be put in a pants pocket (make a tiny hole to put the tube through). Ankle and leg carriers for that pump are also available.

Christie is an epoprostenol user and the mother of two. She says it helps her to think more positively when she doesn't have to keep answering questions about her disease. She really likes the smaller 8-hour cassettes because they let her "fit PPH in my pocket."

Handicapped parking placards and license plates. These are the blue or red signs with the white outline of a wheelchair that you see dangling from the rearview mirrors of cars in handicapped parking slots. The symbol also appears on license plates.

The rules governing the availability and use of these placards varies from state to state. In the state of Washington, for example, you can pick up an application form at any Vehicle Licensing Office. The placard and license plates not only enable you to park in a disabled persons' parking location, but you can also get refueling service at gasoline stations for the self-service price if nobody in the car with you can do the fueling (totally self-service stations and convenience stores with remotely controlled gas pumps do not offer this service). You can even park free for unlimited periods in areas with parking meters (there are some exceptions).

Washington State requires a certificate from a licensed physician stating that one of the following disabilities applies:

♦ Cannot walk 200 feet without stopping to rest.
♦ Is severely limited in ability to walk due to arthritic, neurological, or other conditions.
♦ Cannot walk without the use of an assistive device or assistance from another person.
♦ Requires the use of a wheelchair.
♦ Uses portable oxygen.
♦ Ability to walk is restricted by lung disease.
♦ Impairment by cardiovascular disease—falls within the American Heart Association Standard Class III or Class IV.
♦ Has a disability resulting from an acute sensitivity to automobile emissions that limits or impairs the ability to walk.

There is a fee for special license plates, but not for one or two placards. A placard may be used in any car transporting you, so most people are better off just getting a placard.

Amazingly, there is currently one placard for every 10 licensed vehicles in Washington! Obviously, the system is being abused. On the University of Minnesota campus, members of a sorority passed around a disabled placard that had belonged to an old woman who died. Other states are having trouble, too, and are cutting back on privileges. In Florida, you can now park free for only 4 hours, not all day, and you must be recertified by a doctor every 4 years. In Texas, there are no more temporary permits, no free parking, and fewer people are considered disabled. Here are a couple of other examples of how states approach the problem.

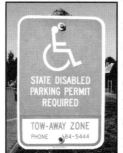

California requires:

♦ Heart or circulatory disease.
♦ Lung disease.
♦ A diagnosed disease or disorder that significantly limits the use of lower extremities.
♦ Specific documented visual problems including low-vision or partial-sightedness.
♦ Loss, or permanent loss of the use of one or both legs or both hands.

With a disabled person placard in California you may park in slots with the wheelchair symbol, next to a blue curb, next to a green curb (which healthy folks may only park in for a limited time) for as long as you wish, in on-street metered parking at no charge, or in an area that requires a resident or merchant permit.

New York State issues plates or parking permits for the disabled through city, town, and village clerks, and Nassau County. New York City does NOT set aside reserved spaces for the disabled on its streets. There is some off-street disabled parking in lots for malls, campuses, buildings, etc. However, if you are a NYC resident or work or attend school in NYC and "have a permanent disability that so severely affects [your] ability to walk that [you] require the use of a private automobile," you can get a "City permit" to put on your dashboard to park on NYC streets.

Because PH is usually an invisible disability, and because so many people who are not disabled use the placards illegally, some PH patients have gotten nasty comments from bystanders who think they are not really disabled. Wear your PH pin or ribbon; instead of scowling, strangers might ask you what the pin or ribbon is for. Put a PHA sticker in your car window by the permit. A PH support group had some bumper stickers printed up with "Support the Pulmonary Hypertension Association" on them. Another support group got some custom-made license plate holders. If someone actually questions your right to use the slot, hand him or her a PHA brochure. One guy we know fakes a limp if others are watching. Better to shrug off the nasty looks—you know you're doing nothing wrong. You also know you can be more independent if you accept a little help when you need it, like parking in a handicapped slot or using an electric cart in grocery stores.

Above all, do not abuse the parking privilege yourself. Not everyone with PH is disabled all of the time. On your good days, let the truly disabled have that close-in spot, so those of us with heavy oxygen tanks or wheelchairs can get around more easily.

Katla, a woman with long, shiny blonde hair and the soul of a flower child, pulled into a handicapped slot at the supermarket and a man put his face in hers and said, "It's healthy people like you who make it impossible for my dad, who's in a wheelchair, to park." Before she could reply, he ducked into the store. Breathless with anger and exertion, Katla tracked him down in the produce section. She told him about PH and flung up her blouse so he could see where the epoprostenol catheter entered her chest. The poor man was reduced to tears. (Katla's son was relieved his mom had worn a bra that day.)

On reflection, Katla isn't sure her revenge was worth the stress. But the story gave her support group a good chuckle. Laughter heals.

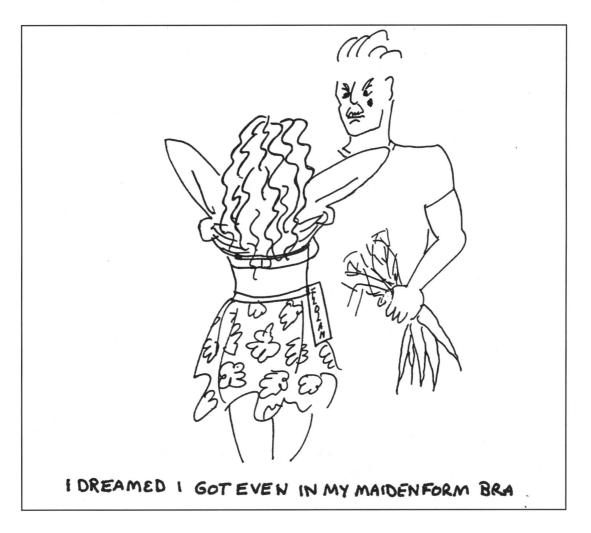

I DREAMED I GOT EVEN IN MY MAIDENFORM BRA

12

The Active Life: Working, Exercising, Traveling, Living

Can You Have PH and Work?

Most PH patients are probably not able to hold down regular jobs. For those with the ability to do so, however, the benefits of working (such as companionship, the rewards of accomplishment, money, and health and disability insurance) may outweigh the extra fatigue.

The Americans with Disabilities Act is a law with teeth (although the Supreme Court has pulled a few) that protects people like us. It states that employers may not ask job applicants about the existence, nature, or severity of a disability. For example, they can't ask you about your family's health, or if you've had any illnesses or operations. They may, of course, ask you if you are able to perform the essential functions of a particular job. An employer must make reasonable accommodations to allow you to do your job. But if a potential employer knows you have PH, he/she might be reluctant to hire you for fear of being hit with workman's compensation claims and higher group medical insurance rates. He/she might also be afraid that you would be unable to carry a full load or will ask for special accommodations. If you can *prove* this sort of discrimination, you can sue for damages or a job. For details go to the Equal Opportunity Employment Commission website: www. eeoc.gov. Here is some information pulled right off their website:

A qualified employee or applicant with a disability is an individual who, with or without reasonable accommodation, can perform the essential functions of the job in question. Reasonable accommodation may include, but is not limited to:

- Making existing facilities used by employees readily accessible to and usable by persons with disabilities.
- Job restructuring, modifying work schedules, reassignment to a vacant position;
- Acquiring or modifying equipment or devices, adjusting or modifying examinations, training materials, or policies, and providing qualified readers or interpreters.

An employer is required to make a reasonable accommodation to the known disability of a qualified applicant or employee if it would not impose an "undue hardship" on the operation of the employer's business. Undue hardship is defined as an action requiring significant difficulty or expense when considered in light of factors such as an employer's size, financial resources, and the nature and structure of its operation.

An employer is not required to lower quality or production standards to make an accommodation; nor is an employer obligated to provide personal use items such as glasses or hearing aids.

The U.S. Supreme Court has ruled that the Act does not require employers to employ people whose *own* health or safety might be put at risk.

Self-employment: the Choice of Some Disabled Persons

In the U.S., roughly one-third of disabled persons are employed (contrasted with 79 percent of non-disabled persons). Fourteen percent of these are self-employed (contrasted with 8 percent of the non-disabled workers). This isn't really surprising, considering the discrimination against the disabled. The advantages are you can work at your own pace in an environment you choose. The disadvantages are the increased risk and the difficulty or impossibility of finding a health insurance pool you can join. You also need a marketable skill or a product that's in demand.

Melanie Astaire Witt has written a book, *Job Strategies for People with Disabilities* (Peterson's Guides, Princeton, NJ, 1992), that may be of help. It covers adapting your work environment to your disability, finding a job that you can do, whether to disclose your disability to your prospective employer, and more. You might also check out Alice Weiss Doyel, *No More Job Interviews: Self-Employment Strategies for People with Disabilities* (2000). Alice, herself an entrepreneur, offers business start-up strategies tailored to people with disabilities.

The U.S. Small Business Administration spends millions every year supporting micro-businesses and has formed a relationship with the Department of Labor, "The New Freedom Small Business Initiative," to help people with disabilities get the skills and resources they need.

True Stories of PH Patients Who Work

When Penny was diagnosed with PPH late in 2000, she and her husband David knew they would need extra income to pay her health-related expenses. They began a business, PennyWise Computer Supplies (www.inkjets4unow.com), which sells ink cartridges over the web and elsewhere. While they were getting the business up and running, David had a heart attack and needed six bypasses. Their new business has had what David calls "a measure of success," and is growing. They donate a percentage of their gross to PHA.

Francella was diagnosed way back in 1979 and takes CCBs. She has two jobs, managing a doctor's office and working at a department store (she took the latter job for the health insurance and because she enjoys the company of her coworkers). The jobs keep her away from the house from 7:30 A.M. to 9 P.M. Yes, she's tired when she gets home (who wouldn't be?).

Miriam and her husband are professional clowns. "It makes you forget your problems when you help other people," she says. "We do have times of pity party...but it helps to have something to look forward to."

Jeff is an instrument and control technician at a big power generating plant. Before going on epoprostenol (he was reluctant to try it) he used to have to sneak off to the welding shop now and then for a hit of oxygen. He could hardly walk across the room and had to rest every 20 feet. Now he does the physical aspects of his job much more easily, although his boss has helped him modify his job so he avoids heavy physical stuff. "Getting up and going to work each day means a lot to me," he says (he gets up at 5:15 A.M.). On weekends he's tired, but he loves his job.

Diane was unable to climb even two steps before starting on epoprostenol. Afterwards, she could travel 50-60,000 miles a year when not working out of her home (she handles 17 floor covering showrooms across the south). Diane is now using sildenafil, not epoprostenol, but back when she used epoprostenol she swore by a Merle Norman base powder that covered her epoprostenol flushing and didn't rub off.

Jerry, a teacher, had to quit when he got too short of breath just walking a short distance. After going on epoprostenol he went back to work within a year to teach fifth and sixth grade. Although he can no longer play basketball and racquetball, sports he enjoyed, he developed skills as a computer geek (the kids love seeing what he can do) and he thinks he is a better teacher than he was before.

Sally Maddox, a PHA board member who has had PPH for 14 years, finished her college graduate program and now teaches at an alternative school. Sally keeps her PPH under control with nifedipine. In the last several years she has missed only one day of work because of illness—a stomach virus, not PH, was responsible. When she is not working, Sally tries to keep off her feet and rest. Sometimes that's hard: in addition to teaching she helps raise her stepson, volunteers for the Red Cross and the Local Crisis Pregnancy Center, and edits *PHA News* (sign up for this on-line service if you haven't).

Suzi, a 60-year-old grandmother, was diagnosed with PPH several years ago. A former nurse, she enrolled in Athens State University to earn her bachelor degree, a long-time goal. She wants to teach. Although her medicine costs $150 a day, it is covered by her truck-driving husband's medical insurance.

Jan, who underwent a bi-lateral lung transplant for PH in 2000, began a successful business selling handcrafted jewelry. Her work is displayed in galleries throughout North Carolina. You can find her PH-ribbon bracelets in the PHA store or at www.rareelegance.com. She will custom design a piece for you.

Finally, there's a famous example worth mentioning: although Laura Hillenbrand suffers from severe chronic fatigue syndrome exacerbated by vertigo, not from PH, she managed to research and write the bestseller *Seabiscuit*, which was turned into a popular movie. Laura spent months and months bedridden, sometimes only able to write while lying in bed with her eyes closed, scribbling on a tablet. Writing the book drained her of energy, and she hadn't fully recovered a year later. But, hey, she'll never have to work again, unless she wants to.

Suggestions from Working PH Patients

♦ If you need a refrigerator or freezer at work for your meds, the Americans with Disabilities Act requires your employer to provide one, as well as to make other reasonable accommodations to allow you to do your job.

♦ If you don't treat your disability like a big deal, others won't either.

♦ If you sign up for health insurance the first time it's offered you may not have to take a physical or worry about preexisting conditions. (Call ACCESS before changing or quitting jobs. See Chapter 13.)

♦ If you run into discrimination because of your PH, your union can help fight for your rights.

As treatments improve, more of us will be able to work. The Ticket to Work and Work Incentives Act of 1999 pays benefit planners (who work for nonprofit groups or state agencies) to advise persons who now receive Social Security disability benefits, but who want to return to work. The planners will explain SSA's work incentives, how going back to work will affect your benefits, and what vocational and rehabilitation and other support might be available. We suggest, however, that you first contact the lawyers at ACCESS if you are thinking of going back to work, and talk to them *before* you talk to a benefit planner.

Is Exercise Dangerous?

There are very few published studies on exercise and PH patients. Doctors used to tell their PH patients not to intentionally exercise. This is because too much exertion causes pulmonary pressures to rise and increases cardiac stress. Repeated overexertion can damage pulmonary blood vessels. But doctors are now taking a second look at the benefits/dangers of exercise for PH patients, and most are saying that at least some exercise is better for nearly all of us PH patients than sitting around doing nothing. (A harder, unanswered, question is how much is too much exercise for active children.) Any exercise program must be individualized to meet a patient's particular needs and limitations. So get your **PH** specialist's approval before starting an exercise program.

Here's why exercise may help: if you experience heart failure and lose your conditioning, all kinds of chemicals that play a role in PH get out of whack. More specifically, the levels of harmful cytokines and endothelin rise, and levels of beneficial nitric oxide fall. You lose muscle mass and strength. But if you can keep your biceps and thighs from shrinking and maybe even expand them a bit, you'll feel stronger and work less hard to accomplish a given task. The chemicals may get back in balance. One way to start is by taking walks, slowly making them longer and faster and never allowing yourself to get more than a little short of breath. You could also do this on a treadmill. As with any exercise, stop if you feel dizzy, or experience palpitations or chest discomfort. If you have a history of fainting during exercise, don't attempt it.

Although there have been very few studies of exercise and PH, there have been lots of studies about exercise and left-heart disease. PH patients tend to have right-heart problems, but it might still be possible to draw some lessons from the left-heart studies about low-grade resistance training and aerobic exercise. A study using pigs found that long-term exercise was associated with thinner walls (that's good) in small pulmonary arteries.

Low-grade resistance training. Don't use heavy weights, and don't strain. If you can, do 10 to 15 repetitions with a 2-pound weight. Slowly, slowly, slowly build up. To repeat, don't strain: if you strain, your heart rate may fall from, say, 80 to 40 and you may pass out. Cardiac outputs can rise in PH patients and increasing yours periodically is probably good.

Light-to-moderate aerobic exercise. Again, build up very slowly and don't push too hard. Bicycling three times a week for 20 minutes may be good for some PH patients (slowly increasing the resistance as you strengthen). But if you are the sedentary type, starting out with a slow walk and progressively increasing is better. You need to get just a tiny bit short of breath, and breathing deeper and faster, for exercise to be doing any good. Swimming is a good aerobic exercise, but don't swim alone if you might pass out. Flotation devices may make it easier to avoid breathlessness.

Unless you are Class I, it's better to exercise just half of your body at a time. While swimming, sit on a flotation device to exercise your arms (with practice you can even sit on a ball), then hug it to kick. Nordic track machines are *not* recommended for most of us.

Don't get hung up on trying to achieve what you think is an "ideal" exercising heart rate limit unless you and your doctor have discussed it. The guidelines set for healthy people (such as 220 beats per minute minus your age) don't apply to most of us, because our meds and illness affect our heart rates. It might be a good idea to have your oxygen measured with a pulse oximeter when you exercise to see if there might be a need for caution or extra oxygen.

PH patients consistently report that they can do more, over time, with exercise training.

Don't expect to see any improvements in what you can do for at least 6 weeks. Each of us is very different as to what amount of exercise we can tolerate. Some of us can jog uphill on a hot day, others can barely punch the remote control buttons. (Actually, it's a good idea for all PH patients to avoid outdoor exercise on hot muggy days.) You must listen to your body, and what it tells you will vary from day to day. If it takes 10 minutes for you to catch your breath after doing something and your heart is thumping in your chest, and you can't speak in full sentences, then cut back. This is also important: if you are going to exercise, do it on a regular basis, not just once a week.

Patient reports. A PH patient from the St. Louis area says that cardiopulmonary rehabilitation turned him from a couch potato into someone capable of driving cross-country and leading an active life. It's true he was in a wheelchair at the PHA 2000 conference, but that's because he hurt his back lifting his oxygen concentrator out of his car.... He uses a little pulse oximeter and doesn't let his saturation get below 93 while exercising (a number he and his doc agreed on). (At least one PH doctor says it's possible that, with rehabilitation, some PH patients may be able to wave bye-bye to their oxygen tanks.)

The author was diagnosed back when doctors told you to camp out on your sofa for the short period until you died. She disagreed, because a little exercise felt good. She got a Newfoundland puppy and started taking it for walks. After building up to a mile a day without too much breathlessness, she and her dog walked an accumulated distance equal to going from San Francisco to Boston and back. The dog grew very old and died. The author adopted another Newfoundland and they have already logged a thousand miles. (The dog wears packs, and carries her groceries home.)

What about sex? The very first call Abigail took when she volunteered to answer the

PHA hot line was from a seventy-something woman, a PH patient using oxygen, who had a new boyfriend and wondered if she could safely "go all the way" with him. We know of many PH patients who make love while using supplemental oxygen and/or while attached to a pump. As a general rule, it's probably okay for most PH patients to have sex, but do check with your doc, especially if you've had a decline in your health since you last had intercourse. Keeping up a loving relationship with your partner can do much to reduce stress and increase happiness. Patients should strive to live as normal a life as possible. If "sex the old way" proves too strenuous, have some fun with being creative. Being sexually active can be good for you physically and emotionally.

The same rules apply as for any other type of exercise. If you're gasping for breath, slow down for heaven's sake. But some increase in heart rate and breathing is part of having sex. National Jewish Medical and Research Center has a 14-page booklet called "Being Close" that offers suggestions for dealing with chronic lung disease and intimacy. It includes diagrams of less strenuous positions and suggestions on how to avoid shortness of breath (e.g., you may want to increase your oxygen flow rate for a bit). If you would like a free copy of "Being Close" call toll-free LUNG LINE (1-800-222-LUNG). Or you can write them at 1400 Jackson St., Denver, CO 80206.

Traveling

Hundreds of PH patients make it to PHA's biennial international conferences. And people with PH travel the globe—with advance planning. You know your limits; don't exceed them. One PHA member who likes to visit exotic places limits her strenuous activities to the mornings. Then she naps, eavesdrops in hotel lobbies, reads up on pyramids or whatever, and rejoins her family for dinner and evening activities. By knowing in advance that she will see only half as many sights as others in her party, she can plan ahead so that she doesn't miss out on what matters most to her. Use common sense: climbing expeditions up Mt. Everest or scuba diving, for example, would be begging for trouble.

Talk over your travel plans with your PH team, who can advise you on whether you will need supplemental oxygen in-flight or at your destination (especially if it's at a significantly higher altitude than your home base). Your doctor can also help you line up enough medication in advance; you'll need to take at least an extra week's worth if you are going on a long trip.

Diane, the floor covering specialist mentioned above, gives herself lots of time when going to the airport so she doesn't need to rush. She checks all her bags and uses a car company that allows her to go directly to a rental car. Back when she used epoprostenol, for trips over a week long she asked her health service company to ship her epoprostenol ahead; when going abroad she carried it with her so it didn't get stuck in customs.

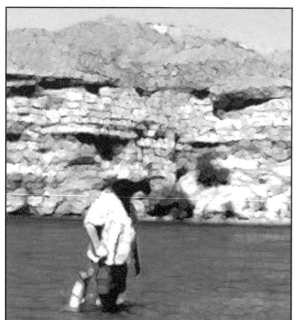

Craig Smith believes in staying active, even if you have to take along a folding chair for those sudden urges to sit down. Here Craig and his tank are out in the Colorado River.

Travel Tips

- Consider having routine blood tests done a few days before your trip so you can get the results before you leave.

- Pack enough medicine to last the trip (including possible delays). If the medicine keeps you alive, try to pack some in at least two places (in case one bag is stolen or lost). Keep a supply of medication on your person (as carry-on baggage) if you are taking public transportation.

- Going through customs is sometimes easier if your meds are in their regularly labeled pharmacy bottles. A letter from your PH specialist describing specific medical requirements often helps simplify the process of obtaining oxygen and taking medications and supplies (like needles) through customs or security checkpoints. Ask your doctor to specify the amounts (e.g., ten 60 cc syringes, 20 vials of epoprostenol). Drug paraphernalia tends to interest customs officials.

- Let your PH specialist know you'll be traveling and review contact numbers. If possible, get the name of a physician familiar with PH at your travel destination whom you can contact in an emergency.

- Carry information on your condition and medications, in case you have to see an unfamiliar doctor.

- Travel with a companion, if possible, someone who knows all about your PH, your meds, and your doctor's name and number.

- Wear your MedicAlert bracelet.

- Patients requiring supplemental oxygen should pack extra tubing.

- Pack light, eat light, don't get dehydrated.

- At theme parks, if you have a letter from your doctor saying it is not good for you to stand for long periods in lines, you can often get a card or sticker that will let you and your party go to the head of lines (you might want to ask you doctor if it's *safe* for you to ride the Drop Dead Daredevil Demon Rollercoaster).

- If you are flying into Mexico City, ask for a wheelchair to be waiting. The high altitude and long, long customs lines pose problems for us. In the wheelchair you reportedly just zip through customs. In fact, whenever you plan to travel to a much higher altitude than you are used to, oxygen needs to be available. You WILL feel poorly, and could otherwise become significantly ill.

- Get all the recommended vaccinations (not just the required ones) for wherever you are going, after checking with your doctor to make sure they won't react nastily with your meds.

- Resolve not to let the inevitable delays, rudeness, and little problems upset you; stress can make PH worse. For example, in some cities people smoke cigarettes all over the place. Just move away from smokers. Don't try to explain to a smoker what a fool he is to endanger his heart and a good set of lungs.

Traveling with a Pump

If you use epoprostenol, take time to plan ahead and arrange for needed refrigeration and freezers. Establish a back-up plan should you not make a scheduled connection or get to your destination on time. If you are going on an extended stay, have your epoprostenol provider ship the majority of supplies to your destination ahead of time. If you use epoprostenol or another pumped drug, it's a good idea to take all the drug paraphernalia that you will need with you, including an extra pump. Pack written instructions on how to use your pump and put a sticker on it with your flow rate, concentration, the telephone number of your medical service company, a warning not to turn the pump off, etc.

Patients treated with epoprostenol should always travel with a small ice chest with 6 to 8 ice packs and a premixed dose of epoprostenol. Always keep your medication, supplies, and back-up pump in the passenger section of a car (not in the trunk). If traveling abroad, it is advisable to check in advance to determine if there are any laws against bringing medical supplies into a specific country or if special documents are needed. Contact your airline, cruise line, tour company, etc. to learn if they have any special requirements or procedures to allow you to use these unique medications.

Air Travel

Air travel can be pure misery for us. PH patients report all kinds of hassles with airports and airlines, including trouble getting wheelchairs, getting oxygen, and finding a row with enough legroom to put their feet up on a bag. (An airline agent told Amanda that she wasn't sick enough to merit a seat with more legroom because such seats were held for "people who need special assistance," but said Amanda was nevertheless too sick to sit in a more spacious exit row!) The only advantage of air travel is that the misery doesn't usually last long.

Think ahead about your oxygen needs. Ask your doctor if you will need supplemental oxygen. (It's hard, often, for even your doctor to really know. He/she would have to know the type of aircraft, how many SOBs [souls on board, for you non-pilots], and whether the captain planned to save fuel by reducing the flow of fresh air.) Many PH patients can fly safely on commercial airplanes without supplemental oxygen. If your doctor says you need in-flight oxygen, let the airline know well in advance. An airline may limit the number of passengers on each flight who use supplemental oxygen. As soon as you arrive at the gate, let the gate agent know you have ordered oxygen. Quite often you'll find it's not ready, and the agent has to call somebody to get it.

Call ahead to find if your flight will leave on time. Allow extra time at the airport in case problems arise. Take along a book or crossword puzzle and a steely determination not to get upset.

Thin airplane air. Jets that travel at altitudes of 35,000 to 42,000 feet are said to be pressurized to between 6,000 and 8,000 feet, or 5,000 and 7,000 feet, depending on whom you believe. (Some non-U.S. airlines are rumored to pressurize less.) This means there is roughly 25 to 40 percent less oxygen in the air than you find at sea level. When considering your needs, remember that airplane air is often stale and polluted. FAA standards for cabin air pressure were not based on any rationale when they were set back in 1964, and may provide inadequate protection for very young children or those with heart and lung problems.

Be alert on airplanes for symptoms of a lack of oxygen. Symptoms of mild hypoxia may remind you of a hangover: headache, breathlessness, lightheadedness, loss of appetite, nausea, and vomiting. For symptoms

of more serious hypoxia, see Chapter 3. It's probably okay for most of us to be a little under-oxygenated for brief periods on airplane trips, but it's probably not good for you to be only 87 percent saturated for the bulk of a coast-to-coast flight. Be conservative. If you're not sure how you're doing, the outdoors store REI (www.rei.com) sells a nifty little SportStat pulse oximeter designed for mountain climbers. You stick your finger into it and in seconds it gives you your pulse and saturation (see photo Chapter 4). The gizmo costs $395 and is about the size of two tubes of lipstick. (JoAnne got one for a lot less on E-bay.) Put a piton or two in your pocket along with the SportStat, and that gal in the middle seat will assume you're a trekker.

Although all airlines carry a tank or two of emergency oxygen, they save it for unexpected emergencies. The oxygen you are arranging for is a separate deal. Your airline might let you pay for round-trip oxygen in advance, with a credit card, at the time you reserve your oxygen. This saves lots of hassle. (Make sure it's refundable if you don't fly.) The airline will mail you your "special equipment" tickets (don't forget to take them with you!). If you have to pay for oxygen at the airport, allow extra time and pay for the entire trip at once. Make sure you get a receipt for every leg of your trip. Look for an alert-looking agent with wrinkles; the young ones don't seem to know the oxygen procedure.

Portable Oxygen Concentrators. Since August 2005, the FAA has allowed passengers to fly on board with certain portable oxygen concentrators. The FAA has approved several POCs (Portable Oxygen Concentrators) for in-flight use. They include the Inogen One, AirSep Lifestyle, AirSep Freestyle, SeQual Eclipse and Respironics EverGo. These are the only POCs approved at this time that patients can bring on board. Most brands are light weight and portable and can be stowed under the seat in front of you during flight. They can be battery powered when not plugged into an electrical socket. However, you MUST check with your airline carrier that they will allow your specific type of POC on your flight. Some airlines require a certificate from your doctor's office to be faxed to the airline well in advance in order to allow you to use your device on board.

Getting Past the Guys with Guns. One widely traveled PHA member using Flolan says she has more trouble over her pump with domestic airport security personnel than she does going through customs (including Israeli customs). Even in wheelchairs, we usually don't look that sick. Barbie ran into problems on her way home from the Dallas conference in 1998: suspicious airport security guards were too scared of her ice packs to even let her take out her Flolan pump to show it to them. Finally they did a hand pat-down (good-natured Barbie didn't mind) and took her to the head of security. Barbie's airplane was leaving in 20 minutes. She was patted down again, and her entire pack and its contents were dusted for explosives. After running the dusting rag through a special machine, the security men just walked off and left her! Although a bit stressed, she made her flight home and wrote up her experience for inclusion in this book. (Barbie, who didn't look sick to the security guys, died of PH not long afterwards.)

The moral? Carry that doctor's letter, on letterhead stationary, explaining about your pump and how turning it off might kill you. Show them your emergency card from your health service company, with a number they can call to ask questions.

Polluted airplane air. Newer models of aircraft recycle up to half their air rather than pulling in 100 percent fresh air. According to the August 1994 issue of *Consumer Reports*,

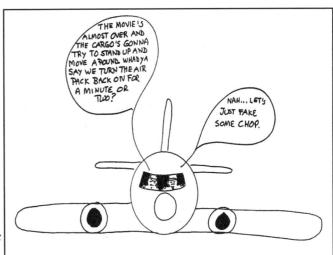

Boeing 757's recycle a lot of air, and have the highest levels of carbon dioxide that their samplers found. The Boeing 747-400, on the other hand, had the lowest levels of carbon dioxide. (The magazine did not take enough samples to provide statistical certainty, and this survey is now somewhat dated.) Carbon dioxide is the gas we humans breathe out, of course, and while it is not toxic to us, as is carbon monoxide, it takes up lung space without providing any benefit.

Airplane air may be at its worst when the craft is sitting on the ground and the filtering and recirculation systems aren't fully up and running. You may need supplemental oxygen during these times.

A study in 2002 by the University of California, San Francisco, found that about 20 percent of passengers catch a cold after a 2-hour flight. The reason, said the researchers, is not that cabin air is recirculated, but that people are crowded together aboard airliners. (The researchers suggest that you frequently cleanse your hands.) Big airliners usually have HEPA filters that (if they are well maintained) can remove some germs. But many viruses, like those that cause colds, are probably usually spread hand-to-hand. Protect yourself by cleaning your hands with a moist towelette or a squirt of alcohol-based gel, such as Purell, before eating the fake nuts.

The Association of Flight Attendants is

our ally in trying to get better cabin air. The union has been complaining for years that the airlines don't always properly maintain the filters. And the National Academy of Sciences agrees with them that there is a problem. The Academy wants more monitoring, and says that available information "suggests that environmental factors, including air contaminants, can be responsible for some of the numerous complaints of acute and chronic health effects in cabin crew and passengers." According to the Academy, airplane ventilation systems "do not appear" to facilitate the spread of infections.

These are some of the contaminants in airplane air that worry the Academy:

Ozone. Only newer airplanes have a gizmo to neutralize it, but ozone irritates the lungs and diminishes their capacity. There's more of it up high where airplanes fly.

Carbon monoxide. It isn't monitored on aircraft, and high concentrations can happen if a ventilation system isn't working well; even low concentrations may cause headaches and dizziness.

Pesticides. In the U.S. they no longer spray cabins and passengers with these toxic chemicals, but it's still done is some countries.

Fumes. Possible exposure to fumes from engine oil, hydraulic fluids, and de-icing liquid is bad for everyone.

The air in the cabin of an airplane is also exceedingly dry, which dries out your breathing passages and makes them less able to filter out germs. So drink lots of water (you'll have to climb over people to get to the loo, but moving around helps keep clots from forming in your legs).

Finally, a few foreign airlines still allow smoking on some flights. Avoid such flights. If you can't, and are using supplemental oxygen, be sure you aren't seated anywhere near a smoker. A cabin attendant should understand why this is dangerous. (In a precedent-setting case, the U.S. Supreme Court ruled that Olympic Airways was liable for the death of a patient with asthma, because an attendant had repeatedly refused to seat him farther away from smokers. The refusal constituted an "accident" under the Warsaw Convention governing airline liability, the Court said.)

Denver: a Rocky Mountain low. You may want to avoid long layovers at high altitudes like Denver, because the airlines don't provide oxygen in terminals. There is 20 percent less available oxygen in the air at Denver than there is at sea level. If it is their fault that you're stuck in their Denver hub, United has been known to scrounge up some oxygen, but don't count on it. To use it, they may make you sit in the room with people in their nineties wearing big name tags. When making reservations, be sure to tell them that you can't be stuck in Denver for long without oxygen. Even if you do not normally need a wheelchair, you may want to request one in Denver to carry you between gates. This service is free.

Airway robbery. Dr. James Stoller and his group (Cleveland Clinic Foundation) did a survey in 1997 of 33 U.S. and international airlines' policies on in-flight oxygen. Practices varied greatly. Seventy-six percent of the airlines surveyed said they would provide oxygen, most requiring 48- to 72-hours advance notice (one, SAS, requires a month's notice). Some type of notification from your doctor is required by all. Nearly all airlines in the U.S. will provide medical oxygen, but America West, Southwest, Midwest Express, and Skyway stubbornly refused to. Nor did many short-hop carriers offer supplemental oxygen (it's rare to find it available on propeller airplanes). All airlines that provided oxygen offered nasal cannulas. There is a great difference among airlines in the liter flow options offered when you want something other than the "standard" 2 or 4 liters per minute. You and your doctor will need to figure out how many liters-per-minute you will need.

There are big price differences, so you need to shop around. Six carriers offer oxygen free. The good guys are: KLM, China Airways, Emirates, Mexicana, Saudi Arabian, SAS, and South African Express.

No U.S.-based carriers offer free oxygen. A loophole in the Air Carrier Access Law, which parallels the Americans with Disabilities Act, allows U.S. airlines not to provide supplemental oxygen. (Some lawyers argue this is illegal; hang on to your oxygen receipts in the [unlikely] event a class action refund is ever offered.) If airlines offer oxygen, they charge a lot: either by the "trip leg" or by the bottle. If you have to stop at a hub, for example, it doubles the cost of your oxygen. The oxygen to fly cross-country to a PHA board meeting cost the author more than her ticket.

Various pricing systems are used, so Dr. Stoller's group calculated the cost of a "standard trip," which they defined as a nonstop, round-trip of 6 hours total flying time at a flow rate of 2 liters per minute. Alitalia was by far the most expensive, charging $1,500. The U.S. airlines' standard trips cost between $100 and $200, with Continental being the most expensive. Prices have gone up, of course, since Dr. Stoller's survey, so call around.

If you also need oxygen waiting for you at the gate when you land, that will cost you extra. You will need to arrange for it in advance with a health agency.

In-flight oxygen is not covered by Medicare or most other insurance. Complain loudly and look for direct flights. Boycott airlines that don't provide oxygen, even if you don't need it yourself. Write to your senator and representative. Join other disabled people and PHA in lobbying for changes in the law, to make it easier to get the oxygen you need

on airplanes. The National Home Oxygen Patients Association is one such group (www.homeoxygen.org). Others are the American Association for Respiratory Care (www.aarc.org), and the American Thoracic Society's Patient Advocacy Roundtable.

What about using my own tank? For safety and anti-terrorist reasons, federal regs do not allow you to carry your own oxygen container on board. Some airlines allow properly packed and labeled empty portable oxygen tanks to be shipped as baggage. A movement is afoot to get airlines to allow the new battery-operated portable oxygen concentrators on board, so stay tuned. This effort has already been partially successful: a recent change is that some airlines will now allow you to use onboard your personal oxygen concentrator. (U.S. Airways told the author this was their policy.) But there's a catch—there is usually no place to plug it in. So when your battery dies, so do you...just kidding. (There's no place to plug in a portable concentrator at your airplane seat to recharge its battery, but in terminals you might spot a socket the guys with laptops aren't using. Some up-front seats on some airplanes have 7-volt DC plugs for computers, but a concentrator requires at least 12 volts. However, airplanes do have electrical outlets that they let other medical devices use.) A last-minute check (May 2004) at United Airlines found they would not allow the concentrators to be used on board, nor would Southwest. The airlines maintain there is a safety issue because compressed gas is still stored in a cylinder in the devices, and this is a hazard. Because policies may change, call ahead of travel and ask.

These days the airlines are really jittery about terrorists. It might be possible, because oxygen burns so well, to turn a tank into some sort of weapon. Abigail was flying home after her brother's funeral, and had ordered oxygen. The airline pre-boarded her and just one other passenger—a muscular young man who took the seat right next to hers. "Just visiting the Twin Cities?" he immediately asked. After a long while, other people boarded. The engines started. The engines stopped. Abigail was asked to get off the airplane along with all her carry-on luggage. She did so and was thoroughly searched in the boarding passage. Embarrassed, she struggled back into her window seat. The fit man stood up to let her by. His jacket fell open and she caught a glimpse of what looked like a badge. The airplane's path took it over the hospital where Abigail's brother had died. She began to weep. The fit man next to her wanted, of course, to know why she was upset. She gave him an earful.

Land Travel

Consider going by train; Amtrak lets you take your own oxygen on board. They have wheelchair accommodations. Some trains have sleeping cars, dining cars, movie cars, cars for kids, lounges, and ports for your computer. On a train no one asks you to put your shade down, and there's a lot of beautiful country to see.

Oxygen can be taken along on car trips. Margie needs supplemental oxygen at high altitudes, so she ordered a huge tank of oxygen and strapped it into the back of her four-wheel-drive truck. She and her daughter then took off for 10 days exploring the Rocky Mountains. Margie filled a small portable tank from the main tank, so she wasn't tethered to the truck. When they encountered forest-fire smoke so thick they could see only a short way down the highway, both Margie and her healthy daughter breathed clean oxygen. (Wood smoke might aggravate PH, so it's generally not a good idea to hang around forest fires.)

Although some PH patients live in high-altitude places like Salt Lake City and Denver and do just fine, for those of us not used to it, the thin air can really suck out our energy. Carol and Lisa, for example, both reported trouble going from sea level to Las Vegas, which is only 2,300 feet above sea level.

If you're not packing a giant tank, arrange ahead of need for oxygen to be delivered to hotel rooms or the airport or wherever. Your local oxygen company can either arrange this for you, or give you numbers to call in the cities where you are going.

Useful Websites for Travelers

+ **Breathin' Easy** offers a guide for travelers with pulmonary disabilities. They can tell you 2,500 places to refill your oxygen tanks in the U.S. and abroad, plus a lot of travel tips. You can order their guide (about $25) by calling 1-888-699-4360. Regular phone: (707) 252-9333. www.oxygen4travel.com.

+ **Centers for Disease Control and Prevention**, Travelers' Health page. Information on disease outbreaks, vaccinations needed, precautions to take, etc. www.cdc.gov.

+ **U.S. Department of State.** Information on passports and crime and civil unrest regions around the world. www. state.gov.

+ **Travel Health Information Service.** Everything British travelers need to know to stay healthy. www.travelhealth.co.uk.

+ **Lonely Planet**, health section. www. lonelyplanet.com.

Prevent Pulmonary Embolisms

There you are, headed off to your dream trip to New Zealand, seated in row 134, seat K, of the mumbo jumbo jet. Your supplemental oxygen is working fine. But you are basically immobilized in that seat, your legs in a down position and your tray jammed up against your gut. If you stay in this position too long, you may form clots in your legs (deep vein thrombosis or D.V.T.) that can break off and travel to your lungs. D.V.T. can result in pulmonary embolisms in about 10 percent of cases, causing death in about 1 percent.

This problem has been given a nickname, "economy class syndrome," although it occurs in first class, too, and it's becoming more common among air travelers because seats are getting more cramped and people are taking longer flights. The DuPont Pharmaceutical Company says that about 5 million Americans a year get clots from air travel, accounting for about 800,000 hospitalizations. (This number sounded high to one doctor, who pointed out that DuPont sells a blood thinning drug to prevent such clots.) Clots can also form in cars, on buses, or in theaters.

They are more likely to form aloft, however, because lower air pressure reduces the anticlotting ability of blood; your blood may be 2 to 8 times more likely to clot. Low air pressure may also relax the walls of veins, making it easier for blood to pool and clot. Dehydration, which is common on long flights because of the dry air, also "thickens" the blood. Those of us who take warfarin are less likely to form clots (but it's still possible). Don't take chances.

Embolisms require emergency medical care. Unfortunately, they can be hard to detect and can be confused with panic attacks or heart attacks or other conditions. Before the leg clot breaks off there may be redness, swelling, or pain in your calf. After a clot lodges in the lungs there is commonly a sudden onset of shortness of breath (worse than our usual). There may be a feeling of apprehension, sharp chest pains when you breathe in, dizziness, or fainting. You may even cough up blood.

You are at a greater risk of forming embolisms if you:

- have blood abnormalities that make you tend to form clots
- have an injury to your legs
- are over 50
- have heart problems or poor circulation
- are obese
- have a personal or family history of D.V.T.
- have cancer
- are short (so there's more pressure against the back of your legs from the seat)
- are dehydrated

Things to do to prevent D.V.T.:

- Wear support hose (compression stockings) on long flights.
- Flex your legs at least a few times every hour. Try to walk around at least once an hour.
- Ask for an aisle seat, which makes it easier to get up.
- Drink a quart of water before or during a 5-hour flight. The water will prompt you to get up every once in a while—to use the biffy.

A Hodgepodge of Good Ideas Suggested by Other Patients

Here are some tips that just didn't seem to fit anywhere else in the book, but were too good to ignore. The warning about general anesthesia really comes from doctors, but PH patients passed along all the rest.

When you feel breathless, pause. Pretend to admire the scenery or look for something in your billfold. Germans call this technique *Schaufenster schauen* (window shopping).

Don't breathe in dust when handling mulch. Mulch contains all kinds of bacteria and fungi that can get into lungs and kick up trouble. The resulting flu-like illness is called "organic dust toxic syndrome." Best way to avoid trouble? Dampen the compost before using it.

Be cautious about using indoor, bubbly hot tubs. There is a disorder called "hot-tub lung," in which a nasty bug, *Mycobacterium avium*, gets into your lungs and drains your energy. National Jewish Medical and Research Center in Denver, and the Mayo Clinic in Rochester, MN, have expertise in this disease.

Avoid smoke and smoking smokers. Smoky fireplaces and forest fires can really get to us, too. Wood smoke can worsen lung disease.

No general anesthesia without consulting your PH doc. General anesthesia can be dangerous for us, especially if our PH is not well controlled. There are some medical procedures, however, that just can't be done with only local anesthetic. Your PH specialist should be involved in any such undertaking, and it should be done at a center with PH experience.

Get a carbon monoxide (CO) detector. CO poisoning is potentially fatal for everyone, but even more likely to kill persons with PH. CO is odorless and colorless. It may leak from a poorly vented furnace or other fuel-burner. A CO detector can be plugged into an electrical outlet in your house. You may even want to visit an aviation shop for private pilots (an "FBO") at an airport, where they sell simple dots you can stick on the dash of your private airplane, Hummer, Honda, or John Deere. The dots change color if CO is present.

Consider starting a project to help pass the time while you wait for a transplant or for your medicine to start working. You'll be happier with something to focus on other than your woes. Things that can be done at your own pace and own place include arts and crafts, organizing photo albums, doing genealogical research on your family (there are oodles of websites that can help), or just sorting through papers. Make a list of the books you've always meant to read, then actually read them. What a luxury!

Lighten kitchen work. Get light-weight plastic dishes and glasses, and have paper plates available for the really bad days. Ask your kids to unload the dishwasher, set the table, and do the bending down necessary to get some pots and pans; just leave the ones you use a lot right on the counter. Look for dishwasher detergent tablets, which are lighter than bottles of liquid or boxes of powder.

Children can help out a lot. Even pre-schoolers can help. They can sort the wash, empty the dryer, and fold the clothes (you can sit on a chair to help). They can carry the folded clothes to their rooms. Older children may be able to make dinner once a week.

A basic weekly dinner menu can save a lot of effort and waste. For example, Sunday is pizza and salad; Monday is grilled chicken, rice, and carrots; Tuesday is tuna casserole, peas, and fruit salad; etc. You'll be surprised how this simplifies buying groceries and saves on food waste. It also makes it easier for everybody in the family to learn to prepare a dinner or two. They won't be running to you and asking where the timer is or how to wash lettuce.

Make your bed from the inside, before you get out of it, by pulling the covers up and straightening them; this can save some bending over.

On-line grocers can be a godsend. You order on their website, pick a delivery time, and they will often put the groceries right on your kitchen counter. Local stores will sometimes let you order by phone and then deliver your groceries for a small fee. If you go to the store yourself, use the electric cart if you're tired—we don't get brownie points for suffering.

Shop online or by catalog rather than running around town. You can do so on PHA's website through iGive and eScript—flowers, fruit baskets, books, clothes, pet supplies—you can buy just about anything, and PHA gets a percentage at no cost to you.

Stock up on staples at a warehouse. This lightens your grocery store load, saves money, and helps you stay prepared for power outages, earthquakes, floods, or snowstorms.

Use dry cleaners, laundries, and pharmacies that pick up and deliver. Many also have a drive-through option.

Pick your favorite charity and get involved. Many PH patients can do work that isn't too strenuous, such as reading to children in day care, visiting the elderly in nursing homes, helping out at a local historical landmark or museum, or making phone calls for the local blood bank. PHA has lots of work for volunteers, too—this book is one such project.

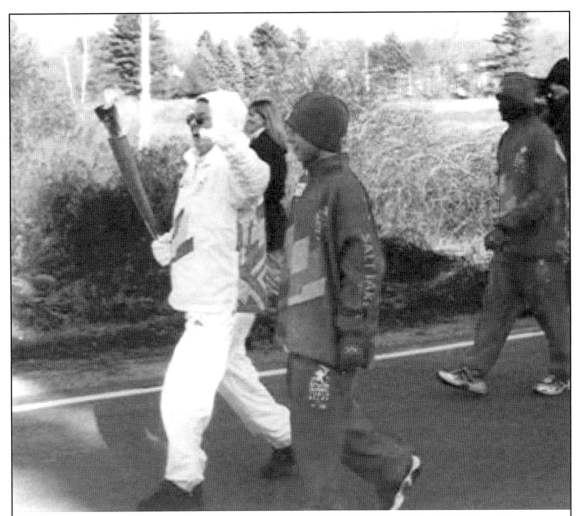

Kathy C. Forrest (in light clothing) carries the Olympic Torch as the relay to the 2002 Winter Games made its way through York, Maine in December 2001.
Kathy was diagnosed with PPH in 1999 and listed for transplant in 2000. Now 65, and a grandmother, she is doing so well on new oral meds that she is no longer thinking about a transplant.
Photo by Gordon Forrest.

13

Tedious Paperwork and Legal Matters

This chapter is intended for PH patients subject to the laws of the United States.
But all patients will want to write wills and make the equivalent of medical directives.

Medical and Disability Insurance

You or your child might be entitled to medical and disability benefits that you don't know about. Finding and understanding those benefits can be ridiculously complicated.

Insurers aren't happy to learn we have PH, because they know we're likely to cost them a bundle. They may deny our claims until we make a fuss. Cynicism is bad for our health, so we believe that most insurance companies and government agencies are honorable, if sometimes misguided. We need to educate them about PH and its treatments.

Medical Insurance

Medicare will pay for infused PH drugs that are FDA-approved for particular types of PH (see below). At present, Medicare itself does not pay for prescription oral medications (such as bosentan, or warfarin). Some types of Medicare supplement ("Medigap") insurance will pay for up to half of the cost of oral FDA-approved PH drugs, and often for drugs that are approved for other illnesses, but prescribed to treat PH (such as calcium channel blockers and sildenafil). (Once the FDA approves a drug, doctors can legally prescribe it for off-label as well as on-label uses, but the more expensive a drug is, the less likely insurers are to pay for off-label uses.) Close to a third of PAH patients are probably eligible for Medicare. Other insurers usually follow Medicare's lead.

In early 2004, perhaps the most effective treatment for many PH patients is epoprostenol (Flolan). It usually costs in the range of $60,000 a year to $120,000. In the past, some health insurers refused to pay for it on the grounds that the insured's PH was secondary to another illness, and that only "*primary* PH" is an on-label use listed under the "Indications and Usage" section of the package insert. Now that Medicare has approved epoprostenol for uses beyond what is on the label (this happened after Dr. David Badesch and colleagues published a landmark article showing the benefits of epoprostenol in secondary PH), it is now unlikely that PH patients who would benefit from it will be denied insurance coverage.

Medicare now covers infused epoprostenol if:

1) The PH is NOT secondary to pulmonary venous hypertension (e.g., left-sided atrial or ventricular disease, left-sided heart valve disease, etc.) or disorders of the respiratory system (e.g., chronic obstructive pulmonary disease, interstitial lung disease, obstructive sleep apnea, or other sleep-disordered breathing, alveolar hypertension disorders, etc.); and

2) The patient has "PPH" or PH that is secondary to one of the following conditions: connective tissue disease; thromboembolic disease of the pulmonary arteries; human immunodeficiency virus (HIV)

infection; cirrhosis; diet drugs; congenital left-to-right shunts; etc. If these conditions are present, the following criteria must be met:

a) The PH has progressed despite maximal medical and/or surgical treatment of the identified condition; and

b) The mean pulmonary artery pressure is greater than 25 mm Hg at rest or greater than 30 mm Hg with exertion; and

c) The patient has significant symptoms from the PH (i.e., severe dyspnea on exertion, and either fatigability, angina, or syncope); and

d) Treatment with oral calcium channel blocking agents has been tried and failed, or has at least been considered and felt not to be indicated.

Medicare also pays for treprostinil (Remodulin) injection therapy (for the medication, the pumps, and supplies) for nearly all PAH patients for whom this drug is recommended.

The situation can still arise where you need a drug other than epoprostenol or treprostinil to treat your PH, but Medicare or your insurance company refuses to pay for it. You can fight a balky insurance company. First, try the free help discussed in the following section. As a last resort, you can hire a lawyer. The lawyer might look for other instances where the insurance company has paid for off-label uses of other drugs, and argue that the company does not have the right to pick which off-label uses it pays for.

The New Medicare Drug Benefit

In January 2006, Medicare launched its Medicare Part D prescription drug plan; one of the biggest changes in Medicare history.

For the first time, Medicare beneficiaries could sign up to obtain prescription drug coverage. The service, however is given through contracted private prescription drug plans. There are several ways to learn about different plans that may be available to you. You can get information from the Medicare web site (www.Medicare.gov), your state insurance office, and through many senior services agencies.

There is a seven month window to sign up for a Part D plan, three months before you are eligible, the month in which you become eligible and three months after you become eligible for any other Medicare benefits. If you do not sign up for when you are eligible, you may pay a penalty and the next time you can join is from November 15 to December 31 of every year.

For the part D plan, you will pay a monthly premium (between $0 to $265 in 2007). You will also pay part of the cost of your medication. This cost will vary depending on which drug plan you choose. Some plans offer more coverage and more drugs at a higher monthly premium. You may have also heard of the "donut hole." This is when the government and you together have spent $2400 a year (in 2007) for your drugs, you enter a period where the part D plan will not cover any of the cost of your drugs. You will be responsible for paying 100% until you have spent a total of $3850 of your own money. Then the part D plan will kick in and pay 95% of any additional costs.

You may be thinking, that $2400 is a lot of money and you will unlikely hit the "donut hole," or maybe even if you do, you will only exceed it by a little bit and have only a small out of pocket expense. Beware of this, as all PH medications are very expensive. Being on one PH oral medication itself can put you in the "donut hole" after only a few months.

Furthermore, in order for you to stay on the medicine, you will have to pay out of pocket for these drugs which can be $1000s of dollars per month and there is generally no maximum out of pocket limit. It is virtually impossible to appeal to lower the cost of your deductible at that point. Therefore, when you choose your plan, be sure to choose one that will cover all the PH oral drugs whether you are on it or not. Plans generally work on a "tier" system where, at least until you hit the donut hole, you may pay different copays for drugs depending on the tier of the drug, the higher the tier the higher the copay.

If you have limited income, when you sign up for the part D plan they will usually include an application for financial assistance. If no such form was included, or if you want to know if you qualify, you can actually apply on-line by visiting www.socialsecurity.gov and click on the Medicare Prescription Drug Plan link, or by calling Social Security at 1-800-772-1213 (TTY 1-800-325-0778). Of course, the policies outlined in this section may be subject to change and so accuracy can't be guaranteed by the time this revision of the Survival Guide goes to print.

Free Help Getting Medical and/or Disability Benefits

When you feel tired and are emotionally overwhelmed by the diagnosis of PH it is really hard to find the strength to argue with your insurer. Insurers know this. They take advantage of your weakness by turning down your claim and hoping you won't appeal. Fortunately, there are smart energetic people out there on our side who will help us without charge. You do not have to be poor or disabled to get the following help. You only need to have PH.

ACCESS

Many PH patients have benefited from a wonderful free service called ACCESS (Advocating for Chronic Conditions, Entitlements and Social Services). A woman whose husband had severe hemophilia founded ACCESS in 1991. It offers its services only to those with hemophilia, PH, and a handful of other rare, chronic diseases. We're lucky to be on their list! ACCESS is now a program of Accredo Therapeutics, and Accredo Therapeutics pays for it, *but you don't have to be a client of Accredo Therapeutics for ACCESS to help you.* All services are provided with the utmost confidentiality; no personal or statistical information is shared with Accredo Therapeutics.

ACCESS focuses on government entitlements. They can advise you on your options and help you every step of the way through the process of applying for Social Security Disability (SSD), Medicare, Medicaid, and Supplemental Security Income (SSI). They also help PH patients who are still working to hang on to their health insurance under COBRA and HIPAA. They collect medical records and other evidence you will need to press your claim, help you fill out forms, and if your application is denied they will help you appeal it and often will appear at your hearing and argue your case before an administrative law judge (at no charge to you). What they cannot do is litigate for you. (To do so, their lawyers would have to be licensed in every state.) They will, however, upon your request, write letters on your behalf to your creditors telling them that you are filing for SSD. They cannot make promises about whether your claim for SSD will be successful. Their specialty is federal law, but they have been known to remind private insurers of their legal obligations.

A booklet you'll want. A free booklet, "ACCESS: Helping Families Cope," explains their program and gives a good overview of federal medical and disability entitlements plus some tips on applying for disability. Call toll free: 888-700-7010. Their local number is 813-806-0800.

Eighteen times to call ACCESS. You can avoid many mistakes by calling them whenever any of these situations apply to you:

1. I quit my job.
2. I lost my job.
3. I got a new job.
4. I'm looking for work.
5. I'm no longer able to work.
6. I'm about to lose my health insurance.
7. I'm about to use up my health insurance.
8. I just lost my health insurance.
9. I can't get health insurance.
10. I just got married.
11. I just had (or adopted) a child.
12. My child has lots of medical bills that I can't pay.
13. My child just turned 18.
14. My spouse stopped working.
15. I'm getting a divorce.
16. I'm moving.
17. I'm considering a transplant.
18. I'm thinking of returning to work.

You lose a lot of potential benefits if you don't act within certain time limits. It is so important to recognize events that can jeopardize your medical coverage (and happiness) that we're offering a second list of additional times to call ACCESS or to do your own research:

♦ Your child is about to leave for college.
♦ You are leaving a job and COBRA or HIPAA is an issue.
♦ You are really too sick to work, but must continue working to survive.

♦ Your spouse dies and you have dependent children.

Your Health Service Company (Accredo Therapeutics, CVS Caremark, Curascript)

Accredo Therapeutics, Caremark, and Curascript have reimbursement specialists to help their clients get private or government insurers to pay for the client's specialty PH medication. While their focus is on helping you get and keep your specialty drug coverage, in the process they can help you get and keep insurance coverage for all your medical expenses. Accredo Therapeutics and Curascript will help you apply for a full spectrum of insurance coverage including SSD, Medicare, SSI, and Medicaid. Your health service company will bill your primary and secondary insurance carriers for you. They will deal with case managers, medical directors, and others within the insurance industry. (Caremark bought TheraCom in spring 2004, and it isn't known yet exactly how their services will be merged.)

Accredo Therapeutics and CVS Caremark (along with the maker of Flolan, GlaxoSmithKline) have patient assistance programs for those who cannot afford co-payments and deductibles. Curascript has a patient assistance program for Remodulin patients who have no insurance or inadequate insurance. As a last resort, it is often possible for your health service company to arrange for free or subsidized medicine if you qualify financially.

At the PHA conference in the year 2000, representatives of Accredo Therapeutics and TheraCom (bought by CVS Caremark in 2004) offered some tips for PH patients:

♦ Be a strong self-advocate.
♦ Tell your employer if your insurer isn't

coming through for you.

- Keep track of your lifetime maximum.
- Document any interactions with your insurer (keep a log of who you talked to, when, and what was said).
- Keep a copy of any written communication with your insurer.
- Maintain your current health insurance until an alternative is found.
- When sending in insurance payments, write the check for the exact amount (COBRA insurance has been discontinued because a check was 50 cents off!), send the payment "signature required" so you have proof it's been received, and mail it on time!
- If you can plan a couple months ahead of the time you will be starting on Flolan, contact your health service company so they can get authorizations for both the hospital stay and home care.
- If your company changes insurers and wants you to go to new doctors, but you don't want to switch from your "center of excellence," you can go to your state insurance commission and argue that you need "continuity of care." Your present doctor will need to back you up. Tell them that if you go to a less experienced doctor it could kill you.

State Agencies

Insurance commissioners, who are often elected, can also be helpful with many types of insurance problems. So can a state attorney general's office, if your problem appears to be part of a larger scam.

Key Federal & Federal/State Medical Insurance Laws

For a more detailed overview of the following laws, ask ACCESS for their booklet, "ACCESS: Helping Families Cope." Also visit the Centers for Medicare & Medicaid Services (CMS) website: www.cms.hhs.gov. It's a portal to all sorts of relevant government services. CMS' toll-free number: 1-877-267-2323. Local number: 410-786-3000. TTY toll-free: 1-866-226-1819. TTY local: 410-786-0727.

COBRA

If a private, state, or local government employer has at least 20 employees and offers a group health plan, COBRA requires that employer to offer employees, their families, and retirees an opportunity to keep their health insurance, at group rates, after leaving the company or reducing the number of hours they work. If you stop work, you can maintain your group coverage for 18 months, but you must notify your employer within 60 days of the qualifying event that you wish to elect COBRA. You will have to pay both your share and your employer's share of the insurance premiums, plus 2 percent. At the end of the 18-month period, you are allowed to enroll in an individual conversion health plan if your employer offers one. There are other deadlines and requirements that must be met.

If you leave work because you are disabled, COBRA gives you an additional 11 months of coverage, bringing the total to 29 months, which will be about when your Social Security Medicare kicks in (if you qualify). This is a reason that you should apply for Social Security and/or SSI immediately if you think you might be disabled for a year or more. Warning: the 11-month extension is not automatic—there are rules you must follow to be entitled to it, and many extensions to the rules. It's best to consult with someone who understands the ins and outs of COBRA or it can *bite* you!

Health Insurance Portability and Accountability Act (HIPAA)

It's sometimes said, "you slide down COBRA and land on HIPAA." HIPAA helps workers keep their group health plan coverage if they change jobs, are laid off, or leave a job to start their own business. It prohibits employers that offer health coverage (see ERISA, below), and insurers that offer coverage in connection with employer-sponsored group health plans, from canceling your policy if you have a high-cost illness such as PH (as long as you pay your premiums, of course). Before HIPAA, people were afraid to change jobs for fear their preexisting conditions would not be covered under their new employer's policy. Although HIPAA sets out minimum standards for portability and preexisting conditions, states can enact greater protections.

If an employer offers group health insurance, it must be offered to new employees as well, if they were previously enrolled in a group health plan and there was not a break in coverage of 63 days or more. Insurers sometimes try to get around this by stalling—by not giving quotes or making a decision until the 63 days have passed. Most applicants appear unaware of the 63-day limit.

ERISA: Health Insurance Provided by Employers and Unions

A federal law called ERISA governs these plans. It applies when your company or employee organization, such as a union, "self-insures." (If your employer does not "self-insure," then your state's laws and HIPAA govern things like how long an insurance company can make you wait before they cover

a preexisting condition.) A very complex law, ERISA is unfair to consumers in many regards, but does provide certain rights, such as the right to appeal a denial of benefits and a right to judicial remedies.

See "Knowing the Rules of the Insurance Game," by Benjamin A. Baker, Esq., in *Pathlight,* winter 1996, or visit the Department of Labor website (www.dol.gov). You can call the Department of Labor at: 1-866-4-USA-DOL. TTY: 1-877-889-5627.

Medicare & Social Security Disability (SSD)

Medicare provides federal health insurance for persons over 65 and disabled people under 65. To qualify, you have to have worked a certain number of quarters and paid Social Security taxes (FICA), and to have contributed to the program within the last 5 years. In other words, if you are in denial about your disability and wait too long after quitting work before you apply for benefits, you miss out. Because those of us with PH are living longer, most of us will eventually use Medicare, even if we don't need it right now.

It is a good thing to qualify for SSD. Not only do you get a monthly benefit check based on the FICA you paid when you were working, but 24 months after you become entitled to your first benefit check (which is 29 months after you become disabled) you can also get Medicare coverage.

SSD and Medicare benefits are also sometimes available in special situations for disabled people who can't qualify on their own work record, but who are still a minor, blind, or the widow or widower of a deceased worker.

With traditional Medicare, you can pick any PH doctor in the country without getting anyone's prior approval. This allows you to consult with that specialist in another city who might save your life.

On their website (www.ssa.gov/dibplan/dqualify5.htm), the SSA says they ask five questions to determine if somebody is disabled for their purposes (and for the purpose of getting Medicare). Benefits are payable only for a total disability that is expected to last at least a year or to result in death. Here's their list:

1. **Are you working?** If you are working in 2004 and your earnings average more than $810 a month, you generally cannot be considered disabled....If you are not working, we go to Step 2. [*Author's note*: Passive income that you get from things other than working—such as interest, annuities, your spouse's job, or benefits from a disability insurance policy or worker's compensation—is not counted.]

2. **Is your condition "severe"?** Your condition must interfere with basic work-related activities for your claim to be considered. If it does not, we will find that you are not disabled. If your condition does interfere with basic work-related activities, we go to Step 3.

3. **Is your condition found in the list of disabling conditions?** For each of the major body systems, we maintain a list of medical conditions that are so severe they automatically mean that you are disabled. If your condition is not on the list, we have to decide if it is of equal severity to a medical condition that is on the list. If it is, we will find that you are disabled. If it is not, then we go to Step 4.

4. **Can you do the work you did previous-**

ly? If your condition is severe but not at the same or equal level of severity as a medical condition on the list, then we must determine if it interferes with your ability to do the work you did previously. If it does not, your claim will be denied. If it does, we proceed to Step 5.

5. **Can you do any other type of work?** If you cannot do the work you did in the past, we see if you are able to adjust to other work. We consider your medical conditions and your age, education, past work experience and any transferable skills you may have. If you cannot adjust to other work, your claim will be approved. If you can adjust to other work your claim will be denied.

A lawyer with ACCESS says this is what it really boils down to: Can you work 40 hours per week, consistently, without an overly accommodating employer, at a type of job that hires a reasonable number of people in the area where you live, and still have a decent quality of life at the end of the day? If you collapse on the couch when you get home, too tired to cook or have a little fun with your family, then you may meet the qualifications for disability.

Don't be discouraged if you apply for SSD and are denied; most disability claims are denied in the first two steps of the process. You may well have to go to a hearing before an administrative law judge. If your doctor says you are disabled because of PH, you are very likely to win in the end.

There are incentives that allow you to retain many of your SSD and Medicare benefits while attempting to return to work. The rules are complex; call ACCESS before making any changes in your status.

Medicare has a policy that allows them to

cover some medications as "durable medical equipment," such as some drugs administered through external infusion pumps. Medicare has agreed that epoprostenol meets the criteria of their external infusion pump policy, for most persons with primary PH (for specifics, see above section on Medical Insurance). Infused treprostenol is also currently covered. (Medicare drug coverage is subject to change, and therefore accuracy cannot be guaranteed as this is being written.)

If you have limited resources, there are little-known and under-utilized programs to exempt you from having to pay the monthly Medicare premium, the 20 percent share of charges for office visits, and hospital deductibles. Ask about the Qualified Medicare Beneficiary program and the Specified Low-Income Medicare Beneficiaries program. There are also some newer programs. What's available varies from state to state. For information call either ACCESS or the CMS. Telephone numbers are above. If you are an AARP member, ask for a copy of their worksheet to help you learn if you qualify (800-424-3410). You can also get the information on AARP's website: www.aarp.org.

Medicare pays for hospice care. If a doctor certifies that a person has a life expectancy of less than 6 months, Medicare will pay for hospice care at a facility that is Medicare-certified. When home care is not feasible, this underused option can save a family from having to deplete its resources on nursing home care. Don't rely on the nursing home to tell you when you or your family member might qualify (they may not want to lose a paying customer). Instead, ask your doctor to let you know when it's the right time to consider the hospice option.

Detailed information on Medicare and SSD can be found at www.medicare.gov, or www.ssa.gov, or by calling 1-800-MEDICARE. You can apply by contacting any Social Security Administration (SSA) office. The general number is 1-800-772-1213. Application forms and directions to your local office (and tons of other information) are available on their website. ACCESS can also help explain the rules (more clearly, often, than the people who answer SSA's lines). ACCESS has a list of tips for persons applying for SSD or SSI. For example, putting a bright face on your illness while visiting your doctor won't help you to get disability benefits. This is the time to whine and keep a log of symptoms.

SSI & Medicaid

Supplemental Security Income (SSI) is a combined state and federal program that gives monthly payments to poor persons who are over 65, blind, or disabled. You don't need to have a work history to qualify for SSI. You do need to be living in the U.S. and be a U.S. citizen or living in the U.S. legally. Medicaid covers prescription drugs. Epoprostenol is usually covered, but coverage varies a bit from state to state. Some people will be eligible for both SSI and SSD and for Medicaid and Medicare. The amount of benefits you receive depends on what state you live in.

Children are usually eligible for disability under SSI (if the child is over 18 only her income and resources are considered, even if she still lives with her parents).

In most states SSI automatically includes medical benefits through a Medicaid program, and benefits start the first month (unlike the long wait to get Medicare). The criteria for being disabled (if you are an adult) are the same as they are for SSD; it's common to apply for both at the same time. There are incentives that let you return to work and still hang on to many SSI and Medicaid benefits. For information contact ACCESS or go to www.ssa.gov. Some states cover hospice care under their Medicaid plans.

Family and Medical Leave Act (FMLA)

This law applies to all private employers with 50 or more employees, state and local governments (including schools) and some federal employees. It says that an employer must allow up to 12 unpaid weeks of leave a year when various situations occur, including a serious health condition of the employee that leaves him/her unable to work, or if a dependent of the employee has a serious medical condition that requires the employee to miss work to care for the dependent. Group health benefits must be continued during the leave. The law is enforced by the U.S. Department of Labor's Employment Standards Administration, Wage and Hour Division. You can get all the details at www.dol.gov/dol/esa/fmla.htm.

How to Keep Up with Changes in the Law

Because federal health care laws change so often, the Employee Benefits Security Administration of the Department of Labor offers a free, regularly updated publication called "Recent Changes in Health Care Laws." Call 1-800-998-7542.

Private Disability Insurance

If you decide you must quit work, find out if your employer carries private disability insurance. If so, get your own copy of the entire policy and any amendments to it to keep at home.

The definition of "disabled" in private insurance policies varies. The relevant clause might read something like this:

"Total disability" and "totally disabled" mean that because of injury or sickness: (1) you cannot perform each of the material duties of your regular occupation; and (2) after benefits have been paid for 24 months, you cannot perform each of the material duties of any gainful occupation for which you are reasonably fitted by training, education or experience.

For professionals like attorneys, the first part might require only that you cannot perform each of the material duties of your specialty.

Before you actually leave your job, call ACCESS to get their advice. Read your policy carefully; know your rights and insist upon them. If you are rejected, appeal the decision. Do not let the company stall too long. Complain to your state insurance commissioner. If you go to court and the insurer loses, in some states it must pay extra damages for its bad behavior.

Do not be surprised if your disability insurance company sends a snoop to your house to check up on you. It's perfectly fair for them to do this; there are cheaters out there, although we, of course, are not among them. Rachel had a man turn up on her doorstep, unannounced. Her disability company had sent him to see if she was really at home during the day, and to question her about what activities she could do. Before letting him in, she called the insurance company to find if he was legit, and let them know her heart rate was soaring!

You do not have to talk to such an unannounced visitor on the spot. It is all right to say you would like to schedule an appointment for another day (this will give you time to reflect, or to consult with your lawyer).

Help! I (or My Kids) Don't Have *Any* Insurance

It's deplorable that the U.S. is almost

alone among top-tier nations in not providing universal health coverage. You might be one of the millions of people with no health insurance at all. Call ACCESS and describe your situation. Many states have high-risk insurance pools, special services for disabled kids, and spend-down provisions that cover people who earn a little too much or have too many assets to qualify for Medicaid. Ask your hospital's social services department if they know of state programs. The health service company that provides your special PH medicine (such as a prostanoid or an endothelin receptor antagonist) can often be helpful. They know their way around various insurance options you might have overlooked, and might have or know of patients' assistance programs for those with no insurance who meet certain financial criteria. They might also know ways you can obtain your medicine at a lower cost.

Many pharmaceutical manufacturers offer uninsured poor patients free or reduced-price medications. Many even claim that no patient in need of their medications will have to go without them. Your pharmacist may know about such assistance, or you can try contacting the maker of your drug. The Google Internet search engine (search terms "medication assistance programs") quickly turned up a lot of information on such plans, including the names of drug companies participating and their criteria. See suggestions in the Resources chapter of this book.

Children's Health Insurance Program. This is a federal/state program to help working parents who otherwise couldn't afford medical insurance for their children to get free or low-cost insurance. It applies to children through 18 years of age. Each state has its own program, so details differ depending on where you live. The web portal for the federal Centers for Medicare & Medicaid Services (CMS) is: http://cms.hhs.gov. You can also go to the U.S. Department of

Health & Human Services: call toll free 1-877-KIDS-NOW (1-877-543-7669), or go to www. insurekidsnow.gov.

Free Life Insurance?

Some life insurance policies contain clauses stating that if the owner becomes disabled, he or she does not have to pay premiums, and the policy will still remain in force. Check your policy! Stan's TIAA term policy has such a clause, and the company has cheerfully honored it to the letter.

Health Care Directives & Durable Powers of Attorney

The U.S. Supreme Court has held that you have a right to refuse medical treatment even if you are comatose, if you have previously made your wishes known. Each state sets its own standards for "clear and convincing evidence" of a patient's wishes. The best way to make your wishes known is through a health care directive and a medical power of attorney. Every adult, not just PH patients, should seriously consider preparing both of these documents. Even family members cannot overturn "clear and convincing" directives.

Health Care Directives
(a.k.a. Living Wills, Health Care Proxies, or Advance Directives)

Whatever you call them, they are a set of instructions to your physician about what you do or do not want done if you experience a medical emergency and are unconscious or otherwise unable to express your wishes. In some states a directive can be viewed as advisory only, or apply only if a doctor determines that you have developed a terminal condition. Without a directive, if you are incapable of making your own medical decisions, in a medical emergency decisions will be made for you according to hospital protocol or by a doctor after discussions with your next of kin. You might not like the results. In many states there is a hierarchy that determines which relatives get to make the decisions: the spouse first; then the offspring; the sibling; the parent; etc. But even with this hierarchy, if your relatives don't agree, big legal messes can occur at your expense (financial, mental, emotional, physical, etc.). *See*, Durable powers of attorney, below.

Donating organs. A health care directive is a good place to say that you want to be an organ donor. Because doctors will still ask family members for permission to remove organs and use them in a living patient, be sure to talk it over with your kin so they will go along with your plans. A driver's license pledge or "donor dot" can be overridden by surviving family members.

Durable Powers of Attorney for Health Care & Financial Affairs

Durable powers of attorney for health care. This type of document gives someone you trust the power to make medical decisions for you, should you become unable to speak for yourself. The power is not limited to situations where you are about to die; it can also apply when you are in what appears to be a permanent unconscious state. It is called "durable" because it remains effective after the maker is incapacitated.

Although a doctor might just go along with what the family of the patient requests, if there is no durable power of attorney for medical care, the doctor might refuse, or an interested person might contest the proposed action, and then the family would have to go to court to get authorization for providing or withholding certain types of care. (Another option might be to petition a court for the appointment of a conservator of the person.)

Once you go to court, the details of your medical condition—and the dispute—become public. Going to court is also a lot more expensive and stressful than making a durable power of attorney.

If you make a living will or a durable power of attorney, you can modify or revoke it at any time. You can get these documents for very little money. Of course, a lawyer would be delighted to draft them for you and may give good advice on some of the finer points, as well as advice on estate planning matters. This is the most costly route to go. Alternatively, you might be able to buy the right forms for your state from your neighborhood stationery store. You can also get a free living will off the web, specific for your state, from www.legaldocs.com. Nolo Press has an excellent website (www.nolo.com) that offers general information for nonlawyers on health care directives, living wills, and durable powers of attorney. They also publish books of legal tools and software for do-it-yourselfers. You can call them at 800-992-6656.

The big decision. How far do you want doctors to go to try to prolong your life if you are in really bad shape and not going to get better? You need to put instructions about this in your durable power of attorney and/or health care directive. Do you want

COURTS FROWN UPON
POST-DEPARTURE WILLS
SO MAKE YOURS NOW!

doctors to do everything possible to keep you alive? If your brain has suffered serious damage, do you still want to be revived? If you are in a coma and unlikely to fully recover, do you want breathing tubes, feeding tubes, hydration, antibiotics, etc.? What about the use of pain medication to ensure your comfort, even if it could hasten your death? It is your choice, and spelling it out (and giving a copy to your doctors) makes things easier for everybody.

A final thought: if you are making the ultimate decision for an unconscious loved one who has left you with written instructions making it clear that after a certain point they want to let nature take its course, think carefully before you ask the doctor, "Is there *any* possibility at all, however small, that he/she will recover?" Because miracles happen, the doctor ethically, and to protect herself/himself legally, has to say yes, there is a chance. If you then stop life support, you will be burdened with undeserved guilt. For every-one's comfort, it is wiser to ask, "Doctor, in your best medical judgment is there anything more that can *reasonably* be done to help this person I love recover and enjoy life?"

Durable power of attorney for financial affairs. It is also possible to prepare a durable power of attorney for financial affairs, which allows a trusted person to manage your money while you are incapacitated. This might be a smart thing to do if you are planning to undergo a procedure like a transplant that could put you out of commission for a while. This is a document where you will probably want a lawyer's guidance. A lawyer can help you think through contingencies and tailor your power of attorney to safeguard your assets and meet your particular needs. The alternative is for a judge to appoint a "conservator," "guardian," or whatever your state calls them to make

decisions for you. This process eats up money and time and exposes your finances to the public eye.

Estate Planning

There is absolutely no evidence that people with wills or estate plans die any sooner than those without. It can take a big load off your mind and (if you have considerable assets) save your heirs a bundle. Look for a lawyer with expertise in the field and discuss fees up front.

Even if you don't own much, a will is a good idea. A will is essential if you have minor children, because you can name a guardian and set up a "testamentary trust" for them, in the event both you and your partner die. You can make your own will yourself if you don't have a large or complicated estate, beneficiaries who are likely to sue one another, or minor children. If you want to leave assets to the children of a previous marriage, or plan to divide your assets in a complicated or uneven way, or put restrictions on when a beneficiary can get his/her inheritance, then you need a lawyer. Simple will forms are available from stationery stores. Books with forms and instructions can be found in libraries and bookstores. Nolo Press offers quality legal advice to nonlawyers on matters like wills and estate planning. You can glean some general information off their web-site (www.nolo.com) and even more from their do-it-yourself books. If you have a computer, Quicken WillMaker Plus 2004 (about $50 (1-800-728-3555; www.nolo.com) is a good choice. The wills it produces will work everywhere but Louisiana. You can also go to a site like www.legaldocs.com and pay less, but know less, too. To be safe, pay an attorney $150 to $200 to look it over before you sign it. If you do something wrong, like forget to sign in the presence of witnesses, your will won't fly.

If PHA has been helpful to you and your family, please consider making it a beneficiary in your will. PHA has very good estate-planning materials available just for the asking (301-565-3004); the Association also offers a confidential estate planning analysis. It is often possible to benefit a charity, such as PHA, while reducing your estate taxes.

There are three basic forms of bequests:

1. A specific dollar amount can be stated with this wording: I give, devise and bequeath to the Pulmonary Hypertension Association, headquartered in Silver Spring, Maryland, $_____.

2. An alternative is to leave a percentage of your estate: I give, devise and bequeath to the Pulmonary Hypertension Association, headquartered in Silver Spring, Maryland _____% of my estate.

3. Another option is to provide for your family first and still leave something for PHA by leaving us the residue of your estate. The residue is simply whatever is left of your assets after your other beneficiaries have received their bequests. The language reads: All the residue of my estate, including real and personal property, I give, devise and bequeath to the Pulmonary Hypertension Association, headquartered in Silver Spring, Maryland.

If your will is already in place but you'd like to add PHA as a beneficiary, a codicil can be added by consulting your attorney. Please consult with your financial or legal advisor if you are considering any form of gift to PHA. PHA is deeply appreciative of such gifts, and relies on them to continue its programs.

Resources

14

Pulmonary Hypertension Association (PHA)

PHA was founded by three patients, a family member, and their husbands in 1990. It quickly grew a strong professional medical arm and expanded into a nation-wide organization with international affiliates. As of 2008, PHA (U.S.) has over 9,000 members and over 160 affiliated support groups.

The mission of PHA is to seek a cure, to provide hope, support, and education, to promote awareness, and to advocate for the pulmonary hypertension community. Patients, family members, and medical professionals all sit on the Board of Trustees. PHA has a dedicated permanent staff at an office in Silver Spring, Md. Volunteers are still at the heart of the organization, however, and contribute to PHA's publications, help raise funds, run support groups, and contribute in many other ways.

PHA fulfills its mission by sponsoring scientific research, helping patients learn about new treatments and ways to cope with PH, and advocating for federal funding, research, and legislation that will improve the lives of PH patients. Because PH is an under-diagnosed and often misdiagnosed condition, PHA promotes awareness of PH both to the medical community and general public. PHA is a nonprofit organization.

To join PHA, call toll-free 1-800-748-7274 and ask for its free brochure, which contains a membership form. Or write PHA at 801 Roeder Road, Suite 400, Silver Spring, MD 20910. A contribution of $15 is suggested, but not required. For those outside the U.S., a donation of $25, in U.S. dollars, is suggested, to help cover the additional expense of mailings. A membership form can also be found at www.PHAssociation.org.

Pathlight. Membership in PHA includes a subscription to its quarterly newsletter, *Pathlight*, which is produced by PHA with input from the PH community and is crammed with useful information on new research, PHA events, networking, support groups, living with PH, ways to get involved in fighting this disease, a page for children with PH, and lots more.

Persistent Voices. This literary periodical is sent to all members. It allows patients, friends, and family members to tell, in their own voices, about their experiences with PH.

Website: www.PHAssociation.org. PHA's site is now getting over 390,000 hits a month. In addition to the popular message boards (where patients trade stories and information, vent steam, and give reassurance), the site offers information on PH and PHA, breaking news related to PH, a bibliography of PH-related research papers, clinical trial listings, PH-related links on the web, support group listings, hosted weekly chat room meetings, listservs, access to old *Pathlights* and to PHA's medical journal *Advances in Pulmonary Hypertension*, links to PH specialists all over the world, a store where you can support PHA while buying just about anything over the web, etc. Current message boards include: the **General Discussion Board, Transplant Board, Parents' Board**, and the **Caregivers' Board**.

PHA listservs include: **PHAnews** (items of interest to PH patients, their families, and medical professionals); **PHAdvocacy** (for activists to share information and learn how to organize advocacy campaigns); **PH Community Leaders; Caregivers; PHA International** (where discussions can be held in whatever language is preferred, and clinical trials and things of interest in countries other than the U.S. can be discussed); and **PH Doctors/Researchers** (to provide information to specialists and generalists).

Research fellowships. As a result of PHA's growing special events program and the generosity of donors, PHA is able to offer grants to researchers looking for a cure. PHA raises funds through golf tournaments, selling holiday cards, and other activities. For more information visit www.PHAssociation.org.

Through PHA's advocacy work with the National Heart, Lung, and Blood Institute and with Congress, $15 million has been earmarked for PH research through the NHLBI.

Clinical research support. PHA partners with the NHLBI to support Mentored Clinical Scientist Development Awards (K08) and Mentored Patient-Oriented Research Career Development Awards (K23). The purpose is to support the development of outstanding clinician research scientists who are committed to a career in research in pulmonary hypertension. For information, visit www.PHAssociation.org.

Support groups. PHA works with individuals, medical professionals, and health care companies to set up patient and caregiver support groups. There are presently over 160 such groups in the U.S., and recently PHA

has helped establish groups in other nations. If you want to start a group, contact the Director of Volunteer Services at: pha@PHAssociation.org. PHA will send out flyers for meetings, reimburse for some copying and postage expenses, and provide a Support Group Leaders' Manual.

Toll-free number. People call 1-800-748-7274 for many reasons. Often a newly diagnosed PH patient just needs somebody to talk to who can tell them a bit more about the disease and what it is like to live with it. You can get names of doctors who treat PH patients, order a packet of information for new patients or PH awareness ribbons, learn how to make a tax-deductible contribution to PHA (always needed and welcomed), find out how to order conference videos, get information on support groups, talk with someone who has had a lung transplant or is knowledgeable about PH treatments, etc. As far as we know, PHA's hot line is unique in that it is staffed by a team of volunteers who are also patients.

PH awareness ribbons. PHA's color is periwinkle blue (a wit remarked that it is the same color as our lips and nails, before treatment). The metal ribbons are available by calling the toll-free PHA number or the PHA office. PHA logo pins are also available.

Biennial International Pulmonary Hypertension Conference. It's held in even-numbered years and is open to all PHA members, patients, their families and caregivers, health care professionals, and researchers. At the year 2006 conference in Minneapolis, Minnesota, over 1,100 people from 11 nations participated in over a dozen support groups, and soaked up information from experts during about 50 general and breakout sessions.

Scientific Sessions are held during the two days before the general conference, at the same hotel, with posters explaining new research. Presentations and discussions from internationally recognized experts as well as selected oral abstracts from PAH experts are included. Patients may watch at no extra charge.

At the main conference will be presentations designed for patients on topics like the diagnosis of PH, drug therapies, surgical removal of pulmonary emboli, transplantation, genetics, the special problems of children with PH, living well in spite of PH, and treatments under development. Workshops, support groups, and entertainment are tailored for both adult and child patients and their families. Watch *Pathlight* and check PHA's website for information. The cost of transportation to a conference and the registration fee may be deductible on your taxes as a medical expense.

Dr. Victor Tapson of Duke University describes PHA conferences as "a new model for a way to approach medicine." The conference is unique in that patients and professionals mingle and learn from one another; it's a great chance to corner that researcher who wrote a paper that might save your life, and it's also a great opportunity for the researcher to ask you for a blood sample or your medical history.

Conference tapes. Because not everyone is able to attend the international conferences, key sessions are recorded. Call PHA's toll-free number to get a list of available tapes. You can also purchase conference tapes from AVEN, (800) 810-8273, or order on-line at: www.aven.com. Please note: this is an external site and does not offer orders through a secure server, so you may wish to telephone instead.

Scientific Leadership Council (SLC). PHA is proud of its Scientific Leadership Council, which is composed of more than 20 leaders in the field of pulmonary hypertension. The members are clinicians, research scientists, and nurses who come from medical centers

recognized for performing outstanding research and providing excellent care for PH patients. An additional member advises the SLC on research at the National Institutes of Health (NIH). The medical centers involved in the SLC (as of August 2007) include the Mayo Clinic, Columbia Presbyterian Medical Center, University of California San Diego, Harbor-UCLA, Duke, University of Colorado, University of Utah, Vanderbilt, Baylor College of Medicine, Stanford University, University of Michigan, University of Alabama at Birmingham, Tufts - New England Medical Center, and Allegheny General Hospital. The SLC also has international members from Italy, France, Australia, Mexico, and Canada.

The mission of the SLC is to provide medical and scientific leadership and guidance to PHA by proactively facilitating the development of new knowledge about PH, actively disseminating knowledge about PH to medical and public audiences, and advocating and raising awareness about PH. Members of the SLC speak at the biennial conference of PHA, provide editorial oversight to PHA's publications as well as to the SLC's medical journal, *Advances in Pulmonary Hypertension*, advise on PHA's research fellowship program and administrate PH Clinicians and Researchers.

PH Resource Network, which has its own website and listserv, is a forum for all healthcare professionals. As part of PHA, PH Resource Network is dedicated to enhancing communication, professional development, and research and education among PH medical professionals who are currently employed caring for PH patients. Membership in PH Resource Network is available to any medical professional who is a member of PHA. For questions about PH Resource Network memberships please call 301-565-3004 ext. 121. PH Resource Network offers peer-to-peer support, CEU educational sessions, PHA's medical journal, *Advances in Pulmonary Hypertension,* patient education tools, administrative support for developing and submitting research proposals, and much more.

PH Clinicians and Researchers (PHCR) is PHA's professional group for physicians and MD/DO/PhD-level researchers interested in pulmonary hypertension. By joining PHCR, physicians and researchers can gain access to information and contribute to the PH community by learning from and educating peers. Learn more, or request a free copy of the PHCR brochure by calling 301-565-3004 ext. 104.

Donations to PHA. PHA deeply appreciates any help you can give. Contributions are tax-deductible, and contributors are thanked in *Pathlight.* Donations may be given in honor of, or memory of, a particular person. Checks should be made out to Pulmonary Hypertension Association. Please mail contributions to: PHA, 801 Roeder Road Suite 400, Silver Spring, MD 20910. Ask, too, for information on PHA's planned giving program and accompanying estate planning advice (for more information see the Estate Planning section of Chapter 13).

PH Patient Organizations Around the Globe

Our goal is to be inclusive—if we missed your group or your information needs updating, please contact pha@PHAssociation.org *and ask for your listing on PHA's website to be corrected.*

Australia
PHA Australia
54 Mimosa Drive
02650 Wagga Wagga
NSW Australia
Email: carmel@phaaustralia.com.au
Website: www.phaaustralia.com.au/

Canada
British Columbia Pulmonary Hypertension Society (BCPHS)
2881 Canyon Park Place
Victoria BC V9B 4Z4
Canada
Email: LGMcCall@shaw.ca
Website: www.bcphs.com

New Brunswick Pulmonary Hypertension Society (NBPHS)
97 Dale Avenue
Hampton NB E5N 5J2
Canada
Email: jgendron@nb.sympatico.ca
Website: www.nbphs.org

The Pulmonary Hypertension Society of Ontario/Canada (PHSC)
3550 Kelly Rd, RR3
Windsor ON N9A 6Z6
Canada
Email: phs@mnsi.net;
lparoian@paroianlaw.com
Website: www.phscanada.com

PPH Quebec
613 Sinclair Rd.
Brownsburg-Chatham
QC J8G 1Y1
Canada
Email: lyndab64@hotmail.com
Website: groups.msn.com/PPHQuebec

The Manitoba Pulmonary Hypertension Support Group
78 Whitehead Crescent
Brandon MB R7B 0W4
Canada
Email: dlmcguire@mts.net
Website:
http://ca.geocities.com/mb_ph_group/

China
PHA China
Center of Pulmonary Vascular Disease,
Department of Medicine,
Fu Wai Heart Hospital
Peking Union Medical College
167 Beilishi Road
100037 Beijing
China
Email: phachina@yahoo.com.cn
Website: www.phachina.com

Europe
PHA Europe
A nonprofit umbrella group that aims to
extablish cooperation among its member
groups and other organizations relevant to PH
Molenvliet 13
3961 MT Wijk bij Duurstede
The Netherlands
Email: info@phaeurope.org
Website: www.phaeurope.org

Austria
Selbsthilfegruppe Lungenhochdruck
Lazarettgasse 19/ 4th Floor
A-1090 Vienna
Austria
Email: info@lungenhochdruck.at
Website: www.phaaustria.com

Belgium
PH vzw [Pulmonale Hypertensie Patienten Vereniging] (Dutch)
Cantincrodelaan 48 b2
02150 Borsbeek
Belgium
Email: ph-vaz@yucom.be
Website: home.tiscali.be/yuc-johan.bastings/

HTAP Belgique (French)
Premiere Avenue 83
B-1330 Rixensart
Belgium
Email: htapbelgique@hotmail.com
Website: www.htap-belgique.be

France
HTAP France [Hypertension Arterielle Pulmonaire France]
31 Rue Jacques Cellier
51100 Reims
France
Email: secretariat@htapfrance.com
Website: www.htapfrance.com

Greece
PHA-Greece
Lokridos 32
Tayros, Athens
Greece
Email: giannoulis_phagr@yahoo.gr;
barlas_phagr@yahoo.gr

Germany
PHeV [Pulmonare Hypertonie e.V.]
Wormser Str. 20
D-76287 Rheinstetten
Germany
Email: info@phev.de
Website: www.phev.de

Ireland
PHA-Ireland
Pulmonary Hypertension Unit, Mater
Misericordiae University Hospital
Eccles St.
Dublin 7
Ireland
Email: sdoherty@mater.ie;materpph@yahoo.ie
Website: www.mater.ie/pha-ireland/html/intro.htm

Italy

AIPI [Associazione Ipertensione Polmonare Italiana]
Via Vigoni 5
20122 Milano
Italy
Email: pisana.ferrari@aliceposta.it
Website: www.aipiitalia.org

AMIP [Associazione Malati Ipertensione Polmonare]
Via Bagnoregio 51
00189 Roma
Italy
Email: mpproia@tiscalinet.it
Website: www.assoamip.net

IRPPH - International Registry of Primary Pulmonary Hypertension
A registry based at the CINECA Institution in Bologna, Italy, to develop and create a uniform and consistent patient population to collect epidemiological, clinical, and therapeutic information
Website: http://irpph.cineca.it/public/welc.htm

Netherlands
PHA Nederland
Kastanjelaan 6
5268 CA Helvoirt
The Netherlands
Email: Info@pha-nl.nl
Website: www.pha-nl.com

Portugal
RESPIRAR-APHP
Avenida Dr. Luis Navega 38-42
03050 Mealhada
Portugal
Email: maria.j.saraiva@clix.pt
Website: www.aphpweb.pt

Spain
Asociación de Hipertensos Pulmonares de España
Avenida de las Artes 7 (Aranjuez)
28300 Madrid
Spain
Email: irene@grapesadsl.com
Website: www.hipertensionpulmonar.com

Switzerland
German, French, Italian - Swiss Society For Pulmonary Hypertension SSPH
SSPH is a group representing experts in pulmonary hypertension (pulmonoglogists, critical care doctors, angiologists, cardiologists, pediatricians and internists) who can serve as a point of reference in PH information for the Swiss medical community and for patients.
Website: www.saph.ch

German - Selbsthilfegruppe Schweiz
im Rossweidli 1
CH- 8045 Zürich
Switzerland
Email: bosshard@lungenhochdruck.ch
Website: www.lungenhochdruck.ch

French - HTAP Revivre
Promenade de la Borgne 23
CH-1967 Bramois
Switzerland
Email: monika.sorgemaitre@hcuge.ch

UK
PHA UK
PO Box 2760
BN8 4WA Lewes, Sussex,
United Kingdom
Email: enquiries@pha-uk.com
Website: www.pha-uk.com

Julia Polak Research Trust
Tissue Engineering & Regenerative
Medicine Centre
Imperial College London
Chelsea & Westminster Hospital
369 Fulham Road
London SW10 9NH

United States
Pulmonary Hypertension Association (PHA)
(See start of chapter.)

PHCentral
A lively, well-designed, and informative
website with material of interest both to newly
diagnosed and "veteran" PH patients. Lists of
helpful books, PH news, scientific articles, and
interesting polls.
P.O. Box 477
Blue Bell PA, 19422
Email: info@PHCentral.org
www.phCentral.org

Israel
PH Israel
33 Inbar St.
30900 Zikhron Ya'akov
Israel
Email: iris_tal@netvision.net.il;
ajberg@gmail.com
Website: http://www.phisrael.org.il/

Japan
PHA-Japan
Village A-209 5-8 Tsukimino, Yamatoshi
242-002 Kanagawaken
Japan
Email: m-yukiko@cf6.so-net.ne.jp
Website: www.pha-japan.ne.jp

Mexico
**Asociacion Mexicana de Hipertension
Arterial Pulmonar (AMHAP)**
Instituto Nacional de Cardiologia
Juan Badiano #1-4 piso
14080 Mexico
D.F. Mexico
Email: pultom@cardiologia.org.mx;
hap_am@yahoo.com
Website: http://hapmx.ods.org/

South Africa
South African PH Support Group
30A-50th Avenue
04092 Umhlatuzana
South Africa
Email: dravid@mweb.co.za

Southeast Asia
PHA SEA (South East Asia)
Blk 46, #10-667, Circuit Road
370046 Singapore
Singapore
Email: smamub@yahoo.com.sg;
KohGM@nuh.com.sg

Venezuela
**Fundacion de Hipertension Pulmonar de
Venezuela**
Av Los Proceres Edif. Mactor 1 PB No 5
San Bernardino
Caracas
Venezuela
Email: phlatinsociety@hotmail.com

Nongovernmental Resources

Note: Many of the diseases that are associated with PH have their own organizations and websites. There are far too many to list here, but you can find such sites easily with a search engine. Go to www.healthfinder.gov for links to over 1,800 health-related organizations. Be wary of the information on sites that aren't well known or government sponsored. Look to see exactly who is behind the site and if the information was recently updated, and by whom. Just because the same information appears on more than one site doesn't make it more likely to be true.

ACCESS Program

Many PH patients have benefited from the services of the ACCESS (Advocating for Chronic Conditions, Entitlements and Social Services) Program. It is operated by Accredo Health (which is run independently from Accredo Therapeutics), *but you don't have to be a client of Accredo Therapeutics for ACCESS to help you.* ACCESS helps families navigate the complex maze of state and federal entitlement programs, as well as eligibility for health insurance through state and health insurance continuation programs (COBRA). All services are provided at no charge. They do not provide direct assistance with co-payments. A woman whose husband had severe hemophilia started ACCESS, and ACCESS' lawyers have devoted years to exploring the benefits and services available for chronically ill patients, including those with hemophilia, PAH, and a handful of other rare diseases. We're lucky to be on their list! For more information contact them at 1-888-700-7010 or www.accredotx.com/access/access.html.

Accredo Therapeutics

Accredo Therapeutics is a for-profit provider of all six FDA-approved medications for PAH (Flolan, Letairis, Remodulin, Revatio, Tracleer and Ventavis). With local pharmacies throughout the U.S., Accredo Therapeutics provides customized services to patients who require immediate access to clinical support and assistance with PAH therapies. Accredo Therapeutics is an active member of the PH community and impacts the lives of PH patients through the ACCESS Program (see above); clinical support and expertise with Flolan, Letairis, Remodulin, Revatio, Tracleer, and Ventavis; and through their financial support of PHA and involvement in PH support groups throughout the country. Patients needing assistance should call: 1-866-344-4874 (1-866-FIGHT PH).

Air and bus transportation, for free

Several groups provide free transportation (usually in small airplanes) to and from medical diagnosis and treatment for patients who cannot afford commercial means of transportation.

Air Charity Network™ (ACN). ACN is an umbrella organization comprised of a series of independent regional nonprofit organizations that together operate nationwide and help, free of charge, not only the financially challenged, but also those who cannot travel by other means because of their condition, the distance to the treatment facility, or threat of contagion on public transportation. Arrangements for oxygen can generally be made. ACN includes Airlift Hope, Angel Flight Central, Angel Flight Mid-Atlantic, Angel Flight Northeast, Angel Flight South Central, Angel Flight Southeast, Angel Flight West, Grace Flight, Mercy Flight Southeast and Mercy Medical Airlift. To reach the ACN organization that services your area, call toll-free phone: 1-877-621-7177. www.aircharitynetwork.org.

Here are three more outfits you can call if the patient is a child:

Miracle Flights for Kids™, 1-800-FLY-1711. www.miracleflights.org. They provide free air transportation to hospitals across America. It takes at least 10 business days to arrange a flight within the U.S. and at least 21 business days to arrange an international flight. An income certification form and other requirements must be met.

Operation Liftoff™, 314-298-9770. www.operationliftoff.com. They provide both treatment and "special" trips (such as to Disney World or a Broadway play) for children between the ages of 3 and 18 who are afflicted with a life-threatening illness and have not had a wish trip from another organization. It takes just a few days to arrange a trip.

Angel Bus™. On a smaller scale than the above air transportation programs, the new national nonprofit Angel Bus program helps children under 18 with a financial need make non-emergency trips to the hospital in comfort. Private coach owners donate their buses. Angel Bus coordinates with Angel Flight and the Make-a-Wish Foundation. www.angelbus.org. Toll-free phone: 1-877-428-4798. Referrals often come from counselors, ministers, or someone affiliated with a hospital.

American Society of Transplantation (AST)

Their website has a public policy library, information on legislation, patient information, and more. www.a-s-t.org. Phone: 1-856-439-9986.

Caremark Specialty Pharmacy

A for-profit company that provides Flolan, Letairis, Remodulin Revatio, Tracleer and Ventavis to PAH patients, along with the supplies needed to use them (Caremark acquired TheraCom, Inc. in 2004). They have a dedicated pulmonary hypertension nurse and pharmacist available 24 hours a day, 7 days a week, in case of emergencies. Their dedicated PAH line is 1-866-879-2348. Caremark will work with you and your insurance carrier to determine benefits, confirm and secure coverage, and assist with getting your PAH medicine covered.

Caring Voice Coalition

Caring Voice Coalition is dedicated to building relationships with charitable organizations founded to help individuals and families affected by serious chronic disorders and diseases. Caring Voice will work together with these organizations to offer outreach and support services that directly benefit the patient community. They can help identify resources for copay assistance for medications for qualified patients and families. They can be reached at 888.267.1440

Clinical Trial Information

While there is no central location for all clinical trials that are underway, there are a few resources for information regarding clinical trials. For information on thousands of federally and privately funded clinical trials, go to www.clinicaltrials.gov. The Rare Diseases Clinical Research Database contains a list of current PH clinical trials underway at the NIH Clinical Center in Bethesda, MD. Phone toll-free: 1-800-411-1222, TTY 1-866-411-1010, http://clinicalstudies.info.nih.gov. For some of the drug-industry sponsored trials go to CenterWatch, an information source for the clinical trials industry (www.centerwatch.com). Additional information can be found at www.phassociation.org/Clinical_Trials.

CuraScript

A provider of Letairis, Remodulin, Revatio, Tracleer, and Ventavis, this for-profit company is a national distributor of specialty pharmaceuticals and related medical supplies to the alternate healthcare market and a provider of patient-specific, self-injectable biopharmaceuticals and disease treatment programs to individuals with chronic diseases. Their PH center number is 1-888.773.7376. A pharmacist and nurse are available (by beeper, after hours) to help answer questions about site pain, pump malfunctions, dosing, etc.

Reimbursement specialists can try to help you with your insurance problems.

INR home testing kits

The advantages of home kits are convenience for the patient (especially those who live far from a clinic) and the ability to test weekly instead of the typical once-a-month test. Medicare covers the devices only for patients with mechanical heart valves and makes your doctor buy them for you through a reimbursement plan strangled in red tape. Private insurers are increasingly paying for them without the red tape. Some training is necessary. The cost is about $1,100-2,000. Several testing kits have been FDA approved: *AvoSure™ (Beckman Coulter)*. Phone: 888-AVOCET1 or 888-286-2381.
CoagCare® system (Zycare). Phone: (919)419-7228.
CoaguChek (Roche Diagnostics). Phone: 1-800-852-8766.
Harmony INR monitoring system (Lifescan). Phone: 1-877-520-8608.
INR@Home (Raytel). Phone: 1-877-729-8350.
INRatio (Hemosense). Phone: 1-800-563-5680.
ProTime Microcoagulation System (International Technidyne). Phone: 1-800-631-5945 or 732-548-6677.

Lung Line

The National Jewish Medical and Research Center provides these toll-free lines. Call: 1-800-552-5864 to reach Lung Facts, which offers prerecorded information on things like asthma, allergies, and COPD. They have some PH information but do not have a PH specialist. To speak to a person (for example to ask for one free copy of their booklet "Being Close: Dealing with Chronic Lung Disease and Intimacy") call 1-800-222-5864.

MedicAlert

A nonprofit foundation operating in 10 nations, MedicAlert provides bracelets, wallet cards, etc., with some of your medical information (diagnosis, drugs you take, dosages, allergies, doctors' names) and provides an emergency number that can be called around the clock, around the world, if someone finds you unconscious and unable to speak for yourself about your medical condition. Information that can't fit on the bracelet or card can thus be supplied over the phone. Yes, these bracelets have really saved the lives of PH patients. You can sign up online. Updates may be made by phone or online. Cost: $39.95 the first year and $25 a year thereafter, which includes free updates (also available is a 3 year membership for $65). 2323 Colorado Avenue Turlock, CA95382. Phone toll free: 1-800-432-5378. From outside the U.S. call: 209-668-3333. www.MedicAlert.org.

Medicare Rights Center

A national nonprofit organization that provides free counseling services on Medicare-related issues to Medicare beneficiaries, especially (but not exclusively) those who cannot afford private assistance. 520 Eighth Ave., North Wing, 3rd Fl., New York, NY 10018. Residents of NY state phone: 212-869-3850. 110 Maryland Ave, NE Suite 112, Washington, DC 20002, Phone: 202-544-5561. National Medicare HMO Appeals toll free: 1-888-HMO-9050. This line assists Medicare HMO members who are appealing HMO denials of care or coverage. www.medicarerights.org.

National Foundation for Transplants

Their goal is to make sure people who need transplants aren't turned away simply because they can't afford one. Phone toll free:1- 800-489-3863. Local phone: 901-684-1697. Email:info@transplants.org. www.transplants.org.

National Home Oxygen Patient's Association

A good group that some oxygen-using PH patients have joined and done volunteer work for. You can find information there on obtaining oxygen aboard airliners. www.homeoxygen.org.

NORD (National Organization for Rare Disorders, Inc.)

A nonprofit federation of voluntary health organizations that helps people with rare "orphan" diseases (such as PH) and assists the organizations serving them. NORD is committed to the identification, treatment, and cure of rare disorders through education, advocacy, research, and service. 55 Kenosia Avenue, PO Box 1968, Danbury, CT 06813-1968. Phone: 203-744-0100; toll free: 1-800-999-6673 (voice mail only); TDD: 203-797-9590. www.rarediseases.org.

Oxygen Users

In addition to the National Home Oxygen Patient's Association (above), check out www.portableoxygen.org. It's run by Peter M. Wilson, an oxygen user with no financial interest in the oxygen business who seems to know *everything* about various forms of portable oxygen.

Prescription drugs for low-income patients
Partnership for Prescription Assistance.

This interactive website by PhRMA and 48 of its member companies is designed to help patients find out if they qualify for patient-assistance programs. PhRMA claims that, in 2002, PhRMA members provided free prescription medicines to over 5.5 million patients in the U.S. www.pparx.org. Individual drug companies also have sites explaining assistance programs. Another place you can find information is at www.needymeds.com.

Prescription drugs: compare prices

To compare prescription drug prices within the U.S., try Google's "Product Search." Just go to Google, click on "Product Search", and type in the drug name. Or try websites like www.destinationrx.com. Also try Costcoand www.drugstore.com.

For Medicare patients: www.medicare.gov (you'll need to supply your zip code and the names of your prescriptions and the system will crank out the best card available for you in your area) or 1-800-Medicare and ask for the free "Guide to Choosing a Medicare-Approved Drug Discount Card."

What about drugs from Canada or Mexico? The legality of U.S. citizens filling their prescriptions in Canada or Mexico is in flux. Presently, a great many U.S. citizens order such drugs over the web or climb aboard a bus "drug tour" headed to Canada or Mexico. Not only are the prices often much lower, but the exchange rate may also boost your savings. (Prices are not *always* lower in Canada, especially on generic drugs, and prices vary from one Canadian pharmacy to another.) If you have insurance that covers drugs, check with your insurance provider to find if they will reimburse you. The reimbursement procedure may be a bit different than for prescriptions filled in the U.S. If you travel to Canada to buy medications, you will need a prescription from a Canadian doctor (clinics in border towns offer such walk-in service for about $20 to $40). The Canadian doctor will want to see an up-to-date prescription and a recent letter explaining your illness from your U.S. doctor. Be sure to declare your meds at U.S. customs; they allow only meds for your personal use. (Be alert for changes in custom laws.) It may be possible to avoid a trip to Canada if your U.S. doctor is willing to order and receive the prescription on your behalf. As of this writing, it is still possible and convenient to order Canadian drugs over the web. You can get the names of reputable online Canadian pharmacies through www.canadiandrugstores.com and other websites. Brand-name and generic prescription medications are closely regulated by the Canadian Health authorities for quality and safety. Still beware, because Canadian pharmacies may have different regulations than U.S. pharmacies. In Mexico you will need a prescription from a Mexican doctor; this is often done at the same time you get your prescription filled. The pharmacist will keep the original. Be sure you get a copy for U.S. customs. Some PH patients have been told by their doctors that the quality of drugs obtained in Mexico is questionable; if your sildenafil (Viagra), for example, is life-sustaining, you shouldn't take the risk.

The website of Consumer' Checkbook, www.checkbook.org, has a very good article on how to save money buying drugs (it's also in the spring/summer 2004 issue of *Puget Sound Consumers' Checkbook)*. AARP has been active in trying to lower the price of medications in the U.S., and their magazine and website have good suggestions.

Professional independent patient advocates for hire

These "hired guns" work for a fee. It may be as low as $50 for an uncomplicated case, or $200 to review a complicated one. Some charge $100 per hour or work on a contingency basis, for a percentage of any insurance payments their efforts obtain.

Always discuss fees up front. Don't confuse these guys with lawyers specializing in insurance cases or patient advocates hired by hospitals. Some employers have an advocate on their payroll to help employees. Advocates don't diagnose or treat you, but can negotiate with your insurance company, locate a specialist or nursing home, advise you on how

to complain about hospitals and insurance companies, etc. Before hiring anyone, try ACCESS first (for government entitlement claims). See, also, the Patient Advocate Foundation (listed below). You will also want to first ask your employer's human resources or benefits department for help, exhaust your insurer's in-house appeals (if you won't endanger your health by waiting for that process to creak along), and look into free state ombudsmen programs. Here are a few hired guns we've read about; undoubtedly there are others.

American Medical Consumers (1-818-957-3508); www.medconsumer.com. A nonprofit outfit.

Care-Counsel (San Rafael, CA)(415-472-2366); www.carecounsel.com.

Healthcare Advocates. Philadelphia, PN (215-735-7711); www.healthcareadvocates.com.

Patient Advocate Foundation. A national, nonprofit group that actively liaisons between patients and their insurers, employers, and/or creditors to resolve matters relative to their diagnosis. 1-800-532-5274. http://patientadvocate.org.

Second Wind Lung Transplant Association, Inc.

A forum to provide "support, love, advocacy, education, information and guidance" for people who have had, or are contemplating, lung transplants. They have a book for purchase, *Information You Should Know About Lung Transplantation: Before, During, and After*, with an extensive resource section and appendix. Second Wind also has a list of all lung and heart/lung transplant centers in the U.S. with information on average waiting times, which centers are Medicare approved, and how many transplants a center has done. 300 South Duncan Ave., Suite 227, Clearwater, FL 33755-6457. Phone toll free: 1-888-855-9463. www.2ndwind.org.

TRIO (Transplant Recipients International Organization)

TRIO offers information and help to people receiving and awaiting transplantation. Phone: 1-800-TRIO-386 (1-800-874-6386) or 1-202-293-0980. www.TRIOweb.org.

UNOS (United Network for Organ Sharing)

UNOS, an independent agency, has a federal contract to administer the National Organ Transplant Act, enacted by Congress in 1984. Data on survival rates for various kinds of transplants, waiting list times, and much more is available on the UNOS website: www.unos.org. UNOS collects and manages data about every transplant event occurring in the United States, facilitates the organ matching and placement process, and helps to develop organ transplantation policy.

Help from Uncle Sam

Centers for Medicare & Medicaid Services (CMS). The federal portal site for a wealth of information on these entitlements. www.cms.hhs.gov. Toll-Free: 1-877-267-2323; local: 410-786-3000; TTY toll-free: 1-866-226-1819; TTY Local: 410-786-0727.

DisabilityInfo.gov. The government's attempt to provide one-stop web shopping for information on federal disability programs. It contains information from 22 government sources. There are so many links it resembles a spider plant. www.disabilityinfo.gov.

Healthfinder. Go to www.healthfinder.gov for links to over 1,800 health-related organizations. This site is sponsored by the Dept. of Health and Human Services along with other federal agencies, to help you find the best government and nonprofit health information on the web. (They have a link to PHA.) Some information is available in several languages.

Medicare-Approved Lung and Heart-Lung Transplant Centers

A list of Medicare-approved transplant centers is available from the Centers for Medicare & Medicaid Services CMS), part of the Dept. of Health and Human Services. http://www.cms.hhs.gov/ApprovedTransplantCenters/01_overview.asp.

MEDLINE (Entrez PubMed), Medline Plus, PubMed Central, Etc.

The National Library of Medicine's exceedingly popular, free, website is a compendium of 14 million references and abstracts. **Entrez PubMed:** www.ncbi.nlm.nih.gov/sites/entrez. You can also get in through **MedlinePlus** (www.medlineplus.gov), a joint project of the National Library of Medicine and the National Institutes of Health. This trustworthy, reasonably up-to-date site offers a medical dictionary, drug information, information on diseases, information in Spanish, and information on clinical trials. Its background information on PH wasn't impressive, however. **PubMed Central** offers free, unrestricted access to the *entire text* of articles in selected journals (or that were contributed by selected authors). It is a digital archive of life sciences journal literature, developed and managed by the National Center for Biotechnology Information (NCBI) at the U.S. National Library of Medicine (NLM). www.pubmedcentral.nih.gov.

Keep this in mind when doing your research: a study reported in 2004 in the *Canadian Medical Association Journal* examined the association between industry funding and published pro-industry findings. The researchers found that "industry-funded trials are more likely to be associated with statistically significant pro-industry findings, both in medical trials and surgical interventions." This could be due to publication bias (journals are often loaded with ads), careful selection by drug companies of trials that are likely to be positive, or many other reasons. Not all medical journals require disclosure of funding sources, but it is becoming more common.

National Center for Biotechnology Information. An awesome website at www.ncbi.nlm.nih.gov. As you might guess from its address, the National Library of Medicine and the National Institutes of Health sponsor it. It has information ranging from genetics 101 to gene testing, gene therapy, and research in progress. One of its links is to the (NCBI's) "Genes and Disease" site, where you can search for our pulmonary hypertension gene to learn about its features and discovery.

National Heart, Lung, and Blood Institute (NHLBI). Part of the NIH, this group is of particular interest to PH patients because in 2007 it put $35.6 million into PH research and $1.9 million into PH-related training. Those are your tax dollars at work—for you! www.nhlbi.nih.gov View a report from their workshop on PH at www.nhlbi.nih.gov/meetings/wrokshops/pah-wksp.htm.

National Institutes of Health (NIH); NIH Office of Rare Diseases. There are 19 institutes and 8 centers that are part of the NIH. Several of them get their separate listings in this section. An A-Z index of NIH health resources, clinical trials, health hotlines, drug information and more can be found at www.nih.gov. For information on thousands of federally and privately funded clinical trials, go to www.clinicaltrials.gov. The Office of Rare Diseases site has information about more than 6,000 rare diseases, but not much on PH! http://rarediseases.info.nih.gov. The Rare Diseases

Clinical Research Database contains a list of current PH clinical trials underway at the NIH Clinical Center in Bethesda, MD. Phone toll-free: 1-800-411-1222, TTY 1-866-411-1010, http://clinicalstudies.info.nih.gov.

National Registry for Familial Primary Pulmonary Hypertension. Begun in 1994, this program is funded by the NIH, with research being done at Vanderbilt University in collaboration with geneticists at Indiana University and Ohio Children's Hospital Medical Center. The researchers collect information from families with hereditary "PPH" (now called FPAH) with the goal of learning the basic cause of the disease and developing new treatments. What they find helps identify new genes associated with FPAH, to identify genes that may modify the course of the disease, and to learn about the relationship between FPAH and environmental factors. (Such research helps patients with any kind of PH.) Nearly 100 U.S. families are currently enrolled in the study. Researchers know there are many more FPAH families out there. If you have more than one family member with PH, *please* join this effort! Families will be actively enrolled indefinitely. Your confidentiality is protected. Call toll free: 1-800-288-0378. For more information, contact project coordinator Lisa Wheeler (lisa.wheeler@vanderbilt.edu) or web surf to: www.mc.vanderbilt.edu/root/vumc.php?site=vupphstudy.

Social Security and Medicare. For information call toll-free:1- 800-772-1213 from 7AM to 7PM, Monday to Friday. If you have a touch-tone phone, recorded information and services are available 24 hours a day, including weekends and holidays. Toll-free TTY number:1-800-325-0778. Please have your Social Security number handy when you call. The labyrinthine home web page for the SSA is at www.ssa.gov. For Medicare, also see listing above for Centers for Medicare & Medicaid Services.

How to Find a Good PH Doctor or Clinic

PHA does not endorse some PH doctors or centers over others. Many PH centers have websites, but the quality of a site does not always reflect the quality of medical care. Sometimes your primary care physician can give you a good referral, but all too often PH patients are just referred to a pulmonologist or cardiologist who doesn't specialize in PH. So how can you find a good doctor and center of care? PHA plans to list its member doctors on its web page; if a doc joins PHA he/she probably has more than a passing interest in the disease. You might search PubMed (see above) to find out who has authored important PH research papers. Some doctors have written entire books on the subject of PH. Doctors contribute to *Pathlight,* or are mentioned therein. Another place to learn a little about PH doctors is in PHA's medical journal, *Advances in Pulmonary Hypertension* (past issues are available on PHA's website). Ask other PH patients how they like the center/doctors where they get care. An excellent way to find if you are on the same "wave length" with a doctor is to attend PHA conferences, listen to doctors speak, and ask them questions.

To learn where a doctor went to school, etc., go to www.ama-assn.org and look under "DoctorFinder." To learn if a doctor is board certified try The American Board of Medical Specialties at www.abms.org/newsearch.asp.

Bibliography of PH-Related Research Papers

An extensive bibliography prepared by Kathy Hague, RN, is available at www.PHAssociation.org.

Reference Books of Interest to PH Patients

Gersh, Bernard J., ed. The Mayo Clinic Heart Book, Second Edition, William Morrow & Co., 2000. Useful and easily understood descriptions of heart-related medical conditions including PH/PPH, tests used to diagnose such conditions, and treatment issues. $21, new, on www.Amazon.com.

The Merck Manual of Medical Information, Home Edition (Second Edition), Merck & Co., 2003. A whopping 1,907 pages, this is an excellent source of "everyday language" information on many of the medical conditions that relate to PH. It has a few pages on PH itself. $37.50. You can get it used through Amazon for half that, or for about $3 if a used paperback is okay.

A Glossed-Over Glossary

You can find the definitions of many medical terms online. Two useful sites are MedlinePlus (www.nlm.nih.gov/medlineplus/ency) and Hyperdictionary (www.hyperdictionary.com).

- A -

ACE inhibitors. ACE stands for angiotensin-converting enzyme. ACE inhibitors help prevent the conversion inside our bodies of angiotensin I to angiotensin II (a powerful vasoconstrictor). Drugs in this class (e.g. Accupril) dilate arteries and let blood flow through them with less resistance. It isn't known, yet, if they will help some PH patients.

acute vasodilator challenge. During a right-heart catheterization, drugs like vasodilators or prostacyclin are injected into a catheter (that has been inserted into your heart) to see how your cardiac output and pulmonary vascular pressures respond.

angina (two pronunciations: AN-jin-ah, an-JIGH-neh). The word means a sense of suffocation. It is often used as shorthand for angina pectoris, which means chest pain, or a sense of pain or pressure about the heart. The pain may radiate down the left arm and is caused by an insufficiency of blood to the muscle wall of the right ventricle of the heart. The pain lasts from a few seconds to several minutes. Symptoms are more variable in women.

angiogram (AN-jee-o-gram). An x-ray picture of blood vessels after a radiopaque dye is injected to make the vessels more visible.

anticoagulants. "Blood thinners" that make the blood less likely to clot. Warfarin (Coumadin, Panwarfin) is frequently used. Another is heparin (given by IV).

arginine. We're interested in arginine because it is one of the things our bodies use to make nitric oxide, and because it comes in pill form. Researchers are looking at arginine's possible helpfulness in reducing the symptoms of PH, especially in PH/sickle cell anemia patients. Arginine is an essential amino acid. "Essential" means our bodies can't make their own arginine, so we need to get it from the foods we eat. A normal endothelium makes enough NO to control blood pressure, but the endothelia of PH patients are damaged and might not be up to the task.

atrium. One of the two upper chambers of the heart. **Atria** is the plural of atrium.

atrial fibrillation. When the regular beating of an atrium is replaced by rapid, random twitches. Less blood is therefore pumped.

apnea (AP-nee-uh). Temporary cessation of breathing.

ascites (eh-SIGH-tees). Watery fluids in the abdominal cavity, making you swell up.

- B -

beraprost. *See* **prostanoids**. A synthetic version of prostacyclin taken in pill form.

bosentan. *See* **endothelin receptor antagonists**.

BMPR2. The "PH gene." Its full name is bone morphogenetic protein receptor II, and mutations on it have been linked to both familial and sporadic PAH.

bronchiolitis obliterans (a.k.a. obliterative bronchiolitis, OB). Chronic rejection of a lung or lungs after a transplant.

– C

calcium channel blockers (CCBs). Vasodilating drugs in pill form such as nifedipine (Procardia XL, Adalat), diltiazem (Cardizem), and Norvasc that make perhaps up to 10 to 15 percent of PH patients feel much better by relaxing artery walls, thus increasing blood flow to the lungs.

cardiac catheterization. A catheter is put into a blood vessel and wiggled into your heart so doctors can learn about the pressures in there, how your blood flows, and evaluate structural defects.

cardiac output. The total amount of blood the heart pumps per minute. In a healthy person this is about 5 liters; in someone with severe PH it can be only 2-3 liters. (A human has about 5 liters [roughly 5.3 quarts] of blood per 70 kilograms [about 150 pounds] of body weight.)

catheter. A thin, flexible tube inserted into the body for injecting or removing fluids. A surgeon puts one end of a central line catheter into your heart; the other end stays outside your body so you can put medicine into it.

Cialis. *See* **phosphodiesterase inhibitors**.

Classes I, II, III, and IV. *See* **functional classifications for PH**.

collagen vascular disease (a.k.a. connective tissue disease). Disorders affecting joints (muscles, bones, tendons, cartilage). There is often an autoimmune component. Types associated with PH include SLE (lupus), scleroderma, and mixed connective tissue disease.

COPD (chronic obstructive pulmonary disease). Generalized obstruction of the small airways in the lungs associated with chronic bronchitis, emphysema, asthma, etc.

cor pulmonale. Enlargement of the right ventricle of the heart. It can be caused by PH. See Chapter 1 (and the drawing of the normal and enlarged heart).

CREST syndrome. A trigger of PH, it is a somewhat dated term for a form of scleroderma that includes calcium deposits in the skin, Raynaud's phenomenon, esophageal involvement, swollen fingers with tight skin, and skin reddened/discolored by blood vessels.

CT or CAT scan. An x-ray image of your insides gotten by narrow x-rays beamed at you from several angles and run through a computer so doctors can look at cross sections of you, including soft tissue.

Coumadin. A trade name for warfarin, an **anticoagulant** (see above).

cyanosis (sigh-ah-NO-sis). Blue skin--usually the lips, nails, or tongue--caused by lack of oxygen.

– D

diastole (die-ASS-toe-lee). The period when the heart is relaxed and filling with blood . Diastolic pressure: the bottom, lower number in your blood pressure). *See* **systole**.

digoxin. A drug that seems to help a weak right ventricle of the heart squeeze better.

dilate. To relax, expand.

diuretic. A chemical that helps you lose water by increasing the amount of urine. Sometimes called a "water pill."

dyspnea (DISP-nee-eh). Labored breathing; shortness of breath.

– E –

echocardiogram (echo). A graphic record produced by ultrasonic waves bounced off your heart to show its structures and functioning.

edema (eh-DEE-mah). Swelling.

Eisenmenger's complex. Because of a birth defect in the heart, too much blood goes to the lungs, which results in PH.

electrocardiogram (ECG or EKG). A graphic record produced by a device that detects the electrical activity of the heartbeat.

embolus (EM-buh-les) (plural, **emboli**). A clump of something (usually a blood clot) or a bubble that has plugged up a blood vessel. An **embolism** is the blockage of a vessel by an embolus. It's usually a blood clot that has formed somewhere else and traveled to the lungs. A thrombus is a fibrinous blood clot that obstructs a blood vessel. If a thrombus forms in one place and moves to another, it is called a thrombotic embolus. Sorry you asked? Just think of them all as blood clots.

endothelin. A chemical made by the **endothelium** (see below). It causes the smooth muscles in blood vessel walls to tighten up. PAH patients have too much endothelin in their blood.

endothelin receptor antagonists. Drugs such as bosentan (Tracleer), ambrisentan, and sitaxsentan (Thelin) taken in pill form that keep endothelin from attaching to ET_A and/or ET_B receptors in smooth muscle cells in little pulmonary arteries. This keeps the vessels from tightening up as much. An endothelin receptor antagonist might be dual (such as bosentan) or selective to just one of the receptors (such as sitaxsentan or ambrisentan).

endothelium. The one-cell thick lining of the blood and lymph vessels, the heart, and some other things. If you spread yours out, it would cover a football field! Endothelial cells produce lots of chemical compounds that affect platelets and make vessel walls relax and dilate.

enzymes. Organic catalysts made by cells that can act inside or outside of cells, controlling the rate of chemical reactions without being changed themselves (an enzyme can help the same process along over and over).

epoprostenol sodium (Flolan). A prostanoid (see below) that has several beneficial effects for most PH patients including vasodilatation, slowing or stopping the process of fibrosis inside little pulmonary arteries, making blood less likely to clot, etc. It is administered through a central line catheter.

etiology (ee-tee-AWL-o-gee). The cause of a disease.

– F –

familial pulmonary arterial hypertension (FPAH). This term is used when genetic studies and/or a family history of PPH have shown that members of a family carry the "PH gene," so the disease is inherited. It used to be lumped into the old category of primary pulmonary hypertension (PPH).

fibrin. Thrombin acts on fibrinogen to form this insoluble hunk of protein (part of the blood coagulation process).

fibrosis (fie-BROH-sis). When inflammation or other irritants cause a build-up of fiber-like tissue (scarring).

Flolan. *See* **prostanoids**. Flolan is the trade name for epoprostenol sodium that is administered through a central line **catheter**. The trade name Flolan is not familiar to U.K. patients, who know the drug as prostacyclin.

functional classifications for PH. PH patients are put into one of four possible classes; which class you are in depends on the severity of your symptoms and may affect your choice of treatments. You will find references in the literature to both **WHO class** and to modified **NYHA class** (WHO Class III, for example, or NYHA Class III). The World Health Organization (WHO) simply modified the New York Heart Association (NYHA) categories for generic heart failure to make them specific to PH patients. The WHO and NYHA classes are essentially identical, except that if you are prone to fainting, you automatically go into Class IV under the WHO scheme. See Chapter 1 to learn which patients are in each class.

- G -

Gaucher's (go SHAZE) **disease.** An inherited disease where the lack of an enzyme leads to the accumulation of a fatty substance. If the fatty cells accumulate in the lungs, it can lead to secondary PH.

- H -

hemodynamics. Pressures in the heart, the movements of the blood, and the forces involved in the circulation of blood throughout the entire body or to particular areas of it (the heart and lungs, in our case). Typically, hemodynamics refers to blood pressures, cardiac output, and resistance. Some say you need a degree in physics to fully understand it.

herpesvirus 8 (HHV-8). A newly discovered member of the herpesvirus family, IPAH patients appear to be considerably more likely to be infected with HHV-8 than are members of the general population. Persons with HIV infections are also more likely to also be infected with HHV-8. Kaposi's sarcoma, which afflicts some HIV patients, is similar in some ways to the plexiform lesions found in the small pulmonary arteries of PH patients.

hypertension. Abnormally high blood pressure.

hypotension. Abnormally low blood pressure.

hypoxemia. Too low a concentration of oxygen in the blood. This condition is a potent vasoconstrictor.

hypoxia. A low concentration of oxygen in the air that is breathed, such as occurs aboard an airliner or high on a mountain.

- I -

idiopathic. Without a recognizable cause.

idiopathic pulmonary arterial hypertension (IPAH). Formerly called **primary pulmonary hypertension** (PPH). It means **pulmonary arterial hypertension** (see below) where the cause is unknown. This category used to (and still does, in some literature) include PH that runs in families (FPAH), PH caused by taking various drugs, and PH triggered by diseases not directly associated with the heart and lungs, such as liver dise:

iloprost. *See* **prostanoid**. A stable version of prostacyclin that is usually inhaled, although it is sometimes given by IV, and clinical trials involving an oral form have been undertaken.

INR level. Pro-time (how long it takes your blood to clot) translated into a standardized number, so it doesn't depend on the reagent used and results can be compared among labs.

intravenous. Administered by injection into a vein.

ischemia (is-KEE-mee-eh). A localized, temporary reduction in the number of oxygen-carrying red blood cells because of a blockage of blood flow.

– K –

Kaplan-Meier estimates of survival, a.k.a. Kaplan-Meier survival plot. These phrases appear in the captions on some graphs. It is a statistical technique that allows researchers to estimate survival even when all the patients in a study have not been on a drug for the same length of time.

– L –

lesion (LEE-zhun). An area of diseased or injured tissue.

Levitra. *See* phosphodiesterase inhibitors.

– M –

mean pulmonary artery pressure (mean PAP). When your heart contracts ("beats") blood pressure rises in your pulmonary arteries (this is your systolic artery pressure). Pressure falls when your heart relaxes between beats (your diastolic pressure). Your "mean PAP" is a continuous average of the pressures in your arteries throughout a complete squeeze/relax cycle. You can find your mean PAP by multiplying your diastolic artery pressure by two and adding the product to your systolic artery pressure, and dividing the total by three. The result is always closer to your diastolic pressure than to your systolic pressure.

MRI (magnetic resonance imaging). By using a strong magnetic field and low-energy radio waves, technicians can look wherever they want to inside your body. This is the test that often requires you to lie inside a white tunnel, fight claustrophobia, and listen to what sounds like sneakers tumbling in a dryer.

– N –

NHLBI. The National Heart, Lung, and Blood Institute. This is from their website: "The Institute plans, conducts, fosters, and supports an integrated and coordinated program of basic research, clinical investigations and trials, observational studies, and demonstration and education projects. Research is related to the causes, prevention, diagnosis, and treatment of heart, blood vessel, lung, and blood diseases; and sleep disorders." PHA interacts with the NHLBI through the agency's Public Interest Organizations group. A PHA representative (Judy Simpson, R.N.) has served on the planning committee of this group and lobbied hard to focus attention on PH issues.

NIH. The National Institutes of Health, a part of the U.S. Department of Health and Human Services.

nitric oxide (NO). A potent vasodilator in gas form. (Not the same thing as nitrous oxide, which is laughing gas.) NO is made both in our bodies and in labs. It is being used experimentally on some PH patients and is known to help newborn babies with persistent pulmonary hypertension. The nice thing about NO is that it is selective for the lungs, so it doesn't cause systemic dilation.

– O –

oximeter. A gizmo you put on your fingertip to measure the concentration of oxygen in your blood. It's desirable to be at least 90 percent "saturated."

- P -

palpitation. A sensation of rapid or throbbing heartbeats.

PAP. For our purposes, it means pulmonary artery pressure, not a smear done by a gynecologist. Do not confuse it with your "mean pulmonary artery pressure" (see above).

pathogenesis. The biography of a disease.

persistent pulmonary hypertension of the newborn (PPHN). When a newborn's arteries to the lungs remain constricted after delivery, cutting down on blood flow to the lungs and resulting in PH.

perfusion lung scan. After a dye that shows up on x-rays is injected, your chest is scanned with penetrating radiation to look for blood clots.

PH gene. *See* **BMPR2**. Others may yet be discovered.

phosphodiesterase (PDE-5) inhibitors. Drugs such as sildenafil (Viagra), tadalafil, (Cialis), or vardenafil (Levitra). Approved by the FDA and the regulatory bodies in many other countries to treat erectile dysfunction, such drugs are now being tried (often in combination with other PH drugs) to dilate pulmonary arteries. The drugs are fairly selective for vessels in the penis and lungs, so they have fewer side effects than some other options.

portopulmonary hypertension. PH associated with high blood pressure in the liver.

primary pulmonary hypertension (PPH). Pulmonary arterial hypertension (see below) where the cause is unknown. An imprecise, dated term, it has now been split into two categories: idiopathic pulmonary arterial hypertension (IPAH) (see above), and familial pulmonary arterial hypertension (FPAH). As originally used by doctors and researchers, the category PPH often included other types of PAH patients as well: those who got PAH from certain diet pills or street drugs, or who had PAH associated with the HIV virus. When the author was not certain exactly which groups were included in a study, PPH is put in quotes: "PPH."

prostacyclin, a.k.a. prostaglandin 12 (PG12). A prostanoid (see below), made by our bodies that helps pulmonary blood vessels respond to a lack of oxygen by dilating, and that PH patients don't make enough of. (The name comes from the prostate gland because prostaglandin was first isolated from seminal fluid and was thought to have been made by the prostate!) In addition to being a vasodilator, prostacyclin may inhibit the proliferation of smooth muscle cells.

prostanoid. Technically, a prostanoid is an end product of the cyclo-oxygenase pathway of the metabolism of arachidonic acid. It could be a prostaglandin or a thromboxane. Got that? In this book, we use the term to mean a manufactured substance much like prostacyclin (see above). Members of the prostacyclin family of drugs are chemically very similar to one another (they are analogs). Present analogs include epoprostenol sodium (Flolan), treprostenol sodium (Remodulin), beraprost sodium (Dorner, Procylin), and iloprost (Ventavis). These prostacyclin analogs help many PH patients by dilating blood vessels, reducing clotting, slowing down the growth of smooth muscle cells, and improving cardiac output. Although they are all in the same class of drugs, they are not identical, and their toxicity, side effects, and effectiveness may differ.

pro-time. Prothrombin time; how long it takes your blood to clot. Used to see if you are taking the right amount of warfarin. *See* **INR level**.

pulmonary. Relating to the lungs.

pulmonary artery. The blood vessel carrying blood from the right ventricle of the heart to the lungs, where the blood is oxygenated.

pulmonary artery wedge pressure. A little balloon on the tip of a catheter is inflated (wedged) in the pulmonary artery where it can measure pulmonary vein pressures.

pulmonary arterial hypertension (PAH). PH caused by problems in the small arteries of the lungs. It includes **idiopathic PAH (IPAH)**, **familial PAH (FPAH)**, **persistent PH of the newborn** (PPHN), PH triggered by collagen vascular disease, congenital heart disease, portal hypertension, HIV infection, certain drugs and toxins, etc. It specifically excludes PH due to left-sided heart disease.

pulmonary function tests (PFTs). These are done to find out how much air your lungs can hold, how well they move air in and out, and how well they exchange oxygen. You breathe into a device called a spirometer, or into a flow meter. The tests can help diagnose some conditions that trigger PH.

pulmonary hypertension (PH). High blood pressure in the pulmonary artery because of changes in the small blood vessels in the lungs that make it harder for blood to flow through the vessels. In this manual, the term PH includes all types of PH unless otherwise indicated.

pulmonary thromboendarterectomy. A surgical procedure to remove a blood clot (or clots) in a pulmonary artery in the lungs.

pulmonary vascular resistance (PVR). This is a measure of how difficult it is for the heart to pump blood through the lungs. It is measured by dividing the pressure drop across the lungs (mean pulmonary artery pressure minus left atrial ["wedge"] pressure) by the cardiac output (blood flow per minute). PVR therefore reflects not only PAP, but also cardiac function. If cardiac function is good, the PVR will be lower. Some drugs, such as epoprostenol, may not improve a patient's PAP, but the patient feels better because his/her cardiac output has improved. PVR measurement requires a cardiac catheterization--an echocardiogram can't do it.

pulmonary venous hypertension. PH caused by problems *downstream* from the air sacs in the lungs. It includes problems with the left side of the heart, pulmonary veno-occlusive disease, compression of the central pulmonary veins, etc.

– R –

Raynaud's (RAY-nose) phenomenon. When fingers get blue and cold easily because of a vascular disorder. Persons with Raynaud's are more likely to have PH than someone without this condition.

Remodulin (known as UT-15 and Uniprost in early stages of development). *See* **prostanoid.** A prostanoid that has a longer half-life than Flolan and needn't be refrigerated in the pump. It is pumped into the fat under the skin; studies are underway to get approval to deliver it through central line catheters as well.

right atrial pressure. An index of right-heart failure.

right-heart catheterization. A thin tube with a special tip is inserted into a neck or groin vein and threaded into the pulmonary artery where it measures the pressures.

right ventricle. The chamber of the heart that pumps unoxygenated blood through the pulmonary arteries and into the lungs. In PH patients, this chamber is often enlarged, and its walls thickened.

– S –

scleroderma (skler-eh-DER-mah). Like PH, this is a progressive and possibly fatal disease. The body's tissues slowly harden. In some persons, only the skin is affected; in others even the internal organs harden, including the lungs. It is not known what causes it. Scleroderma is a common cause of PH.

secondary pulmonary hypertension (SPH). Pulmonary hypertension that is caused by a pre-existing disease.

sildenafil. *See* phosphodiesterase inhibitor.

Sitaxsentan. *See* endothelin receptor antagonists.

sleep apnea. A disorder where someone stops breathing long enough, while asleep, to decrease the amount of oxygen in their blood. It can trigger mild PH

syncope (SIN-ko-pee). Fainting because of a temporary insufficiency of blood to the brain.

systemic. Something that affects the body generally.

systemic lupus erythematous (SLE). A progressive autoimmune inflammatory disease of connective tissue. Its cause is unknown and it is often fatal. A skin rash is often present that spreads across the face in a butterfly pattern. The disease often involves the heart and lungs. It is associated with PAH (patients with SLE are much more likely to get PAH than people in the general population-the general incidence of IPAH is only 1 or 2 in a million).

systole (SIS-toe-lee). The period when your heart is contracting and squeezing blood out. **Systolic pressure** is the top, higher number in your blood pressure. *See* **diastole.**

– T –

Thelin. *See* endothelin receptor antagonists.

Tracleer. *See* endothelin receptor antagonists.

– V –

vasoconstrictor. Anything that narrows the blood vessels, thereby increasing blood pressure.

vasodilator. Anything that relaxes and widens blood vessels, thereby decreasing blood pressure.

Viagra. *See* phosphodiesterase inhibitors.

VO2. A measure of the amount of oxygen (O2) that the body takes in (and thus uses). Doctors measure peak VO2 during exercise-the higher the number, the better the condition of your heart and lungs. It is measured in milliliters of oxygen per minute.

– W –

warfarin. *See* anticoagulant.

Acknowledgements

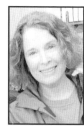

The author: Gail Boyer Hayes

Gail was diagnosed with IPAH in 1983, and treated with CCBs from 1993 to the present. Formerly a magazine editor, speechwriter, TV talk show hostess, book reviewer, and lawyer, and now a writer/editor, she serves on PHA's Board of Trustees. Gail lives in Seattle with her husband and co-conspirator, Denis.

Medical Editor: Dr. Ron Oudiz
Associate Professor of Medicine
David Geffen School of Medicine at UCLA
Director, Liu Center for Pulmonary Hypertension
Clinical Director, Wasserman Cardiopulmonary Exercise Laboratory
Harbor-UCLA Medical Center
Torrance, CA

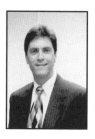

Ron was introduced to PH by Dr. Bruce Brundage in the early 1990s and owes the success of the Harbor-UCLA PH Clinic to Bruce, as well as to his enduring and giving coordinators, Joy and Daisy. He "volunteered" to be the Medical Editor and shares in the pride of contributing to this work. Ron's beautiful wife and two wonderful young children kept him going as the author's chapters kept rolling in for review.

The "Survival Team":
They volunteered to make notes on the tapes from PHA's 2002 International Conference sessions, provide material, answer questions, look up facts, etc.: **Pam Adams, Cindy Caldwell, Anne Caesar** (MD) and her husband **Bruce Gordon, Betsey Crittenden, Rebecca Dworkin, Stephanie Harris** (RN, BSN), **Maureen Keane, Paula Patty, Jessica Poisson, Cathy Severson** (RN, BSN), and **Michelle Smith**.

In tribute to these deceased "Survival Team" volunteers:
Sarah Ing. This remarkable young woman is best described in her own well-written words (www.PHCentral.org).
Lester J. Ishado. Deputy Corporation Counsel, County of Hawaii, Hilo, Hawaii.
Claudia Sample (BSBA, CPDM, and a certified case manager for CasePro). A PPH patient, but her death was caused mostly by an invasive melanoma.
Cynthia Ylagan, M.D. She formerly worked at Far Eastern University in Manila, Philippines, and lived in New Jersey at the time of her death.
Louise Morrison was a business and travel writer and a computer science teacher. Pre-PH,

she climbed high mountains in Tibet and Peru.

Elaine Rubin, an active member and leader of the Connecticut support group, she also worked full-time teaching math to elementary school students in spite of her PH.

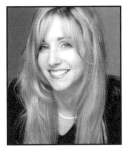

Cover artist and photographer: Michelle Smith

A young graphic artist, illustrator, and web-page designer, Michelle was diagnosed with PH due to a congenital heart defect when she was a year old. She became symptomatic in her twenties and was forced to retire from the work that she loved. She now paints (with a focus on watercolors), designs web sites, reads, gardens, dabbles in interior design, and tries to keep up with her two "neurotic miniature pinschers." You can view more of her art at http://h2oArtist.home.comcast.net. Epoprostenol helps to control her PH. "I'm married to a wonderful and understanding man," she says, "who is also my best friend." Matt and Michelle live in the San Francisco Bay Area.

Co-Revisers of Chapter 5 on PH Drugs:
Glenna Traiger, RN, MSN & Juliana C. Liu, RN, MSN, ANP

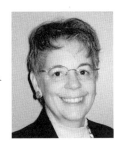

Glenna started caring for patients with pulmonary hypertension in 1999 with Dr. Shelley Shapiro. Currently the PAH program is located at the Greater LA VA Healthcare System/UCLA and the Support Group (West LA) is entering its ninth year. Glenna is reminded daily of the courage, strength and resourcefulness of her PH patients.

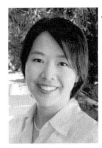

Juliana is the adult nurse practitioner for the Vera Moulton Wall Center for Pulmonary Vascular Disease at Stanford University Medical Center. Juliana received her MSN from the University of California, San Francisco, where she completed both her registered nursing as well as her adult nurse practitioner training. She worked as a cardiac nurse in the acute and critical care setting, where she developed an interest in cardiopulmonary diseases. She is a member of the Research and Publications Committee for the PH Resource Network, serving briefly as committee Chair. Juliana was born in Hong Kong, and grew up in Tokyo. She speaks Japanese fluently and has aural comprehension of Mandarin Chinese. Through PHA, she has been able to partner with PH clinicians in Japan, where she presented at a PH nurses' symposium. She hopes that her background can help play a role in developing understanding and knowledge sharing about PH worldwide.

Author of Chapter 9 on What to Eat: Maureen Keane, M.S.

Marueen is a nutritionist and the best-selling author of 13 books on health, including *Juicing for Life* and *What to Eat If You Have Cancer*. She holds a masters degree in nutrition and is certified by the State of Wash. as a nutritionist. She is also a member of the American Dietetic Assoc. and the Society for Nutrition Education. Diagnosed with PPH in 1996, Maureen first responded to CCBs, but was soon put on epoprostenol. Five years later, she

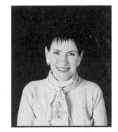

had improved enough to turn off her pump, and for the past two years she has been stable on bosentan. A coveted speaker for PH support groups, she lives with her husband John in Mukilteo, Wash.

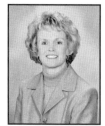

Creator of charts on PH Drugs and Flolan Emergencies:
Cathy J. Anderson-Severson, RN, BSN

Cathy works with Dr. Michael McGoon at the Mayo Clinic. She has been in the PH field for about 20 years, and loves every new challenge that occurs. When pressed, she says she's just a low-key person, a "country bumpkin," who has lived in the Rochester, Minn. area all her life.

Grammar/Style Reviewer & Indexer and Resources Updater: Paula Patty

Paula learned a whole new skill to do the first-ever index for the *Survival Guide.* She is an FPAH patient, who owes much to her gracious mother Esther who lived with PAH for over 15 years using only conventional treatments. Paula is an "Army Brat" who has lived all over the United States and France. She received her degrees in Operations Reseach and worked for American Airlines and Fair, Isaac for over 14 years. Now retired, she continues her studies, focusing on the arts and Spanish. She loves to cook, play poker, and garden. A combination of PH drugs including bosentan and sildenafil make all this activity possible. She and her wonderful husband Bruce live in the San Francisco Bay Area with their two retrievers.

Medical Reviewers:

Poor Dr. Oudiz had little idea what he was getting into, but coped patiently and intelligently, gathering input from his fellow medical professionals (and their staff), all renowned in the field of PH and members (some former, some present) of PHA's Scientific Leadership Council: **David Badesch**, MD (U. of Colo.); **Robyn Barst**, MD (Columbia Presby. Med. Center, N.Y. Presby. Hosp.); **Joy Beckmann,** RN, MSN (Harbor-UCLA); **Todd Bull**, MD (U. of Colo. Health Sciences Center); **Aimee Doran**, RN, CPNP (U. of Colo.); **Gregory Elliott**, MD (U. of Utah); **Alfred P. Fishman** , Prof. of Med. (U. of Pa. Health System); **Adaani Frost**, MD (Baylor Coll. of Med.); **Sean Gaine**, MD (Mater Misericordiae Hospital, Dublin, Ire.); **Nazzareno Galiè** , MD (U. di Bologna, It.); **Nicholas Hill**, MD (Tufts-N.E. Med. Center); **Marc Humbert**, MD (Hôpital Antoine Béclère, Clamart, Fr.); **Dunbar Ivy**, MD (U. of Colo.); **Abby Krichman**, RRT (Duke U. Med. Center); **David Langleben**, MD (Jewish General Hosp., Montreal, Can.); **James E. Loyd,** MD (Vanderbilt U. Med. Center); **Michael McGoon**, MD (Mayo Clinic, Rochester); **Valerie McLaughlin**, MD (U.of Mich.); **John H. Newman**, MD (Vanderbilt U. Med. Center); **Horst Olschewski** , MD (Justus-Liebig U., Ger.); **Harold I. Palevsky**, MD (U. of Penn. School of Med.); **Stuart Rich**, MD (U. of Chicago Hosp.); **Marlene Rabinovitch**, MD (Stanford U.); **Ivan Robbins**, MD (Vanderbilt U.); **Lewis J. Rubin**, MD (U. of Calif. at San Diego); **Cathy J. Severson** , RN, BSN (Mayo Clinic, Rochester); **Shelley Shapiro**, MD (UCLA); **Victor Tapson**, MD (Duke U. Med. Center); and **Allison Widlitz**, PA (N.Y. Presby. Hosp.).

These reviewers provided the patient's perspective:

Linda Carr

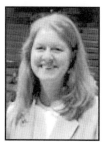

Linda and her husband are parents to three children, one of whom has IPAH and has been treated with epoprostenol since 1994. Before starting a family, Linda worked as a teacher and in the entertainment industry in Los Angeles. She has served on PHA's Board of Trustees since 1997, as President of PHA, and a great deal more. She is currently the 2008 PHA International Conference co-Chairperson. Linda and her family live in Miami Springs, Florida.

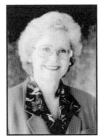

Susan Salay

A former corporate executive in the computer industry, Susan is a PAH patient and long-term survivor (10 years and counting). Now retired, she served on PHA's Board of Trustees until 2007 and was Chairperson of the PHA International Conference in Irvine, Calif., in 2002. Susan's the proud mother of two grown sons, a caregiver to her parents, and is the delighted mom to Marcel (a baby poodle!). She lives in Irvine, Calif.

Judy Simpson

A nurse, Judy became interested in PH when her sister, Pat Paton, was diagnosed with IPAH 20 years ago. Pat and Judy and their husbands (Jerry and Ed) have been active in PHA from the beginning. Judy was founding president. She has been a PHA volunteer and advocate ever since, serving on the Board of Trustees and in many other roles. She was a member of the National Health, Heart, Lung and Blood Institute Advisory Council as a patient advocate. Judy and Ed live in Holiday Island, Arkansas.

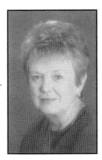

Help on updating legal information:

Lawyers Penni Potter and Bill Leach of ACCESS (operated by Accredo Health) reviewed Chapter 14. Penni also reviewed Chapter 13's section on the Medicare Part D prescription drug plan for the Fall 2007 reprint.

Others who contributed:

Many patients also gave permission to use their stories, and doctors and nurses not listed above answered queries. The author's own doctor, David Ralph (University of Washington) cheerfully answers her endless questions. The professional staff of PHA was, as always, extremely helpful. Particular thanks go to Rino Aldrighetti for looking into and facilitating many issues, and to Kaaryn Sanon, who formatted this book. Thanks also to all those who volunteered their help on the first two editions of this book, because their mark is still visible. In particular, thank you, Dr. Bruce Brundage, for serving as medical consultant, Dr. Stuart Rich for your invaluable comments, and Andrea Rich for your illustrations.

New as of Fall 2007:

As we begin revisions to the third edition of this book, a new system has been implemented so that *A Patient's Survival Guide* can be produced for the PH community for many years to come. Gail Boyer Hayes has been a tremendous author and organizer in taking on all previous editions - words cannot express our gratitude. Since no single writer, reader, or thinker can fill Gail's shoes, the book will now be updated on a rolling basis, chapter by chapter, twice per year. Teams of medical professionals and patients have begun the process of researching and updating this book. For the September 2007 reprint, a well-deserved "thank you" goes to:

Paula Patty, for updating the governmental and non-governmental resources sections of *Chapter 14 - Resources.*

Juliana Liu, RN, MSN, ANP, for updating the *Chapter 5 - PH Drugs* section on ERAs, the medications chart, and contributing to various "spot updates" throughout the book.

Index

Anorexia. *See also* appetite, decrease in
  digoxin, 67
  epoprostenol, 95, 98
Antacids, 67, 191
Anthracosis, 53
Antibiotics, 101, 173, 203
  digoxin, 67
  INR and children, 170
  prophylactic, 196
  transplantation, 160
  warfarin, impact on, 65
Antibody, 27, 179
Anticoagulants, 61–66, 62, 195. *See also*
  Warfarin
  aspirin, in addition to, 63
  children, 166
  conventional therapy, 59
  CTEPH, 57
  dosing, 62
  epoprostenol, drug interaction with, 104
  precautions, 66
  pulmonary thromboendarterectomy, 124
  side effects, 64–65
Antidepressants, 44, 46, 181, 186, 205
Anti-dumping statute, 198
Antifungal agents, 65
Antigen, 27
Antihistamines, 203
Antinuclear antibody, 27
Antioxidants, 181, 182, 185, 189
Antiplatelet drug, 104
Antipyretics, 153
Anti-rejection medications, 140, 141
Antiretroviral therapy, 148
Anxiety, 2, 67, 78
  children, 165
  epoprostenol, 97
  magnesium, 182
  sleep apnea, 54
APAH, 4, 27, 34–50, 45, 46, 60–61, 95. *See
  also* PAH
  autoimmune disease, link to, 27
  calcium channel blockers, 76
  nitric oxide, 86
  transplantation, 129
Apgar score, 167
Appetite suppressant, herbal. *See* diet pills
Appetite, decrease in, 2, 67, 167, 181, 182,
  184, 189, 222
Appetite, increase in, 142
Archibald, Carol J., 155
Archives of Internal Medicine, 207
Arginine, 20, 87–88
ARIES I, 79
ARIES II, 79
Arrhythmia, 3, 5, 135, 195
  caffeine, 195
  calcium, 182
  diet, 181
  digoxin, 67
  diuretics, 67
  ephedrine, 184
  magnesium, 182
  magnesium, deficiency, 68
  sibutramine, 47
  sleep apnea, 54
Arterioles, 16–19

Artificial heart valves, 63
Asbestos, 52–53
Asbestosis, 53
Ascites, 2, 5, 67
  congestive right-heart failure, 21
  epoprostenol, 96
  portopulmonary hypertension, 42
  transplantation survival, 150
  treprostinil, 109
ASD. *See* atrial septal defect
Aspirin, 63
  children, 165, 166
  colds and flu, 195
  epoprostenol, 104
  potassium, 183
  treprostinil site pain, 111
  Warfarin, 65
Ass.ne Malati di Ipertensione Polmonare,
  250
Assistance Publique-Hôpitaux de Paris, 76,
  96
Association HTAP France, 249
Association of Flight Attendants, 223
Associazione Ipertensione Polmonare
  Italiana, 250
AST, 81. See also liver functiuon tests.
Astaire Witt, Melanie, 216
Asthma, 1
  children, 159, 160
  chronic obstructive pulmonary disease,
    52
  CTEPH, 57
  occupational, 53
AstraZeneca, 63
Athens State University, 217
Atherosclerosis, 19
Atkins diet, 181
Atria, 39
Atrial fibrillation
  ephedrine, 184
  ximelagatran, 63
Atrial septal defect, 39–40
  non-surgical closure, 121–22
Atrial septostomy, 130, 152, 172
Atrial ventricular canal, 40
Atrioventricular septal defect, 164
ATS. *See* American Thoracic Society
Attention Deficit Disorder, 168
Atz, Andrew, 89
Autoantibody, 27, 36
Autoimmune disease, 34, 37
Autologous cell-based gene therapy, 116
AVC. *See* atrial ventricular canal
AVEN, 207, 247
Avian flu, 196
Azathioprine, 134
Azithromycin, 133
B9972, 115
Back pain, 65, 91
Bactrim, 65
Badesch, David, 95, 223
Baker, Benjamin A., 228
Balance, sense of, 67
Balloon angioplasty, 122
Barbiturates, 65
Bariatric surgery, 124

Barst, Robyn, 83, 84, 93, 96, 113, 137, 142,
  146, 160, 161, 164
BASF, 79
Bayer, 90
Baylor College of Medicine, 82, 110
Beano, 184
Behçet's disease, 58
Benadryl, 203
Benzodiazepine, 78
Bequests, 243
Beradrak. *See* beraprost
Beraprost, 92, 93–94, 96
  bosentan, 82
  children, 160
  dosages, 94
  inhaled, 94
  side effects, 94
Bergamottin, 192
Bertakis, Klea, 199
Berylliosis, 53
Beryllium, 52–53, 58
Beryllium poisoning. *See* berylliosis
Beta blockers, 186, 191
Bextra, 119
Bicycle tests, 169
Bicycling, 83, 218
Bilirubin, 81, 156, 158
Biofeedback, 39, 207
Biomarkers, 149–50
Biopatch, 101
Birth control, 44, 157–58, 158, 167
  Consensus Statement, 158
Birth defects, 66, 165
Birth weight, low, 165, 167
Bitter orange, 48, 192
Black, Carol, 81
Black, Debbie, 176
Bleeding, 65, 119
Bloating
  calcium channel blockers, 78
  Coumadin, 65
  diet, 176
  epoprostenol, 98
Blood
  coagulation of, 6, 182
  coughing up, 187
Blood clots, 7, 9, 13, 20, 56–57
  aspirin, 63
  detection of, 9
  fibrin, 61
  intravenous drug use, as a result of, 45
  magnesium, 182
  myelofibrosis, 50
  pulmonary thromboendarterectomy, 122
  surgery, 121
  thromboxane, role in, 20
  treprostinil, 111
Blood flukes, 58
Blood pressure. *See* systemic blood pressure
Blood tests, 6
  children, 159
  transplantation, 131
Blood thinner. *See* anticoagulants
Blood transfusion, 49, 135
Blood vessels
  prostacyclin, effect on, 92
  thickening, reversal of, 85

University of Minnesota, 158, 212
University of Minnesota, Veterans'
    Administration Hospital, 48
University of Pennsylvania, 93, 247
University of Southern California, 135, 159
University of Toronto, 116, 117
University of Utah, 29, 247
University of Vienna, 160
University of Washington, 12, 69, 78, 192
University of Wisconsin, 205
UNOS, 136, 157, 159, 257
Up Your Gas, 192
Uprima, 90
Urinary tract infection, 91
Urine, red or brown, 65
Uroplus, 65
Ussetti, P., 141
UT-15. *See* treprostinil
V/Q scan. *See* nuclear scan
Vaccinations, 220
Vaginal cream, 65
Vagus nerve, 141
Valdecoxib, 111
Valerian, 193
Valium, 78
Valsartan, 115
Vanderbilt University, 30, 32, 115, 153, 247,
    257
    familial PAH family research, 29
Vane, John, 92
Vardenafil, 89, 90, 91
Vascular occlusive disease, 17
Vascular tree, pruning of, 7, 13
Vasculitis, 35, 38
Vasectomy, 166
Vasoconstrictors, 20
Vasodilator, 3, 13, 14, 44, 79, 115
    ACE inhibitors, 114
    beraprost, 93
    prostanoid, 93
    types of, 20
Vasodilator study. *See* acute vasodilator
    challenge
Vasopressin, 20
Vegetarian, 184
Vehicle Licensing Office, 211
Venlafaxine, 48
Veno-occlusive disease. *See* pulmonary
    veno-occlusive disease
Ventavis. *See* iloprost
Ventilation/perfusion mismatch, 134
Ventricular septal defect, 39, 40, 164. *See
    also* heart disease
Verenining van Vaatpatienten, 250
Viagra. *See* sildenafil
Vioxx, 111
Vision
    calcium channel blockers, 78
    corticosteroids, 134
    digoxin, 67
    impairment due to hypoxemia, 56
    sildenafil, 91
    tadalafil, 91
    vardenafil, 91
Vitali, Massimiliano, 249
Vitamin A, 189, 193

Vitamin B1. *See* thiamine
Vitamin B6. *See* pyridoxine
Vitamin C, 186, 189, 204
Vitamin D, 189, 191
Vitamin E, 189–90, 193
Vitamin K, 63, 65, 186, 189, 192, 193
    injection, 64
Vitamin supplements, 182, 189, 191
Vitamins, 182, 189–91
    children, 165
    INR, impact on, 65
Voelkel, Norbert, 16, 20, 44
Voice change after transplantation, 141
Voltaren, 65
Vomiting, 194
    alcohol abuse, 167
    anticoagulants, 65
    azathioprine, 134
    calcium channel blockers, 78
    carnitine, 178
    epoprostenol, 97
    hypoxemia, 56
    hypoxia, 214
    liver toxicity, 81
    magnesium, 182
    potassium, 183
    weight loss, 174
Von Willebrand factor, 149
VSD. *See* ventricular septal defect
Walking, 180, 218
Walter Reed Army Medical Center, 53
Warfarin, 62–63. *See also* anticoagulants
    acetaminophen, 195
    birth-control pills, 158
    blue or purple digits, 64
    bosentan, 81
    children, 162
    clots, preventing, 62
    conventional therapy, mortality on, 139
    dose, missed, 64
    drug interactions, 65
    DVT, 219
    green tea, 184
    how to use, 63–64
    NSAIDs, 195
    precautions, pre-surgery, 64–65
    pregnancy, 157
    survival using, 152
    teenager, 167
    vitamin E, 182
    vitamin K, 178, 181
Warsaw Convention, 224
Washington University in St. Louis, 137,
    157
Water, 174, 175
Wayne State University, 167
Wegener's granulomatosis, 38
Weight
    control, 179–80
    gain due to liquid retention, 67
    how to gain, 173–76
    hypothyroidism and gain, 193
    under-, 171–72
Weight loss, 2, 47, 180, 181–82, 182, 184
    calcium, 183
    exercise, 172

histiocytosis X, 58
hyperthyroidism, 193
INR, 64
obesity surgery, 124
protein, 176–77
transplantation, 130
vomiting, 186
Weight Watchers, 181
Weightlifting, 180
Weirs, Ken, 48
Weiss Doyel, Alice, 216
Well Spouse Foundation, 210
Wensel, Roland, 150
Wessel, David, 89
Wheeler, Lisa, 32, 257
WHO. *See* World Health Organization
Whooping cough, 53
Wilson, Peter M., 253
Wojciechowski, Betty Lou, 208
Woo, Marilyn, 171
Workman's compensation, 215
World Health Organization, 27. *See also*
    functional class
    classification of PH, 4, 11, 28
    World Symposium on PH, 4, 44
Xenadrine, 192
Ximelagatran, 63
X-Ray, 9, 13
Yamron, Sharren, 142
Yanagisawa, Masahi, 20
Yaws, 58
Yeast infections, 141
YellowSubs, 192
Yoga, 83, 207
Yung, Gordon, 7
Zanamivir, 204
Zaroxolyn, 67
Zhao, Yidan, 117
Zinc, 189, 204
Zithromax, 141, 170
Zocor. See simvastatin
Zoloft, 205
Zonalon, 111
Zone diet, 184, 185

Special Section:
How to Handle Flolan Emergencies

Chart prepared by Cathy J. Anderson-Severson, RN, BSN, Mayo Clinic

Situation	Action
Your Hickman catheter falls out or is pulled out. **What is happening:** You are not getting your Flolan. This is an emergency.	1. If someone else is around have them call for help. 2. Call 911 or your local emergency number. 3. While waiting for help to arrive minimize physical activity and put oxygen on if you have it at home. Cover the area where the catheter fell out with your hand and apply pressure if bleeding. 4. When emergency help arrives, advise them of your condition and that an IV must be started in your arm. Your pump tubing will connect directly to the IV they put in your arm. Make sure that the pump is running. 5. If the emergency personnel are reluctant to place IV or connect medicine, show them the warning sticker on your pump and call your Flolan provider's emergency number. 6. Remember to take your back-up medication cassette and supplies to the hospital. 7. Once you get to the hospital, have them call your PH center or call them yourself for how to proceed.
You notice a fuzzy raised area on the catheter where it comes out of your skin. **What is happening:** The catheter has a small "cuff" (balloon) under your skin that is designed to hold the catheter in place. Over time, this cuff sits under your skin and forms a bond between the skin and muscle. Sometimes the catheter can start coming out, and the cuff will start to appear outside your skin. This is a problem because it means that your catheter is not secured well in your chest, and thus there is an increased chance that it may fall out. Do not push the catheter back it; it cannot safely be "pushed" back in and may need to be replaced.	1. Secure the catheter with your dressing using extra tape and make several "safety loops" so it does not accidentally get pulled. 2. Call your PH center.
You have a fever. **What is happening:** You may be developing an infection	1. Call your PH center. 2. Be prepared to tell them any new symptoms you might have, what your catheter site looks like, and any other symptoms or feelings that you have.

Situation	Action
You notice drainage or oozing from your catheter. **What is happening:** You may be developing an infection.	1. Call your PH center. 2. Be prepared to tell them any new symptoms you might have, what your temperature is, any allergies you have, when your last infection may have been, and the number for your local pharmacy. 3. Also be prepared to visit your PH center or local **MD** if they need to see the catheter or take a sample of the drainage. 4. Do **NOT** start taking any antibiotics that you may have at home before talking to your PH center.
Your catheter is leaking or has a crack. Blood or medicine may be leaking out. **What is happening:** You are not getting your Flolan and this is an emergency. The catheter might be able to be repaired or might need to be replaced. Until this can be done, you need get your Flolan infusion through a vein in your arm.	1. If someone else is around call for help. 2. Call 911 or your local emergency number. 3. If blood is backing up in the catheter or leaking out, use your clamp to close off the catheter to stop blood from backing up. You may attempt to wrap the crack or hole tightly with tape, but if it is still leaking badly you might need to clamp off the line. You must assess the situation and use your best judgment-is enough Flolan still getting infused that it is helping you? Is so much running out that it is doing you little good? 4. While waiting for help to arrive minimize physical activity and put oxygen on if you have it at home. If you can, get your Flolan emergency kit and have it by your side (see p. 103). 5. When emergency help arrives, advise them of your condition and that an IV must be started in your arm. Your pump tubing will screw directly on to the IV they put in your arm. Make sure that the pump is running. If the emergency personnel are reluctant to place IV or connect medicine, show them the warning sticker on your pump and call your Flolan provider's emergency number. 6. Remember to take your back-up medication cassette and supplies to the hospital. 7. Once you get to the hospital, have them call your PH center or call them yourself for how to proceed.

Treatment Updates

Check PHA's website (www.PHAssociation.org.) for new updates. You will also find more complete information there on these and other developments.

Pediatric Trials Are Underway for Many Drugs

Check the website now and then for new information on the use of various **PAH** drugs in kids.

Sickle Cell Anemia and PAH

Two large trials will soon look at the usefulness of sildenafil (Revatio) and of bosentan (Tracleer) to treat sickle cell disease. It's high time, because of the large number of patients with PH secondary to this condition.

Calcium Channel Blockers

It seems that as new **PAH** drugs are approved, the definition of who truly responds well to CCBs grows less and less inclusive. Doctors now say that less than 10 percent of **PAH** patients are true responders. Verapamil, a CCB that can depress heart function, should not be used in **PAH** patients.

Diuretics

They are used in **PAH** patients with or without evidence of heart failure and fluid retention (e.g. swollen legs, fluid in the abdomen).

Warfarin (Coumadin)

The use of warfarin in diseases associated with the development of **PAH** has not been systematically studied. Warfarin therapy should be considered in patients using **IV** epoprostenol (Flolan) and very seriously considered in patients using **IV** treprostinil (Treprostinil) because it can help prevent clots forming in catheters.

The New UNOS Lung Transplantation Allocation System

As we warned in the 3rd edition of the *Survival Guide*, UNOS has changed the criteria for deciding who gets a transplant when, and the changes are not particularly favorable to PAH patients. The following excerpt on page 292 is from an article that was printed in the Summer 2005 issue of PHA's medical journal, *Advances in Pulmonary Hypertension*. The complete article may be read at *www.PHAssociation.org*.

Written by Gundeep S. Dhillon, MD, and Ramona L. Doyle, MD
Heart-Lung and Lung Transplantation Program
Stanford University Medical Center, Stanford, California

Under a directive from the Department of Health and Human Services to the United Network for Organ Sharing (UNOS), a new lung allocation system has been developed and recently implemented.[3,4] ....

The Lung Allocation Score

The new system is based on a lung allocation score. All individuals in need of lungs who are over the age of 12 years will receive lungs on the basis of his or her lung allocation score. The higher the score, the greater the likelihood of being offered donor lungs. The lung allocation score is derived from multiple clinical variables. These clinical variables (Table 1) are used to calculate the following:

• The waitlist urgency measure (WLi), which predicts the number of days an individual with a specific set of characteristics is expected to live during the next year on the waiting list (range 0-365).

• The post-transplant survival measure (PTi), which predicts the number of days an individual is expected to live during the first year after the lung transplantation (range 0-365).

Table 1. Clinical Variables Used for Lung Allocation Score Calculation.

Characteristics for Waiting List Model	Characteristics for Post-transplant Model
Age (years)	Age at transplant (years)
Body mass index (kg/m^2)	Creatinine at transplant (mg/dL)
Diabetes	New York Heart Association functional class
New York Heart Association functional class	Forced vital capacity for groups B and D (% predicted)
Forced vital capacity (% predicted)	Pulmonary capillary wedge pressure mean 20 mm Hg for group D
Pulmonary arterial systolic pressure for diagnosis groups A, C, and D	Mechanical ventilation
Oxygen requirements at rest (L/min)	Diagnosis groups*
Six-minute walk distance (feet)	Diagnosis detailed**
Continuous mechanical ventilation	
Diagnosis groups*	
Diagnosis detailed**	

* Diagnosis groups
  A = Obstructive lung disease
  B = Pulmonary vascular disease
  C = Cystic fibrosis or immunodeficiency disorder
  D = Restrictive lung disease

** Diagnosis detailed
  Bronchiectasis
  Eisenmenger syndrome
  Lymphangioleiomyomatosis
  Obliterative bronchiolitis
  Pulmonary fibrosis, other
  Sarcoidosis and pulmonary arterial pressure mean ≦30 mm Hg
  Sarcoidosis and pulmonary arterial pressure mean 30 mm Hg

The raw allocation score is calculated using the following equation:

$$\text{Raw Score} = PTi - 2WLi$$

The raw score can range from -730 to 365. A final lung allocation score (0-100) is obtained by normalization of the raw score.

$$
\begin{aligned}
\text{Lung Allocation Score} &= 100[\text{Raw Score} - \text{minimum}]/\text{Range} \\
&= 100[\text{Raw Score} - (-730)]/1095 \\
&= 100[\text{Raw Score} = 730]/1095
\end{aligned}
$$

Under this system the clinical variables listed in Table 1 need to be updated once every 6 months in transplantation candidates, but can be updated more frequently at the discretion of the transplantation center.

Impact of the New Lung Allocation System on Pulmonary Hypertension Patients

It is unclear how the new lung allocation system will impact patients with pulmonary arterial hypertension without or with congenital heart disease (Eisenmenger syndrome)[5]. It is also not known how patients in need of combined heart-lung transplantation will fare under the new system. In addition, the lung allocation system does not account for clinical events such as hemoptysis or syncope, generally accepted poor prognostic factors in pulmonary hypertension. In cases where the transplantation center feels that an individual's lung allocation score underestimates his or her clinical severity, an appeal can be made to a lung review board for adjustment of the score. Thus, although the new system introduces greater uniformity across transplantation centers, it does not replace the need for centers to exercise clinical judgment regarding the need for and timing of transplantation in individual patients.

The old system of selecting patients for lung transplantation required that physicians identify the "transplant window," the time when a patient is sick enough to warrant lung transplantation yet well enough to survive the transplant operation, and this still holds true. Under the new system, the burden of factoring in nonclinical decisions such as waiting time has, presumably, been eliminated. Ideally the new lung allocation algorithm will reduce variability among various centers as to the severity of the illness of patients who receive transplantation thus improving the fairness of the system.

A potential limitation of this new algorithm is that it has not been prospectively validated.[6,7] However, the UNOS plans to update this algorithm every 6 months using the most recent 3-year cohort of patients on the waiting list and lung transplant recipients. In conclusion, the need for change in the way donor lungs are allocated in the United States has been recognized and undertaken. It is hoped that this new system will optimize the utilization of this precious resource....

References

3. Department of Health and Human Services. Organ Procurement and Transplantation Network; Final Rule. 42 CFRPart 121: Federal Register; 1999:56649-61.
4. Organ Procurement and Transplantation Net-work.Policy 3.7. Allocation of Thoracic Organs. 2004.
5. Vongpatanasin W, Brickner ME, Hillis LD, Lange RA. The Eisenmenger syndrome in adults. Ann Intern Med.1998; 128(9):745-55.
6. Justice AC, Covinsky KE, Berlin JA. Assessing the generalizability of prognostic information. Ann Intern Med.1999;130(6):515-24.
7. McGinn TG, Guyatt GH, Wyer PC, Naylor CD, Stiell IG, Richardson WS. Users' guides to the medical literature: XXII: how to use articles about clinical decision rules. Evidence-Based Medicine Working Group. JAMA. 2000;284(1):79-84.

Notes:

Notes: